CANCER ETIOLOGY, DIAGNOSIS AND TREATMENTS

EFFECTIVENESS OF CORE-NEEDLE AND OPEN SURGICAL BIOPSY IN BREAST CANCER EVALUATION

Cancer Etiology, Diagnosis and Treatments

Additional books in this series can be found on Nova's website under the Series tab.

Additional E-books in this series can be found on Nova's website under the E-books tab.

CANCER ETIOLOGY, DIAGNOSIS AND TREATMENTS

EFFECTIVENESS OF CORE-NEEDLE AND OPEN SURGICAL BIOPSY IN BREAST CANCER EVALUATION

LESLIE D. SCHMIDT
EDITOR

Nova Biomedical Books
New York

For permission to use material from this book please contact us:
Telephone 631-231-7269; Fax 631-231-8175
Web Site: http://www.novapublishers.com

Additional color graphics may be available in the e-book version of this book.

Library of Congress Cataloging-in-Publication Data

Effectiveness of core : needle and open surgical biopsy in breast cancer evaluation / [edited by] Leslie D. Schmidt.
p. cm.
Includes index.
ISBN 978-1-61209-799-2 (hardcover)
1. Breast--Biopsy. 2. Breast--Cancer--Diagnosis. I. Schmidt, Leslie D.
RC280.B8E35 2011
616.99'4490758--dc22
2011005656

Published by Nova Science Publishers, Inc. † New York

Contents

Preface

Open surgical biopsy is the "gold standard" or "reference standard" method of evaluating a suspicious breast lesion because it is thought to be very accurate in diagnosing these lesions. While generally considered safe, it is a surgical procedure that, like all surgeries, places the patient at risk of experiencing morbidities and, in rare cases, mortality. However, only 20 to 30 percent of women who undergo breast biopsy procedures are diagnosed with cancer. A less invasive method for evaluation of suspicious breast lesions would be preferable if it were sufficiently accurate. This new book examines the effectiveness of core-needle and open-surgical biopsy in breast cancer evaluation.

Chapter 1- Breast cancer is the second most common malignancy of women, with over 180,000 new cases diagnosed each year in the United States. Survival rates depend on the stage of disease at diagnosis. Women diagnosed with early stages of breast cancer have a 5-year survival rate near 100 percent. However, early breast cancer is asymptomatic, and the only way to detect it is by population-wide screening programs that include regular mammography and physical examination.

Chapter 2- Journals and supplements maintained in ECRI Institute's collections were routinely reviewed. Nonjournal publications and conference proceedings from professional organizations, private agencies, and government agencies were also screened. Other mechanisms used to retrieve additional relevant information included review of bibliographies/reference lists from peer-reviewed and gray literature.

In: Effectiveness of Core-Needle and Open Surgical Biopsy... ISBN: 978-1-61209-799-2
Editor: Leslie D. Schmidt

Chapter 1

Comparative Effectiveness of Core-Needle and Open Surgical Biopsy for the Diagnosis of Breast Lesions

Agency for Healthcare Research and Quality

Acknowledgments

The Evidence-based Practice Center would like to thank Eileen Erinoff, M.S.L.I.S., and Helen Dunn for providing literature retrieval and documentation management support and Lydia Dharia for her assistance with the final preparations of the report.

Executive Summary

Background

Breast cancer is the second most common malignancy of women, with over 180,000 new cases diagnosed each year in the United States. Survival rates depend on the stage of disease at diagnosis. Women diagnosed with early stages of breast cancer have a 5-year survival rate near 100 percent. However, early breast cancer is asymptomatic, and the only way to detect it is by population-wide screening programs that include regular mammography and physical examination.

Mammography uses x-rays to examine the breast for calcifications, masses, or other abnormal structures. Currently, most professional organizations recommend that all women 50 years of age and over receive a mammogram every 1 to 2 years. Many professional organizations recommend that routine breast cancer screening begin earlier, at age 40, although x-ray mammography screening is less effective in younger women. Most experts believe that regular x-ray mammographic screening of all women ages 50- 70 can reduce mortality from breast cancer.

The American College of Radiology has created a standardized system for reporting the results of mammography, the Breast Imaging Reporting and Data System (BI-RADS®). There are seven categories of assessment and recommendation:

0 Need additional imaging evaluation and/or prior mammograms for comparison.
1 Negative.
2 Benign finding.
3 Probably benign finding. Initial short-interval followup suggested.
4 Suspicious abnormality. Biopsy should be considered.
5 Highly suggestive of malignancy. Appropriate action should be taken.
6 Known biopsy-proven malignancy. Appropriate action should be taken.

After identification of an abnormality on screening mammography or physical examination, women typically undergo additional imaging studies (diagnostic mammography, ultrasound, magnetic resonance imaging [MRI]) and a physical examination. If these studies suggest the abnormality may be malignant, a biopsy of the suspicious area may be recommended. Biopsy material may be obtained by fine-needle aspiration, core-needle biopsy, or open surgical procedures.

Open surgical biopsy involves removing a sample of tissue from the suspicious area through a surgical incision. To aid in location of a nonpalpable lesion, it may be marked with a wire, dye, or carbon particles using an imaging method (mammography, ultrasound, MRI) to guide placement of the marker. The procedure may be performed under general anesthesia, sedation plus local anesthesia, or local anesthesia only. The surgeon may attempt to remove the entire lesion during the biopsy procedure (excisional biopsy) if the lesion is fairly small. After the tissue sample is removed, the incision is closed with sutures.

Open surgical biopsy is the "gold standard" or "reference standard" method of evaluating a suspicious breast lesion because it is thought to be very accurate in diagnosing these lesions. While generally considered safe, it is a surgical procedure that, like all surgeries, places the patient at risk of experiencing morbidities and, in rare cases, mortality. However, only 20 to 30 percent of women who undergo breast biopsy procedures are diagnosed with cancer. Exposing large numbers of women who do not have cancer to invasive surgical procedures may be considered an undesirable medical practice. A less invasive method for evaluation of suspicious breast lesions would be preferable if it were sufficiently accurate.

A core-needle biopsy is a procedure that involves removing small samples of breast tissue through a hollow core needle inserted through the skin. Basic core-needle biopsy uses a special 11-, 14-, or 16-gauge needle (the smaller the gauge, the larger the diameter of the needle). The suspicious lesion may be located by palpation or by imaging (stereotactic mammography, ultrasound, MRI). The procedure is usually performed under local anesthesia. Multiple core-needle samples may be taken from the suspicious area.

A variant on core-needle biopsy is vacuum-assisted biopsy. After locating the suspicious area by stereotactic mammography or ultrasound, the probe of the device is inserted into the suspicious area. The device uses vacuum suction to help remove tissue samples. Multiple samples may be taken from the suspicious area without reinserting the needle.

The primary goal of initial biopsy of any abnormality is to diagnose the abnormality as benign or malignant. Generally, only malignant lesions require invasive followup procedures such as surgical excision or lymph node evaluation. As discussed above, the majority of women who are sent for breast biopsy do not have malignant lesions and do not require followup surgery. Thus an accurate initial core-needle biopsy would in most cases allow women to avoid any open surgical procedure. If the core- needle biopsy suggests the lesion is malignant, lymph node exploration and lesion excision to clear margins could be performed during the follow-on surgical procedure. Women who are diagnosed with malignant lesions by open surgical biopsy are often subject to an additional surgical procedure to ensure the lesion has been completely removed and, in some cases, for lymph node evaluation. Therefore, an accurate method of performing core-needle biopsies may enable many women to avoid surgery altogether and reduce the number of surgical procedures women with malignancies must undergo.

Medical indications—such as size and location of the lesion, imaging characteristics of the lesion, and likelihood of eventual surgical excision—may direct the preference of one type of breast biopsy procedure over another. However, other factors— such as patient preferences, access, and practice and referral patterns—also influence decisions about which procedure should be performed.

The large number of possible methods of performing breast biopsy can be bewildering to patients and health care providers alike. Which method should one choose? Is a particular method clearly superior, or does the method of choice depend upon individual patient characteristics? We have performed a systematic review intended to evaluate the accuracy of different methods of performing breast biopsy and to explore what factor(s) may impact the accuracy and possible harms of different methods of performing breast biopsy.

Methods

The topic of this systematic review was nominated in a public process. The Key Questions were developed by a technical expert panel assembled by the Scientific Resource Center for the Agency for Healthcare Research and Quality (AHRQ). The medical literature was systematically searched for articles from December 1990 through September 11, 2009, that addressed the Key Questions.

Medical personnel usually want to see the results of at least one randomized controlled trial demonstrating that a medical procedure is safe, effective, and beneficial to patients before adopting the procedure into general clinical practice. However, it is generally acknowledged that early diagnosis and treatment of breast tumors leads to improved survival rates and quality of life. Women found to have benign lesions on biopsy are able to avoid unnecessary treatment and receive reassurance that they do not have breast cancer. Given the currently available alternatives, there is no need to conduct randomized controlled trials of breast biopsy procedures. Establishing that a type of breast biopsy is safer than open surgical biopsy while being as accurate or almost as accurate as open surgical biopsy is sufficient to justify its routine use.

Studies of diagnostic test performance compare the results of the experimental test to a reference test. The reference test is intended to measure the "true" disease status of each patient. For the diagnosis of breast cancer, the "gold standard" reference test is open surgery and pathological examination of the removed tissue. However, a difficulty with the use of this reference standard in large cohort studies of screening-detected breast abnormalities is that many women with lesions that are probably benign will be subjected to open surgery. The principle of clinical equipoise means that there is genuine uncertainty over whether or not the intervention will be beneficial, and therefore it is acceptable to study the intervention in a clinical research trial. Subjecting women with lesions that are probably benign to open surgery does not meet the principle of clinical equipoise. Therefore we have chosen to include studies that used a combination of followup and open surgical biopsy as the reference standard in our analyses.

Studies of diagnostic test performance were examined to see if they met the inclusion criteria. In brief, the inclusion criteria were: the study directly compared core- needle biopsy to pathological examination of tissue obtained by open surgery and/or patient followup for at least 6 months; the study enrolled 10 or more patients at average risk of primary breast cancer who were referred for breast biopsy after discovery of a possible breast abnormality on screening mammography, routine physical examination, or routine self-examination; the study was a full-length article published in English; and 50 percent or more of the enrolled subjects completed the study.

In our analysis of biopsy accuracy, we focused on measures that evaluate the extent of false-negative errors (cancers falsely diagnosed as benign): sensitivity and negative likelihood ratio. Sensitivity is expressed as a percentage. A biopsy method with a sensitivity close to 100 percent will miss very few cancers. A negative likelihood ratio can be used to calculate an individual woman's risk of having a malignancy following a "benign" diagnosis on breast biopsy. In general, the smaller the negative likelihood ratio, the more accurate the diagnostic test is in predicting the absence of disease. However, each individual woman's post-test risk varies by her individual pre-test risk of malignancy.

We also analyzed the "underestimation rate." Lesions diagnosed by core-needle biopsy as ductal carcinoma in situ (DCIS, a noninvasive early stage of breast cancer) that were found to be invasive by the reference standard were counted as DCIS underestimates. Similarly, lesions diagnosed by core-needle biopsy as benign atypical ductal hyperplasia (ADH) that were found instead to be invasive by the reference standard were counted as ADH underestimates. The underestimation rate was then calculated as the number of underestimates per number of DCIS (or ADH) diagnoses. In the primary analysis of sensitivity and negative likelihood ratio, underestimates were not considered to be missed cancers because current clinical practice is to suggest surgical removal of ADH and DCIS lesions, and thus underestimates would not have been "missed."

The quality of the included studies was evaluated using an internal validity rating instrument for diagnostic studies. The studies were rated as low, moderate, or high in quality for the assessment of accuracy outcomes. Data from the included articles were abstracted and analyzed. Where possible, the data were combined using a bivariate mixed-effects binomial regression meta-analysis model. Underestimation rates were combined using a random-effects meta-analysis. The summary likelihood ratios and Bayes theorem were used to compute post-test probabilities of a malignancy.

The strength of evidence supporting each major conclusion was graded as high, moderate, low, or insufficient. The grade was developed after consideration of the quality of the evidence base, the size of the evidence base, the consistency of the findings, and the robustness of the findings to sensitivity analyses.

Conclusions

Key Question 1. In women with a palpable or nonpalpable breast abnormality, what is the accuracy of different types of core-needle breast biopsy compared with open biopsy for diagnosis?

Our literature searches identified 107 studies of 57,088 breast lesions that met the inclusion criteria. All of the studies were diagnostic cohort studies that enrolled a population of women found to have suspicious breast abnormalities on routine screening (mammography and/or physical examination). The women were sent for various types of breast biopsies, and the accuracy of the breast biopsy was determined by comparing the results of the breast biopsy to the results of a combination of open surgery and patient followup. We graded the supporting evidence for these conclusions as low based on the low quality of the evidence base (i.e., greater potential for bias), although we rated the quantity, consistency, and robustness of the evidence base as sufficient. Our conclusions for Key Question 1 are summarized in Table Table A and Figures Figure A through D. Our key conclusions are stated below.

- Stereotactically guided vacuum-assisted core-needle biopsies have a sensitivity of 99.2 percent (95-percent confidence interval [CI]: 97.9 to 99.7 percent). Strength of evidence: Low.
- Stereotactically guided automated gun core-needle biopsies have a sensitivity of 97.8 percent (95-percent CI: 95.8 to 98.9 percent). Strength of evidence: Low.
- Ultrasound-guided vacuum-assisted core-needle biopsies have a sensitivity of 96.5 percent (95-percent CI: 81.2 to 99.4 percent). Strength of evidence: Low.
- Ultrasound-guided automated gun core-needle biopsies have a sensitivity of 97.7 percent (95-percent CI: 97.2 to 98.2 percent). Strength of evidence: Low.
- Freehand automated gun core-needle biopsies have a sensitivity of 85.8 percent (95-percent CI: 75.8 to 92.1 percent). Strength of evidence: Low.

There was insufficient evidence to estimate the accuracy of MRI-guided core- needle biopsies.

The included studies assumed that open surgical biopsy was 100-percent accurate. We obtained information about the actual accuracy of open surgical biopsy from a review article, and therefore a formal conclusion and strength of evidence rating was not derived for estimates about the accuracy of open surgical biopsy.

Key Question 2. In women with a palpable or nonpalpable breast abnormality, what are the harms associated with different types of core-needle breast biopsy compared with open biopsy for diagnosis?

We recorded the complications and harms reported by the 107 studies that met the inclusion criteria for Key Question 1. Our results are summarized in Table B. Severe complications following core-needle biopsy of any type are very rare, affecting fewer than 1 percent of procedures. Vacuum-assisted procedures may be associated with slightly more severe bleeding events than automated gun core-needle biopsies. The strength of evidence supporting the quantitative estimates of the frequency of complications is low. Information about harms of open surgical biopsy was scanty in the included studies, and we supplemented it with information from recent review articles. Therefore, the strength of the evidence was not rated for conclusions about the safety of open surgical biopsy. However, it is clear that core-needle biopsies have a lower risk of complications than do open surgical procedures.

In Figure E we present a simplified model of what might happen if the same cohort of 1,000 women underwent various types of breast biopsy. The theoretical cohort of women includes 300 women with malignant tumors and 700 women with benign lesions. The model is based on the point estimates of accuracy from our analyses and do not incorporate estimates of uncertainty of the point estimates. Refer to Figure A through D for a visual representation of the degree of uncertainty in the point estimates. The model assumes that all women with nonbenign diagnoses on their first biopsy procedure, including all women who had open surgical biopsy as their first biopsy procedure, will be subject to an open surgical excisional procedure.

We also performed a number of meta-regressions exploring the impact of various factors on the accuracy and harms of core-needle biopsies. Our findings from these meta- regressions are summarized in Table C. Use of image guidance and vacuum assistance improved the accuracy of core-needle biopsy; however, vacuum assistance increased the percentage of procedures complicated by severe bleeding and hematoma formation. Performing biopsies with patients seated upright increased the incidence of vasovagal reactions.

Our meta-regressions did not identify a statistically significant effect of the following factors on the results: needle size, method of verification of biopsy (open surgery, open surgery and at least 6 months' followup, or open surgery and at least 2 years' followup), whether the studies were conducted at a single center or at multiple centers, whether the studies were conducted in general hospitals or dedicated cancer clinics, or the country in which the study was conducted. The studies reported insufficient information about lesion characteristics, patient characteristics, or the training or experience of the persons performing the biopsies to explore the effect of such factors on the accuracy or harms of the biopsies.

Key Question 3. How do open biopsy and various core-needle techniques differ in terms of patient preference, availability, costs, availability of qualified pathologist interpretations, and other factors that may influence choice of a particular technique?

Due to the nature of Key Question 3, we did not use formal inclusion criteria, nor did we come to many formal evidence-based conclusions. We collected information relevant to the topic from many sources, including interviews with experts. There was general agreement that core-needle biopsy costs less than open surgical biopsy, consumes fewer resources, and is preferred by patients. Women were generally satisfied with the cosmetic results of core-needle procedures. Women who underwent a core-needle biopsy as their first invasive test to diagnose a breast cancer had, on average, fewer surgical procedures than women who underwent an open biopsy procedure as their first invasive test. One particularly important finding was that women diagnosed with breast cancer by core-needle biopsy were usually able to have their cancer treated with a single surgical procedure, but women diagnosed with breast cancer by open surgical biopsy often required more than one surgical procedure to treat their cancer (odds ratio 13.7, 95- percent CI: 5.6 to 34.6). Due to the consistency, robustness, and extremely large strength of association between the type of biopsy and the requirement for more than one surgery for treatment, we rated the strength of evidence supporting this conclusion as moderate. There was insufficient information available to evaluate the impact of equipment or pathologist availability.

Discussion

When making decisions about what type of biopsy to use, individual women and their health care providers will need to weigh the pros and cons of each type of biopsy for each individual woman. Open surgical biopsies are highly accurate; however, core-needle biopsies are associated with a much lower incidence of harms and morbidity. In addition, women who are diagnosed with cancer by core-needle biopsy undergo fewer surgeries during treatment than do women who are diagnosed with cancer by open biopsy. The crux of the decision then becomes the question, "Is core-needle biopsy accurate enough?" The answer to this question may vary depending on the individual woman's estimated prebiopsy chance of having cancer (an estimate derived from mammography results and other prebiopsy examination information) and an individual woman's desire to avoid risk. For some women, core-needle biopsy will never be accurate enough to satisfy their desire to know, for sure, whether they do or do not have cancer. For others, the greater safety and less invasive nature of core-needle biopsy are worth a small sacrifice in accuracy. During decisionmaking, women and health care providers also need to consider the clinical implications of a cancer missed on core-needle biopsy. In many cases, the cancer will be detected on subsequent mammography. Women with negative core-needle biopsies should have careful diagnostic followup with clinical correlation as appropriate for the individual patient.

The ratings of low strength of evidence apply to the individual estimates of accuracy for each type of core-needle biopsy. Due to the poor reporting and low internal validity of the included studies, we are concerned that the studies may be consistently biased toward finding that core-needle biopsies are more accurate than they actually are. We have performed sensitivity analyses (Table D) of the impact of this possibility on our conclusions. For each biopsy method, we have estimated the post-test probability of a woman actually having cancer after a negative core-needle biopsy result (assuming the woman had a prebiopsy probability of having cancer of 30 percent). We calculated probabilities using the summary estimate of the negative likelihood ratio from our analysis, and for summary estimates calculated after assuming our analysis had overestimated the sensitivity of the procedure by 1 percent, 5 percent, and 10 percent. We are moderately confident that our analysis has not overestimated the sensitivity by as much as 10 percent, but we present the results of this sensitivity analysis as a "worst case" scenario. For example, for ultrasound (US) guidance vacuum-assisted core-needle biopsy, we estimated the probability of a woman actually having cancer after a negative core-needle biopsy result to be 2 percent. Sensitivity analyses using overestimation of the sensitivity by 5 percent and 10 percent suggest that this probability would increase to 3 percent and 6 percent, respectively.

Table A. Summary of key accuracy findings (key Key question Question 1).

Type of biopsy	Number of missed cancers expected for every 1,000 biopsies[1]	Risk of malignancy following a "benign" test result[2]	Number of malignancies expected per 1,000 biopsy diagnoses of "high risk" lesion[3]	Number of invasive cancers expected per 1,000 biopsy diagnoses of DCIS	Strength of evidence supporting the conclusion
Open surgical[4]	3 to 6	0 to 1%	0	0	Not rated
Freehand automated gun	24 to 73	3.4 to 10%	Insufficient data to estimate		Low
US guidance automated gun	6 to 9	1 to 2%	234 to 359	271 to 450	Low
Stereotactic guidance automated gun	3 to 13	0.5 to 2%	357 to 517	180 to 321	Low
MRI guidance automated gun	Insufficient data to estimate				Insufficient
US guidance vacuum-assisted	2 to 56	0.3 to 8%	Insufficient data to estimate		Low
Stereotactic guidance vacuum-assisted	1 to 6	0.1 to 1%	177 to 264	111 to 151	Low

[1] For a population of women with a prevalence of malignancy of 30%, assuming a 100% specificity (no false positives).

[2] For a woman with a BI-RADS® 4 score following mammography expected to have an approximate prebiopsy risk of malignancy of 30%. Note that an individual woman's risk may be different from these estimates, depending on her own individual characteristics.

[3] Primarily ADH lesions.

[4] Estimates based on other literature reviews.

Abbreviations: ADH=atypical ductal hyperplasia; DCIS=ductal carcinoma in situ; MRI-=magnetic resonance imaging; US=ultrasound.

Table B. Summary of key harms findings (key Key Question 2).

Type of biopsy	Number of deaths expected for every 1,000 biopsies	Number of cases of severe bleeding[1] expected for every 1,000 biopsies	Number of cases of hematomas requiring treatment expected for every 1,000 biopsies	Number of infections expected for every 1,000 biopsies	Strength of evidence supporting the conclusion
Open surgical[2]	0	Insufficient data to estimate	20 to 100	38 to 63	Not rated
Automated gun core needle	0	6	1	1	Low
Vacuum-assisted core needle	0	9	1	1	Low

[1] Although not all studies provided a definition of severe bleeding, those that did included episodes of bleeding necessitating treatment, including hospitalization or surgery.

Table C. Summary of impact of various factors on accuracy and harms.

Category	Factor	Impact on accuracy	Impact on harms	Strength of evidence supporting the conclusion
Patient characteristics	Insufficient data for any patient characteristics			Insufficient
Lesion characteristics	Insufficient data for any lesion characteristics			Insufficient
Biopsy methods	Patient position	Insufficient data	Vasovagal reactions occur more often in patients seated upright	Low
	Needle gauge	Does not affect accuracy	Insufficient data	Low
	Insufficient data for any other factor related to biopsy methods			Insufficient
Clinician characteristics	Operator experience	Accuracy improves with experience	Insufficient data	Insufficient
	Insufficient data for any other factor related to clinician characteristics			Inconclusive
Facility type	Type of facility	Does not affect accuracy	Insufficient data	Low
	Geographic location of facility	Does not affect accuracy	Insufficient data	Low

Table D. Sensitivity analysis of impact of low quality evidence on the conclusions.

	Post-biopsy probability of having cancer after a negative core-needle biopsy result[1]			
Type of biopsy	**Analysis results**	**Analysis overestimated sensitivity by 1% (e.g., sensitivity 97% rather than 98%)**	**Analysis overestimated sensitivity by 5% (e.g., sensitivity 93% rather than 98%)**	**Analysis overestimated sensitivity by 10% (e.g., sensitivity 88% rather than 98%)**
Freehand automated gun	6%	6%	8%	9%
Ultrasound guidance automated gun	1%	1%	3%	5%
Stereotactic guidance automated gun	1%	1%	3%	5%
Ultrasound guidance vacuum- assisted	2%	2%	3%	6%
Stereotactic guidance vacuum-assisted	0.4%	0.8%	3%	5%

[1] For a woman with a BI-RADS® 4 score following mammography expected to have an approximate prebiopsy risk of malignancy of 30%. Note that an individual woman's risk may be different from these estimates, depending on her own individual characteristics.

Remaining Issues

Our systematic review has found that both stereotactically guided vacuum- assisted and US-guided core-needle biopsies are safer than open surgical biopsy and are almost as accurate as open surgical biopsy, justifying their routine use. However, well- reported retrospective chart reviews, retrospective database analyses, or prospective diagnostic accuracy studies are needed to address the as-yet-unanswered questions as to what factors affect the accuracy and harms of core-needle breast biopsy. Answers to such questions are important for both patients and clinicians when faced with the decision of what type of breast biopsy is best for each individual patient. In addition, our conclusions are rated as being supported by a low strength of evidence. The low rating is almost entirely due to the fact that the evidence base, while large, consists of universally poorly reported studies. The studies omitted important details about patients, methods, and sometimes results. The studies presented results in an often confusing and haphazard manner. The poor reporting made it difficult to determine whether or not the studies were likely to be affected by bias, and therefore we rated the evidence base as being of low quality. Publication of better reported diagnostic accuracy studies would permit verification that our conclusions are accurate and not influenced by biases in the studies included in this assessment. Additional studies of MRI-guided biopsy are necessary in order to evaluate the accuracy and safety of MRI guidance.

Summary

An overall summary of the findings and level of evidence for each biopsy type is presented in Table E. Based on currently available evidence, it appears reasonable to consider choosing certain core-needle biopsy procedures given the comparable sensitivity and lower complication rates for some of the percutaneous methods. Our analyses found the highest sensitivity for methods utilizing stereotactic guidance, particularly in conjunction with vacuum assistance. The appearance of breast lesions on imaging and the location within the breast may affect the type of core needle/imaging combination chosen for any particular woman. In general, women undergoing core needle biopsy are subjected to fewer surgical procedures overall than women who initially are diagnosed by open surgical biopsy, and they express satisfaction with the cosmetic results. However, the available studies suffered from poor reporting of important details that would help to identify patient and lesion characteristics that might impact the validity of this conclusion for individual women. We rated the strength of evidence as low for the accuracy outcomes, in large part because the absence of these details also compromised our ability to assess the risk of bias in the published studies. We have identified a number of questions that should be answered by future studies in order to improve individualized decisionmaking.

For a woman with a BI-RADS® 4 score following mammography expected to have an approximate prebiopsy risk of malignancy of 30%. Note that an individual woman's risk may be different from these estimates, depending on her own individual characteristics.

Table E. Summary of all findings on comparative effectiveness of core-needle biopsy methods.

Accuracy			
Type of guidance	**Method of biopsy**	**Level of evidence**	**Sensitivity (95% CI)**
Any or none	Open surgical	Not rated	98 to 99%
Stereotactic	Automated gun	Low	97.8 (95.8 to 98.9)
	Vacuum-assisted	Low	99.2% (97.9 to 99.7)
Ultrasound	Automated gun	Low	97.7% (97.2 to 98.2)
	Vacuum-assisted	Low	96.5% (81.2 to 99.4)
MRI	Automated gun	Insufficient	83.3% (43.5 to 96.5)
Freehand	Automated gun	Low	85.8% (75.8 to 92.1)
Type of guidance	**Method of biopsy**	**Level of evidence**	**Negative likelihood ratio (95% CI)**
Any or none	Open surgical	Not rated	0.00 to 0.025
Stereotactic	Automated gun	Low	0.022 (0.012 to 0.043)
	Vacuum-assisted	Low	0.0090 (0.003 to 0.023)
Ultrasound	Automated gun	Low	0.030 (0.022 to 0.040)
	Vacuum-assisted	Low	0.036 (0.0060 to 0.21)
MRI	Any	Insufficient	0.23 (0.05 to 0.95)
Freehand	Automated gun	Low	0.14 (0.082 to 0.25)
Type of guidance	**Method of biopsy**	**Level of evidence**	**DCIS underestimation rate (95% CI)**
Any or none	Open surgical	Not rated	0.0%
Stereotactic	Automated gun	Low	24.4% (18.0 to 32.1)
	Vacuum-assisted	Low	13.0% (11.1 to 15.1)
Ultrasound	Automated gun	Low	35.5% (27.1 to 45.0)
	Vacuum-assisted	Insufficient	Not possible to calculate
MRI	Any	Insufficient	Not possible to calculate
Freehand	Automated gun	Insufficient	Not possible to calculate
Type of guidance	**Method of biopsy**	**Level of evidence**	**ADH underestimation rate (95% CI)**
Any or none	Open surgical	Not rated	0.0%
Stereotactic	Automated gun	Low	43.5% (35.7 to 51.7)
	Vacuum-assisted	Low	21.7% (17.7 to 26.4)
Ultrasound	Automated gun	Low	29.2% (23.4 to 35.9)
	Vacuum-assisted	Insufficient	Not possible to calculate
MRI	Any	Insufficient	Not possible to calculate
Freehand	Automated gun	Insufficient	Not possible to calculate
Factors potentially affecting accuracy			
Factor category	**Factor**	**Level of evidence**	**Conclusion about impact of factor on accuracy**
Patient characteristics	Patient age	Insufficient	No conclusion possible
	Breast density	Insufficient	No conclusion possible
	Patient comorbidities	Insufficient	No conclusion possible

Table E. (Continued).

Factor category	Factor	Level of evidence	Conclusion about impact of factor on accuracy
Lesion characteristics	Palpable vs. nonpalpable	Insufficient	No conclusion possible
	Microcalcifications vs. masses	Insufficient	No conclusion possible
	Distortions vs. masses	Insufficient	No conclusion possible
	Size of lesion	Insufficient	No conclusion possible
	Location of lesion	Insufficient	No conclusion possible
Biopsy methodology	Number of cores	Insufficient	No conclusion possible
	Patient position	Insufficient	No conclusion possible
	Reference standard	Not rated	The type of reference standard (open surgery, 2 years of followup, or only 6 months of followup) had no impact on the data reported by the studies about the accuracy of core- needle biopsy
	Use of vacuum	Low	Vacuum assistance improved accuracy
	Use of image guidance	Low	Use of image guidance improved accuracy; stereotactic guidance was more accurate than US guidance
	Size of needle	Not rated	The size of the needle did not affect the accuracy of the procedure
Clinician and facility factors	Experience of operator	Insufficient	No conclusion possible
	Training of operator	Insufficient	No conclusion possible
	Facility location	Not rated	The location of the facility had no impact on the accuracy of core-needle biopsy
	Facility type	Not rated	The type of facility had no impact on the accuracy of core-needle biopsy
Harms			
Harm category	**Harm**	**Level of evidence**	**Conclusion**
Number of surgeries required	Undergoing surgery	Moderate	Women diagnosed with breast cancer by core-needle biopsies are more likely to be able to be treated with a single surgical procedure than women diagnosed with breast cancer by open surgical biopsies
Complications	Any	High	Core-needle biopsies have a lower risk of complications than open surgical procedures
Severe complications	Any	Low	2 to 10% of open surgical procedures may be affected by severe complications; 0.09 to 0.72% of core-needle biopsy procedures may be affected by severe complications
	Deaths	Low	No deaths were reported in association with any type of breast biopsy procedure
	Bleeding severe enough to require treatment	Low	0.72% of core-needle procedures were affected by severe bleeding

Harm category	Harm	Level of evidence	Conclusion
	Hematomas requiring treatment	Low	0.09% of core-needle procedures were affected by hematomas requiring treatment
	Infections	Low	0.15% of core-needle procedures were affected by infections requiring antibiotic treatment
	Severe pain	Low	1.7% of patients reported experiencing severe pain during core-needle procedures
Minor complications	Bruising	Low	Bruising following core-needle procedures was reported to be common
	Vasovagal reactions	Low	1.0% of patients had vasovagal reactions during core-needle procedures
	Pain	Low	3.7% of patients required pain medications following core-needle procedures
Factors potentially affecting harms			
Factor category	**Factor**	**Level of evidence**	**Conclusion about impact of factor on harms**
Patient characteristics	Patient age	Insufficient	No conclusion possible
	Breast density	Insufficient	No conclusion possible
	Patient comorbidities	Insufficient	No conclusion possible
Lesion characteristics	Palpable vs. nonpalpable	Insufficient	No conclusion possible
	Microcalcifications vs. masses	Insufficient	No conclusion possible
	Distortions vs. masses	Insufficient	No conclusion possible
	Size of lesion	Insufficient	No conclusion possible
	Location of lesion	Insufficient	No conclusion possible
Biopsy methodology	Number of cores	Insufficient	No conclusion possible
	Patient position	Low	Vasovagal reactions occur more often in patients seated upright
	Reference standard	Insufficient	No conclusion possible
	Use of vacuum	Low	Use of vacuum increased the percentage of procedures complicated by severe bleeding and hematoma formation
	Use of image guidance	Insufficient	No conclusion possible
	Size of needle	Insufficient	No conclusion possible
Clinician and facility factors	Experience of operator	Insufficient	No conclusion possible
	Training of operator	Insufficient	No conclusion possible
	Facility location	Insufficient	No conclusion possible
	Facility type	Insufficient	No conclusion possible

Abbreviations: ADH=atypical ductal hyperplasia; CI=confidence interval; DCIS=ductal carcinoma in situ; MRI=magnetic resonance imaging; US=ultrasound.

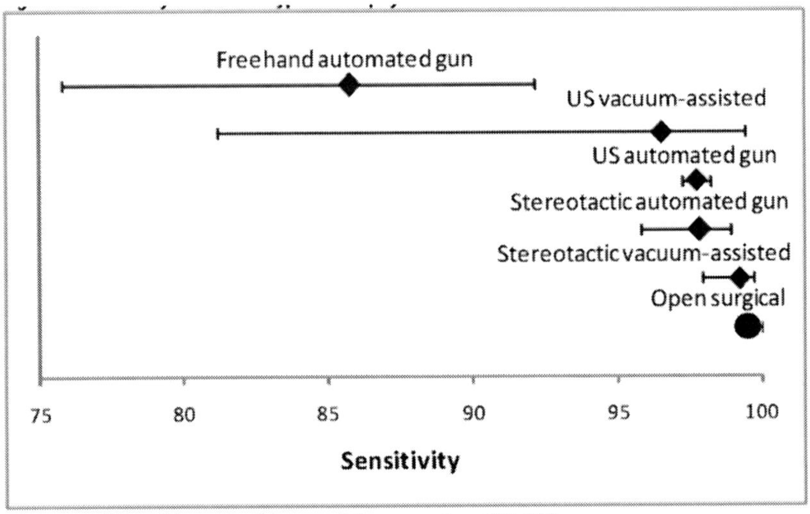

Sensitivity = (true positives/ (true positives + false negatives))* 100.
Freehand automated gun: 5 studies of 610 biopsies.
US vacuum-assisted: 7 studies of 507 biopsies.
US automated gun: 16 studies of 7, 124 biopsies.
Stereotactic automated gun: 33 studies of 7,135 biopsies.
Stereotactic vacuum-assisted: 22 studies of 7512 biopsies.
Open surgical estimate based on other literature reviews.
Abbreviation: US=ultrasound.

Figure A. Sensitivity of different types of biopsy.

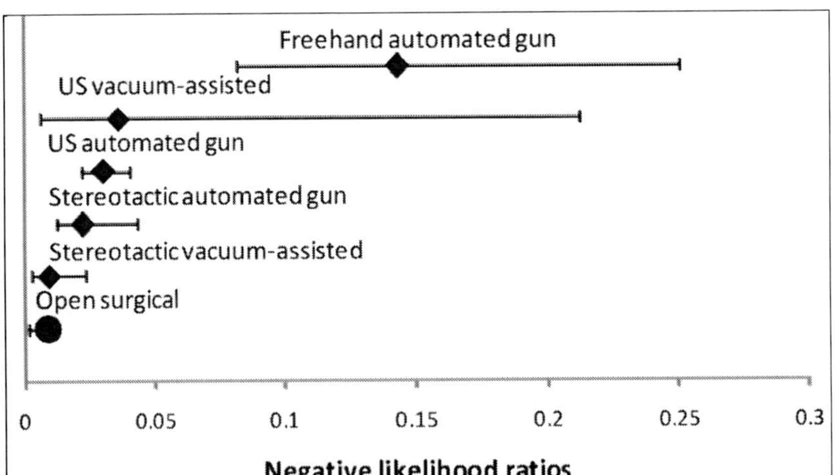

Negative likelihood ratio = (false negatives/(true positives + false negatives)/(true negatives/ false positives + true negatives).
Freehand automated gun: 5 studies of 610 biopsies.
US vacuum-assisted: 7 studies of 507 biopsies.
US automated gun: 16 studies of 7, 124 biopsies.
Stereotactic automated gun: 33 studies of 7,135 biopsies.
Stereotactic vacuum-assisted: 22 studies of 7,512 biopsies.
Open surgical estimate based on other literature reviews.
Abbreviation: US=ultrasound.

Figure B. Negative likelihood ratios of different types of biopsy.

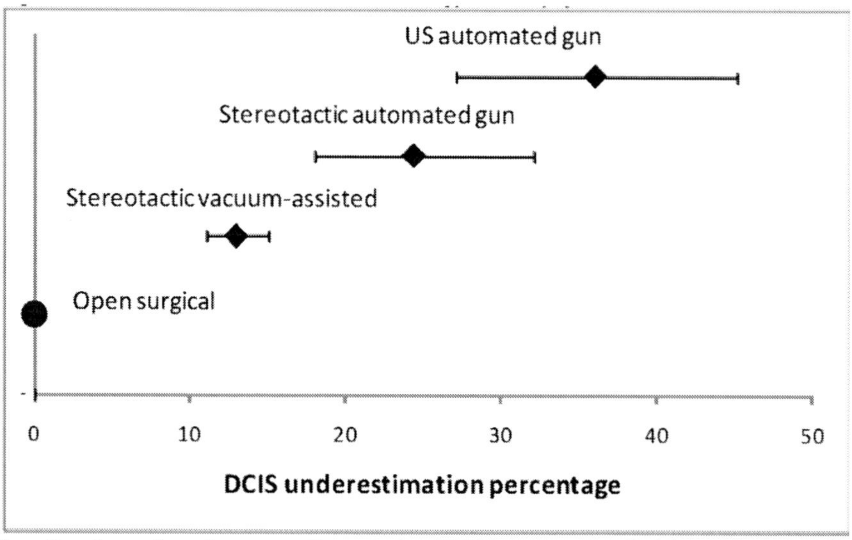

DCIS underestimation = (number cases diagnosed as DCIS on core-needle biopsy that were found to be invasive cancer by the reference standard)/ (total number cases diagnosed as DCIS on core-needle biopsy)*100.

US automated gun: 12 studies of 208 core-needle diagnoses of DCIS.

Stereotactic automated gun: 19 studies of 694 core-needle diagnoses of DCIS.

Stereotactic vacuum-assisted: 21 studies of 1,224 core-needle diagnoses of DCIS.

Open surgical estimate based on other literature reviews.

Abbreviations: DCIS=ductal carcinoma in situ; US=ultrasound.

Figure C. DCIS underestimation rates of different types of biopsy.

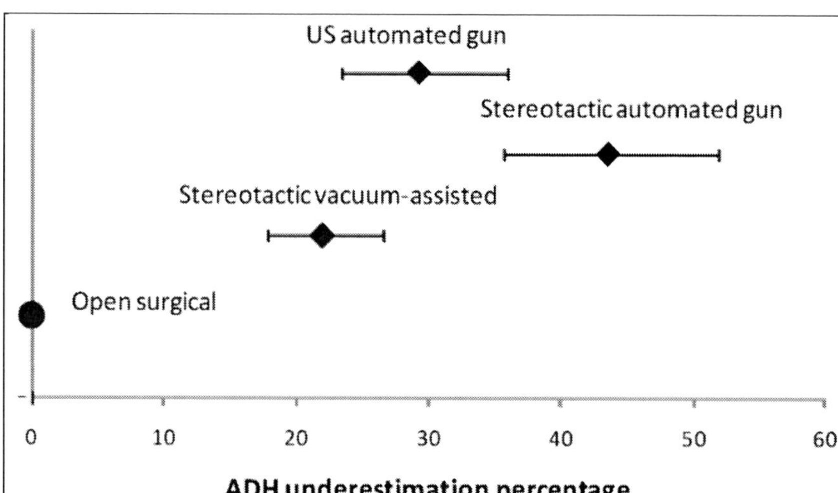

ADH underestimation = (number cases diagnosed as ADH on core-needle biopsy that were found to be invasive or in situ cancer by the reference standard)/ (total number cases diagnosed as ADH on core-needle biopsy)*100.

US automated gun: 13 studies of 207 core-needle diagnoses of ADH.

Stereotactic automated gun: 26 studies of 321 core-needle diagnoses of ADH.

Stereotactic vacuum-assisted: 21 studies of 380 core-needle diagnoses of ADH.

Open surgical estimate based on other literature reviews.

Abbreviations: ADH-=atypical ductal hyperplasia; US=ultrasound.

Figure D. ADH underestimation rates of different types of biopsy.

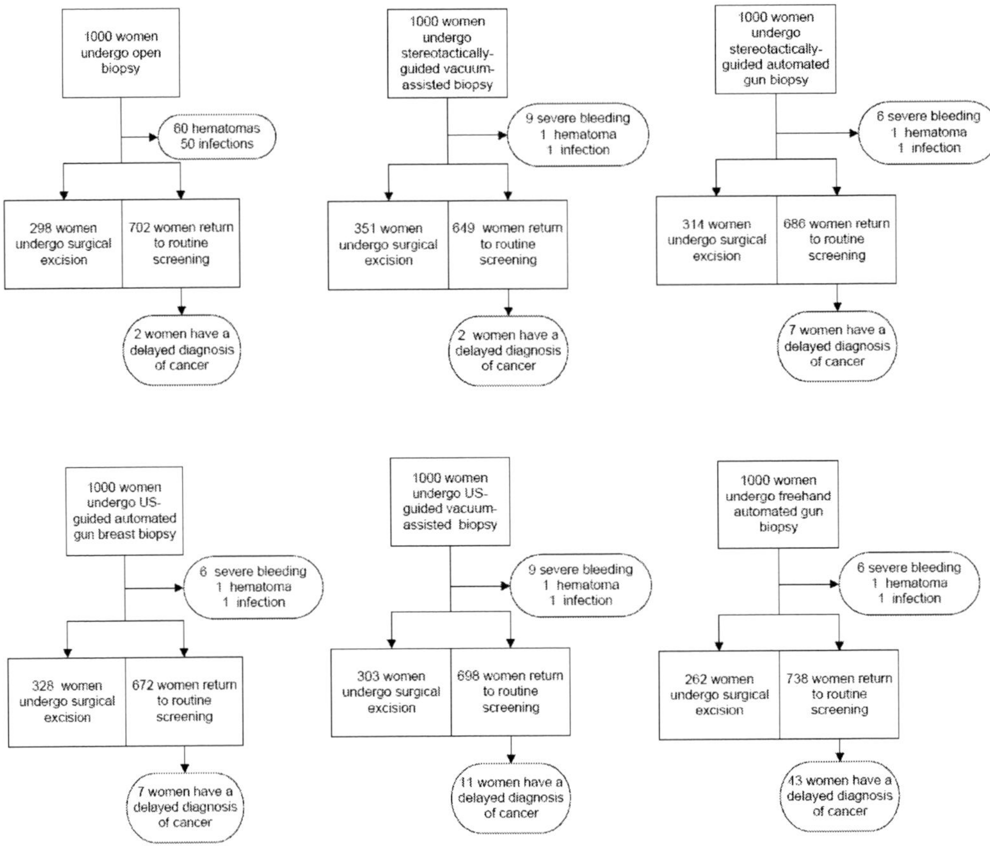

Abbreviation: US=ultrasound.
The numbers may not sum to exactly 1,000 due to rounding.

Figure E. Models of 1,000 women undergoing breast biopsy

1. Introduction

Background

Breast Cancer

Breast cancer is the second most common malignancy of women.[1] The American Cancer Society estimates that in the U.S. in 2009, 67,280 women will have been diagnosed with new cases of *in situ* cancer, 192,370 women will have been newly diagnosed as having invasive breast cancer, and there will be 40,170 deaths due to this disease.[2] In the general population, the cumulative risk of being diagnosed with breast cancer by age 70 is estimated to be 6% (lifetime risk of 13%).[3,4]

Ductal carcinoma, including ductal carcinoma *in situ* (DCIS), is the most common malignancy of the breast. It arises within the ducts of the breast. DCIS is early breast cancer confined to the inside of the ductal system, and invasive (also called infiltrating) ductal carcinoma is a later stage that has broken through the walls of the ducts and invaded nearby tissues. Lobular carcinoma is similar to ductal carcinoma, first arising in the terminal ducts of the lobules and then invading through the walls of the ducts and into nearby tissues. Atypical lobular hyperplasia (ALH) and lobular carcinoma in situ (LCIS) are caused by abnormal cellular proliferation within the terminal ducts of the lobules. The two conditions are distinguished primarily by the degree to which the ducts are filled by cells, and some pathologists have suggested the use of the term lobular neoplasia to describe a continuum of disease from ALH to LCIS.[5] LCIS is not usually detectable by routine clinical exam or mammograms; it is, however, occasionally detected as an incidental finding at the time a breast biopsy is performed for other reasons. Women diagnosed with ALH or LCIS are at elevated risk of developing an invasive carcinoma in the future.

Other types of benign breast abnormalities that have been linked to an elevated risk of invasive carcinoma or a finding of associated invasive carcinoma upon excision are atypical ductal hyperplasia (ADH), papillary lesions, and radial scars.[5]

Breast Biopsy

Breast cancer is usually first detected by feeling a lump on physical examination (either self-examination or an exam conducted by a health practitioner) or by observing an abnormality during x-ray screening mammography. Survival rates depend on the stage of disease at diagnosis. At stage 0 (carcinoma *in situ*) the five-year survival rate is close to 100%. The five-year survival rate for women with stage IV (cancer that has spread beyond the breast) is only 27%.[6] These observations suggest that breast cancer mortality rates can be significantly reduced by identifying cancers at earlier stages. Because early breast cancer is asymptomatic, the only way to detect it is through population-wide screening. Mammography is a widely accepted method for breast cancer screening.[7,8]

Mammography uses x-rays to examine the breast for clusters of microcalcifications, circumscribed and dense masses, masses with indistinct margins, architectural distortion compared with the contralateral breast, or other abnormal structures. Currently, most professional organizations recommend that all women older than fifty years of age receive an annual or biennial mammogram.[6,9] Some professional organizations recommend that routine breast cancer screening begin earlier, at age 40, although x-ray mammography screening is less effective in younger women.[7] Most experts believe that regular x-ray mammographic screening of all women who are between the age of 50 and 70 can reduce mortality from breast cancer.[6-8] The United States Preventive Services Task Force (USPSTF) recommends screening mammography every 2 years for women aged 50 to 74.[10]

The American College of Radiology has created a standardized system for reporting the results of mammography, the Breast Imaging Reporting and Data System (BI-RADS®).[11-13] There are seven categories of assessment and recommendation:

0 Need additional imaging evaluation and/or prior mammograms for comparison
1 Negative
2 Benign finding
3 Probably benign finding. Initial short interval follow-up suggested

4 Suspicious abnormality. Biopsy should be considered.
5 Highly suggestive of malignancy. Appropriate action should be taken.
6 Known biopsy-proven malignancy. Appropriate action should be taken.

After identification of a possible abnormality on screening mammography or physical examination, women typically undergo additional imaging studies (e.g., diagnostic mammography, ultrasound, possibly magnetic resonance imaging (MRI)) and a physical examination. If these studies suggest the abnormality may be malignant, a biopsy of the suspicious area may be recommended. Biopsy material may be obtained by fine-needle aspiration, core-needle biopsy, or open surgical procedures. The combination of physical examination, imaging studies, and fine-needle aspiration is sometimes referred to as the "triple assessment."[14] Fine-needle aspiration is not the topic of this report and is not discussed further.

Open surgical biopsy involves removing a sample of tissue from the suspicious area through an open incision. To aid in location of a non-palpable lesion, it may be marked with a wire, dye, or carbon particles using an imaging method (e.g., mammography, ultrasound, MRI) to guide placement of the marker. The biopsy procedure may be performed under general anesthesia, sedation plus local anesthesia, or local anesthesia only. The surgeon may attempt to remove the entire lesion during the biopsy procedure (excisional biopsy) if the lesion is fairly small. After removing the tissue sample, the incision is closed with sutures.

Open surgical biopsy is the reference standard for evaluating a suspicious breast lesion because it is thought to be very accurate in diagnosing these lesions. However, it is a surgical procedure that, like all surgeries, places the patient at risk of experiencing morbidities and, in rare cases, mortality. Lacquement et al. examined a series of 668 women who underwent biopsy, and reported that only 23% of these women were diagnosed with breast cancer after biopsy.15 Exposing large numbers of women who do not have cancer to invasive surgical procedures may be considered an undesirable medical practice. A less invasive method for evaluation of suspicious breast lesions would be preferable if it were sufficiently accurate.

A core-needle biopsy is a procedure that involves removing small samples of breast tissue through a hollow core needle inserted through the skin. Basic core-needle biopsy uses a special 11-, 14-, or 16-gauge needle (the smaller the gauge the larger the diameter of the needle). The suspicious lesion may be located by palpation or by imaging (e.g., stereotactic mammography, ultrasound, MRI). The procedure is usually performed under local anesthesia. Multiple core-needle samples may be taken from the suspicious area.

A variant on core-needle biopsy is vacuum-assisted biopsy. After locating the suspicious area by stereotactic mammography, ultrasound, or MRI, the probe of the device is inserted into the suspicious area. The device uses vacuum suction to help remove tissue samples. Multiple samples may be taken from the suspicious area. Some vacuum-assisted devices, unlike traditional core-needle biopsy devices, can collect multiple samples while only needing to be inserted through the skin once.

Another variant on core-needle biopsy is large core breast biopsy. Large core breast biopsy is intended to be a minimally invasive method of removing a fairly large sample of breast tissue, or even to remove an entire small lesion. After locating the suspicious area by stereotactic mammography a wire is inserted to mark the location. The device then removes a large core of breast tissue through a cannula. Sutures are required to close the skin at the entry site. There were no large core biopsy devices commercially available in the United States at the time this report was prepared.

Initial biopsy of any breast abnormality has a primary goal of making a diagnosis of the abnormality as benign or malignant. Generally, only malignant lesions require invasive follow-up procedures such as surgical excision or lymph node evaluation. As discussed above, the majority of women who are sent for breast biopsy do not have malignant lesions and do not require follow-up surgery. Thus an accurate initial core- needle biopsy would allow women with benign findings to avoid an open surgical procedure. If the core-needle biopsy suggests the lesion is malignant, lymph node exploration and lesion excision to clear margins could be performed during a subsequent open procedure. Women who are diagnosed with malignant lesions by open biopsy are often subjected to additional follow-up surgical procedures to ensure the lesion has been completely removed and, in some cases, for lymph node evaluation. Therefore, an accurate method of performing core-needle biopsies may enable many women to avoid surgery altogether and reduce the number of surgical procedures women with malignancies must undergo.

Prognostic and Predictive Factors

Pathological prognostic and predictive factors are used in clinical practice to guide treatment planning. One of the major concerns about core-needle biopsy techniques is under-sampling of important areas of the lesion. If important areas are missed, the pathology report may be misleading. Categories of prognostic and predictive factors include tumor type, histological grade, and immunophenotype of the tumor. These categories are briefly discussed below.

Tumor typing is evaluation of type of the tumor, e.g., DCIS, infiltrating ductal carcinoma, medullary carcinoma, infiltrating lobular carcinoma, tubular carcinoma, mucinous carcinoma, inflammatory breast cancer, or other. Tumor typing of mixed-type tumors by core-needle biopsy may be incorrect due to the inability of needle biopsy to sample all parts of the tumor.

Histological grade is used to describe invasive tumors and other breast abnormalities. The grade is based on how closely cells in the sample tissue resemble normal breast tissue. Different grading systems are in use, but in general the higher the grade, the more abnormal the tissue structure and cells. Interpretation of grade from core- needle biopsy material has been reported to commonly underestimate the grade by one level as compared to surgical specimens.[16] Rakha and Ellis have suggested that the discrepancy is often due to the fact that core-needle samples are generally taken from the interior of the tumor and surgical specimens for grading are usually taken from the periphery of the tumor, where the most active growth is occuring.[16]

Immunophenotype of the tumor refers to determining the status of certain biomarkers. The presence of estrogen receptors, progesterone receptors, and HER-2 overexpression are important features of tumor biology that need to be incorporated into treatment decisions. For example, estrogen receptor positive tumors may be effectively treated with hormone-blocking medications such as tamoxifen, and tumors that over- express HER-2 may be treated with trastuzumab (Herceptin) or lapatinib (Tykerb). Core- needle specimens can be utilized in tests to determine the immunophenotype of the tumor.

Staging

Final treatment decisions are based on the stage of the tumor. Breast cancer is most commonly staged with the American Joint Committee on Cancer (AJCC) TNM system.[17] The "T" stands for tumor, and is assigned a number from 0 to 4 to describe the size and local spread of the primary tumor, determined by imaging studies such as mammography, MRI, and CT scanning. The 'N" stands for lymph nodes, and is assigned a number from 0 to 3 to indicate whether the cancer has spread to the lymph nodes and to how many lymph nodes, determined by sentinel lymph node biopsy or axillary lymph node dissection. The "M" stands for distant metastasis, and is assigned either 0 or 1 to indicate whether the cancer has spread to distant locations, determined by imaging studies such as CT scanning and bone scintigraphy.[18] Breast cancer stage may also be expressed as a number from 0 to IV, where stage 0 is ductal carcinoma in situ (DCIS) and stage IV is metastatic cancer.[17,18]

Negative Surgical Excision after after Core-Needle Biopsy

Sometimes a core-needle biopsy specimen suggests that a tumor is present, and thus an open surgical procedure is performed, only to find no tumor present. Many experts suggest that in these cases the core-needle biopsy procedure removed the entire tumor.[16] This may be the case. It is also possible that the pathology report for either procedure was incorrect, or that the open procedure missed the lesion.

Choice of Biopsy Method

Medical indications may direct the preference for one type of procedure over another. For example, the size and location of the lesion, imaging characteristics of the lesion, and likelihood of eventual surgical excision could be important to the choice of method. However, other factors such as patient preferences, access, and practice and referral patterns also influence decisions about which procedure should be performed.

The large number of possible methods of performing breast biopsy can be bewildering to patients and healthcare providers alike. Which method should one choose? Is a particular method clearly superior, or does the method of choice depend upon individual patient or lesion characteristics? We have performed a systematic review intended to evaluate the accuracy of different methods of performing breast biopsy, and to explore what factor(s) may impact the accuracy and possible harms of different methods of performing breast biopsy.

Conceptual Framework

The analytical framework (Figure 1) demonstrates the links between patients, tests, interventions, and outcomes. The numbers on the diagram refer to the Key Questions (see next section) and their placement in Figure 1 exhibits the many links separating the Key Questions from the patient-oriented outcomes. Fryback and Thornbury have proposed a six-level model of assessing diagnostic efficacy.[19] Level 1 is analytic validity; level 2 is diagnostic accuracy; level 3 is diagnostic thinking; level 4 is impact on choice of treatment; level 5 is patient-important outcomes; and level 6 is societal impact. Demonstration of efficacy at each lower level is logically necessary, but not sufficient, to assure efficacy at higher levels. This systematic review is primarily concerned with Level 2, the diagnostic accuracy of various methods of performing breast biopsies.

We have expanded the section of the analytical framework that is relevant to the questions addressed in this systematic review in a patient flow diagram (Figure 2). The numbers on the diagram refer to the Key Questions (see next section). We have simplified the diagram for clarity by combining all types of core-needle procedures together into one pathway.

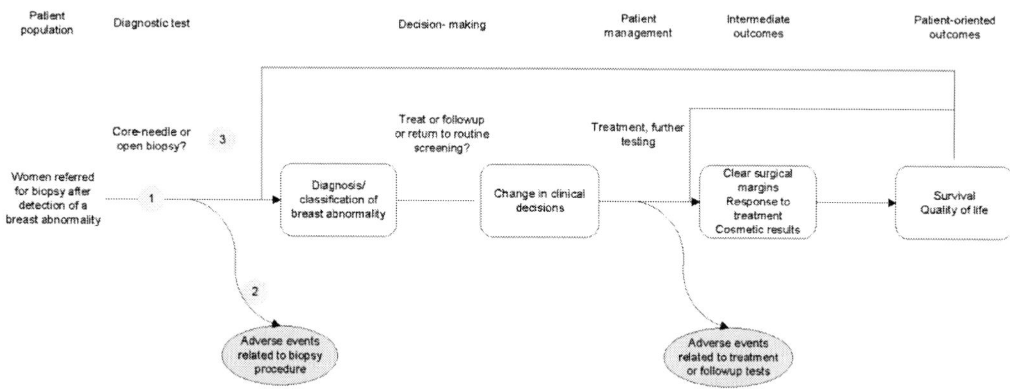

The numbers in the figure depict where the three Key Questions addressed in this report are located within the flow of the analytical framework.

Figure 1. Analytical framework.

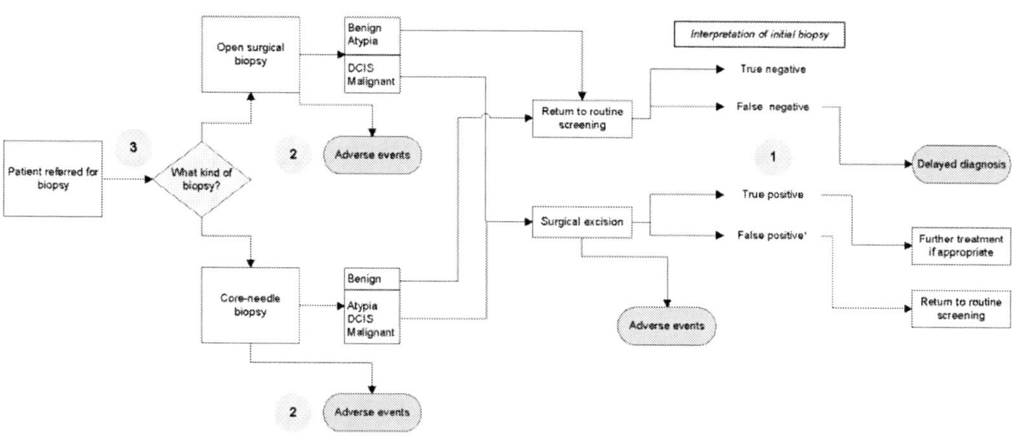

The numbers in the figure depict where the three Key Questions addressed in this report are located within the patient flow diagram.

*If initial core-needle biopsy indicates malignancy but surgical excision is negative for malignancy, many would assume that the initial biopsy removed the lesion rather than to label it a false positive. Patients may then undergo close surveillance or further treatment.

Figure 2. Patient flow diagram.

Diagnostic Test Characteristics

No diagnostic test is perfect. Studies of test performance compare test results on a group of individuals, some of whom have the disease and some of whom do not. Each individual undergoes the experimental test as well as a second reference test to determine "true" disease status. The relationship between the diagnostic test results and disease status is described using diagnostic test characteristics. It is important that the reference test is very accurate in measuring "true" disease status, or else the performance of the experimental diagnostic test will be poorly estimated.

Sensitivity and Specificity

The results of the experimental and reference standard test and their relationship are commonly presented as two-by-two (2x2) tables (see Table 1). From the 2x2 table, sensitivity and specificity are readily calculated:

Sensitivity = TP/(TP+FN)
Specificity = TN/(FP+TN)

Sensitivity and specificity are properties of a test that are useful when deciding whether to use a test. Sensitivity is the proportion of people with the disease who have a positive test for the disease. A test with high sensitivity will rarely misclassify people with the disease as not having the disease (the test has a low rate of false-negatives). Specificity is the proportion of people without the disease who have a negative test. A test with high specificity will rarely misclassify people without the disease as diseased (a low rate of false-positives).

Predictive Values and Likelihood Ratios

To make sense of a diagnostic investigation, a clinician needs to be able to make an inference regarding the probability that a patient has the disease in question according to the result obtained from the test. Sensitivity and specificity do not directly provide this information. The predictive values and likelihood ratios can also be directly calculated from a 2x2 table:

Positive predictive value = TP/(TP+FP)
Negative predictive value = TN/(FN+TN)
Positive likelihood ratio = (TP/(TP+FN))/(FP/(FP+TN))
Negative likelihood ratio = (FN/(TP+FN))/(TN/(FP+TN))

Table 1. Example of a 2x2 table.

	Disease		
		Present	**Absent**
Test Results	Positive	True positives (TP)	False positives (FP)
Negative	False negatives (FN)		True negatives (TN)

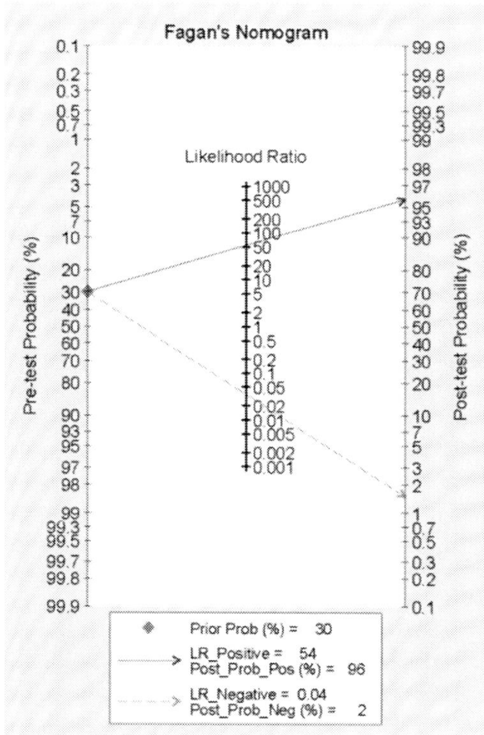

Figure 3. Example of a nomogram.

The positive predictive value of a test is the probability of a patient having the disease following a positive test result. The negative predictive value is the probability of a patient not having the disease following a negative test result. Predictive values describe the probabilities that positive or negative results are correct for an individual patient. However, predictive values depend on the prevalence of disease in the population. A study that enrolled a patient population with a disease prevalence of 70% may report a positive predictive value of 80%. If a clinician tests a patient from a population with a disease prevalence of 70%, and the test comes back positive, the clinician knows the patient has an 80% chance of having the disease in question. However, if the patient comes from a population with a disease prevalence of 20%, the clinician cannot apply the results of the study directly to this patient.

Because sensitivity and specificity are difficult to directly apply to clinical situations, and predictive values vary markedly as a function of disease prevalence (i.e., may be different for each patient subpopulation) a combined measure of diagnostic performance, the likelihood ratio, is a clinically useful diagnostic test performance measure. Negative likelihood ratios measure the ability of the test to accurately "rule out" disease, and positive likelihood ratios measure the ability of the test to accurately detect disease.

Likelihood ratios are independent of prevalence and therefore can be directly applied in the clinic to update an individual's estimated chances of disease according to their test result. Likelihood ratios can be used in Bayes' theorem to calculate post-test odds of having a disease from the pre-test suspicion of the patient's odds of having that disease. Clinicians may be familiar with simple nomograms that allow a direct visualization of post-test chances of disease given a positive or negative test result, without the need to go through the tedious calculations of Bayes' theorem; see, for example, Figure 3 or the interactive form of the nomogram provided by the Center for Evidence-based Medicine at http://www.cebm.net.

In Figure 3 a nomogram using the negative likelihood ratio for ultrasound-guided vacuum-assisted biopsy is shown. A typical woman with a mammogram described as BI-RADS 4 pre-biopsy has an approximate 30% probability of having a malignant tumor. The dotted blue line in the nomogram can be drawn with a straight-edge from 30% on the left side of the figure, through the negative likelihood ratio of 0.04, and continue in a straight line to the right side of the figure to 2%, indicating that if this woman has a "benign" finding on her core-needle biopsy her post-biopsy probability of having a malignant tumor is approximately 2%.

Scope and Key Questions

This systematic review was commissioned by the Agency for Healthcare Research and Quality (AHRQ) to address the following Key Questions:

1. In women with a *palpable* or *non-palpable* breast abnormality, what is the accuracy of different types of core-needle breast biopsy compared with open biopsy for diagnosis? (*The primary outcomes for determination of accuracy are missed cancers [the false negative rate, or sensitivity] and the underestimation rate*).

   1a. What factors associated with the *patient* and her *breast abnormality* influence the accuracy of different types of core-needle breast biopsy compared with open biopsy for diagnosis of a breast abnormality?

   Patient and lesion-associated factors include, but may not be limited to:
   Age, characteristics of lesion on mammography or other imaging, breast density, tissue type(s) and architecture of breast lesion, location of breast lesion, or other patient clinical health issues that may affect biopsy (i.e., clotting disorder).

   1b. What factors associated with the *procedure* itself influence the accuracy of different types of core-needle breast biopsy compared with open biopsy for diagnosis of a breast abnormality?
   Procedure-related factors include, but may not be limited to:
   Equipment used, gauge of core-needle needle used, number of cores, area/amount of specimen obtained, use of vacuum, specific device used, and use of imaging guidance (e.g., MRI, US, stereotactic techniques).

   1c. What *clinician and facility* factors influence the accuracy of core-needle breast biopsy compared with open biopsy for diagnosis of a breast abnormality?
   Clinician and facility factors include, but may not be limited to:
   Training and experience of clinicians performing the diagnostic procedure and interpreting breast specimen (e.g., specialized breast team, pathologist), annual volume of each procedure performed at facility, geographic location (where in country/world), practice setting (e.g., group, solo), facility setting (e.g., office, ambulatory surgical center, hospital)

2. In women with a *palpable* or *non-palpable* breast abnormality, what are the harms associated with core-needle breast biopsy compared to the open biopsy technique in the diagnosis of breast cancer? (*The primary outcomes for determination of harms are inconclusive findings and the re-biopsy rate, dissemination of cancerous cells along needle track, complications, patient centered outcomes including satisfaction, quality of life metrics, time to recover, use of pain medications and subsequent false positive and false negative rate on mammography.*)
   2a. What factors associated with the *patient* and her *breast abnormality* influence the harms of core-needle breast biopsy compared with the open biopsy technique in the diagnosis of a breast abnormality?
   Patient and lesion-associated factors include, but may not be limited to:
   Age, characteristics of lesion on mammography or other imaging, breast density, tissue type(s) and architecture of breast lesion, location of breast lesion, or other patient clinical health issues that may affect biopsy (i.e., clotting disorder).
   2b. What factors associated with the *procedure* itself influence the harms of core-needle breast biopsy compared with the open biopsy technique in the diagnosis of a breast abnormality?
   Procedure-related factors include, but may not be limited to:
   Equipment used, gauge of core-needle needle used, number of core samples, area/amount of specimen obtained, use of vacuum, specific device used, and use of imaging guidance (e.g., MRI, US, stereotactic techniques).
   2c. What *clinician and facility* factors influence the harms of core-needle breast biopsy compared with the open biopsy technique for diagnosis of a breast abnormality?
   Clinician and facility factors include, but may not be limited to:
   Training and experience of clinicians performing the diagnostic procedure and interpreting breast specimen (e.g., specialized breast team, pathologist), annual volume of each procedure performed at facility, geographic location (where in country/world), practice setting (e.g., group, solo), facility setting (e.g., office, ambulatory surgical center, hospital)
3. How do open biopsy and various core-needle techniques differ in terms of patient preference, availability, costs, availability of qualified pathologist interpretations, and other factors that may influence choice of particular technique?

This report focuses on the use of core-needle biopsies to evaluate suspected cancer confined to the breast. Fine-needle aspiration is outside the scope of this report. Other uses of biopsy for diagnosing and managing breast cancer, or any other issue not mentioned in the Key Questions, are outside the scope of this report.

2. Methods

Topic Development

In response to Section 1013 of the Medicare Modernization Act, AHRQ requested an evidence report to synthesize the evidence on the comparative effectiveness of core needle and open surgical biopsy for diagnosis of breast cancer. The topic was nominated in a public process. The Scientific Resource Center (SRC) for the AHRQ Effective Health Care Program recruited a technical expert panel (TEP) to give input on key steps including the selection and refinement of the questions to be examined. The expert panel membership is provided in Appendix A.

Upon AHRQ approval, the draft Key Questions were posted for public comment. After receipt of public commentary, the SRC finalized the Key Questions and submitted them to AHRQ for approval. These Key Questions are presented in the Scope and Key Questions section of the Introduction.

Our EPC created a work plan for developing the evidence report. The process consisted of working with AHRQ, the SRC, and the technical experts to outline the report's objectives, performing a comprehensive literature search, abstracting data, constructing evidence tables, synthesizing the data, and submitting the report for peer review.

In designing the study questions and methodology at the outset of this report, the EPC consulted several technical and content experts. Broad expertise and perspectives were sought. Divergent and conflicted opinions are common and perceived as healthy scientific discourse that results in a thoughtful, relevant systematic review. Therefore, in the end, study questions, design and/or methodologic approaches do not necessarily represent the views of individual technical and content experts.

Search Strategy

The medical literature was searched from December 1990 through November 10, 2008, and the PubMed and EMBASE searches were updated to September 11, 2009. The full strategy is provided in Appendix B. In brief, we searched 14 external and internal databases, including PubMed and EMBASE, for clinical trials addressing the Key Questions. To supplement the electronic searches, we also examined the bibliographies/reference lists of included studies, recent narrative reviews, and scanned the content of new issues of selected journals and selected relevant gray literature sources.

Study Selection

We selected the studies that we consider in this report using *a priori* inclusion criteria. Some of the criteria we employed are geared towards ensuring that we used only the most reliable evidence. Other criteria were developed to ensure that the evidence is not derived from atypical patients or interventions, and/or outmoded technologies.

Studies of diagnostic test performance compare results of the experimental test to a reference test. The reference test is intended to measure the "true" disease status of each patient. It is important that the results of the reference test be very close to the truth, or the performance of the experimental test will be poorly estimated. For the diagnosis of breast cancer, the "gold standard" reference standard test is open surgical biopsy. However, an issue with the use of open surgical biopsy as the reference standard in large cohort studies of screening-detected breast abnormalities is the difficulty of subjecting women with probably benign lesions to open surgical biopsy. Furthermore, restricting the evidence base to studies that used open surgery as the reference standard for all enrolled subjects would eliminate the majority of the evidence. Therefore, we have chosen to use a combination of clinical and radiologic followup as well as open surgical biopsy as the reference standard for our analysis.

For Key Question 1 we used the following formal criteria to determine which studies would be included in our analysis. Many of our inclusion criteria for Key Question 1 were intended to reduce the potential for spectrum bias. Spectrum bias refers to the fact that diagnostic test performance is not constant across populations with different spectrums of disease. For example, patients presenting with severe symptoms of disease may be easier to diagnose than asymptomatic patients in a screening population; and a diagnostic test that performs well in the former population may perform poorly in the latter population. The results of our analysis are intended to apply to a general population of women at average risk of breast cancer participating in routine breast cancer screening programs (mammography, clinical examination, and self- examination programs) and therefore many of our inclusion criteria are intended to eliminate studies that enrolled populations of women at very high risk of breast cancer due to family history, or populations of women at risk of recurrence of a previously diagnosed breast cancer.

1. The study must have directly compared core-needle biopsy to open surgery or patient followup for six months or longer in the same group of patients.
   Although it is possible to estimate diagnostic accuracy from a two-group trial, the results of such indirect comparisons must be viewed with great caution. Diagnostic cohort studies, wherein each patient acts as her own control, are the preferred study design for evaluating the accuracy of a diagnostic test.[20] Retrospective case-control studies and case reports were excluded. Retrospective case-control studies have been shown to overestimate the accuracy of diagnostic tests, and case reports often report unusual situations or individuals that are unlikely to yield results that are applicable to general practice.[20,21] Retrospective case studies (studies that selected cases for study on the basis of the type of lesion diagnosed by core-needle biopsy) were also excluded because the data such studies report cannot be used to calculate the overall diagnostic accuracy of core-needle biopsy. Studies may have performed open surgical procedures on all patients, or may have performed open surgical biopsy on some patients and followed the other patients with clinical examination and mammograms for at least six months.
2. The study enrolled female human subjects.
   Animal studies or studies of "imaging phantoms" are outside the scope of the report. Studies of breast cancer in men are outside the scope of the report.
3. The study must have enrolled patients referred for biopsy for the purpose of primary diagnosis of a breast abnormality.

Studies that enrolled women who were referred for biopsy after discovery of a possible breast abnormality by screening mammography or routine physical examination were included. Studies that enrolled subjects that were undergoing biopsy for any of the following purposes were excluded as being out of scope of the report: breast cancer staging, evaluation for a possible recurrence of breast cancer, monitoring response to treatment, evaluation of the axillary lymph nodes, evaluation of metastatic or suspected metastatic disease, or diagnosis of types of cancer other than primary breast cancer.

Studies that enrolled patients from high-risk populations such as BRCA 1/2 mutation carriers are also out of scope. If a study enrolled a mixed patient population and did not report data separately, it was excluded if more than 15% of the subjects did not fall into the "primary diagnosis of women at average risk presenting with an abnormality detected on routine screening" category.

4. Fifty percent or more of the subjects must have completed the study.
   Studies with extremely high rates of attrition are prone to bias and were excluded.
5. Study must be published in English.
   Moher et al. and Holenstein et al. have demonstrated that exclusion of non-English language studies from meta-analyses has little impact on the conclusions drawn.22,23 Although we recognize the possibility that requiring studies to be published in English could lead to bias, it is insufficiently likely that we cannot justify the time and cost of translations.
6. Study must be published as a peer-reviewed full article. Meeting abstracts were not included.
   Published meeting abstracts have not been peer-reviewed and often do not include sufficient details about experimental methods to permit one to verify that the study was well designed.[24,25] In addition, it is not uncommon for abstracts that are published as part of conference proceedings to have inconsistencies when compared to the final publication of the study, or to describe studies that are never published as full articles.[26-30]
7. The study must have enrolled 10 or more individuals per arm.
   The results of very small studies are unlikely to be applicable to general clinical practice. Small studies are unable to detect sufficient numbers of events for meaningful analyses to be performed, and are at risk of enrolling unique individuals.
8. When several sequential reports from the same patients/study are available, only outcome data from the most recent report were included. However, we used relevant data from earlier and smaller reports if the report presented pertinent data not presented in the more recent report.
9. Studies of biopsy instrumentation that are no longer commercially available were excluded.
   The ABBI device, the MIBB device, and SiteSelect have been discontinued by their manufacturers. Studies of the accuracy and harms related to the use of these devices are no longer clinically relevant.

To address Question 2, we recorded any harms information reported in the studies included to address Question 1. In addition, we collected any articles, regardless of design, that addressed part of Question 2, namely the dissemination of cancer cells by the biopsy procedure. To address Question 3, we consulted a variety of information sources, including published literature, cost-effectiveness analyses, evidence-based clinical practice guidelines, published expert panel consensus statements, and consultations with experts. We did not use formal inclusion criteria for Question 3 due to the nature of the question; instead, we approached the question as an "opinion/discussion" type of question.

To address the accuracy of open surgical biopsy, we first searched for clinical studies that performed open surgical biopsy, followed patients for six months or longer, and met the above listed inclusion criteria. However, we identified no clinical studies that met the inclusion criteria, so we searched for systematic and narrative reviews that addressed the accuracy and harms of open surgical biopsy.

The abstracts of articles identified by the literature searches were screened in duplicate for possible relevance by three research assistants. The first fifty abstracts screened by each research assistant were also screened in duplicate by the lead research analyst, and all exclusions at the abstract level were approved by the lead research analyst. The full-length articles of studies that appeared relevant at the abstract level were then obtained and three research assistants examined the articles in duplicate to see if they met the inclusion criteria. All conflicts were resolved by the lead research analyst. The excluded articles and primary reason for exclusion are shown in Appendix C.

Data Abstraction

Standardized data abstraction forms were created and data was entered by each reviewer into the SRS© 4.0 database (see Appendix D). Three research assistants abstracted the data. The first fifty articles were abstracted in duplicate. All conflicts were resolved by the lead research analyst.

Study Quality Evaluation

We used an internal validity rating scale for diagnostic studies to grade the internal validity of the evidence base (Table 2). This instrument is based on a modification of the QUADAS instrument.[31] Each question in the instrument addresses an aspect of study design or conduct that can help to protect against bias. Each question can be answered "yes", "no", or "not reported," and each is phrased such that an answer of "yes" indicates that the study reported a protection against bias on that aspect. A summary quality score was computed in order to reduce the subjectivity of the assessment of the potential for bias present in the evidence base. A summary score was computed with each "yes" given a +1, each "no" a -1, and each "not reported" a zero. As all of the factors captured by the questions on the quality instrument were thought to be of equal importance for this topic, no weighting was utilized in computing the summary score. This summary score was then normalized[a] to a scale from 0 to 10, with the lower the score the greater the risk that the study was affected by biases. Consequently, a study employing all 14 features would score +10, a study employing none would score 0, and a study simply not reporting any of these features would score 5, thus acknowledging that published studies may not provide information on all study procedures that were actually carried out.

To evaluate the overall quality of the evidence base for each conclusion, we computed the median quality score of the studies contributing to that conclusion. An evidence base with a median score higher than 8.4 was considered to be of high quality; an evidence base with a median score 8.4 or less but greater than 6.7 was considered to be of moderate quality; an evidence base with a median score 6.7 or less but greater than 5.0 was considered to be of low quality; and an evidence base with a median score less than 5.0 was considered to be of insufficient quality. Internal validity assessment findings are summarized for each outcome in the Results section. Responses to the questions in the quality assessment instrument for each study are presented in the Evidence Tables in the Appendix.

Strength of Evidence

The strength of evidence supporting each major conclusion was graded as High, Moderate, Low, or Insufficient. The grade was developed by considering various important domains as suggested in the CER Draft Methods Guide and in accordance with a strength and stability of evidence grading system developed by ECRI Institute.[32] Four domains were evaluated: the quality (potential risk of bias, or "internal validity") of the evidence base, the size of the evidence base, the consistency (agreement across studies) of the findings, and the robustness of the findings (as determined by sensitivity analysis). The domain of "directness" was incorporated into our analytic framework, but not into the grade, as downstream patient health outcomes are rarely reported in diagnostic studies. The domain of "precision" was incorporated into our assessment of the size of the evidence base.

Table 2. Quality assessment instrument.

1. Was patient recruitment either consecutive or random?
2. Were more than 85% of the patients approached for recruitment enrolled in the study?
3. Were the patient inclusion/ exclusion criteria consistently applied to all patients?
4. Was the study free from obvious spectrum bias? Obvious spectrum bias was defined as more than 40% or less than 10% of the breast lesions were diagnosed as malignant; and/or the mean or median age of the enrolled population was less than 50 or greater than 70.
5. Was the study prospective in design?
6. Was a complete set of data reported for at least 85% of enrolled lesions?
7. Were the patients assessed by the reference standard (open surgical procedure) regardless of the initial biopsy results?
8. Were patients assessed by a reference standard regardless of the biopsy results?
9. Was funding for this study provided by a source that doesn't have an obvious financial interest in the findings of the study?
10. Did the study account for inter-reader/scorer differences?
11. Were the reader(s) of the biopsies blinded to the results of the reference standard?
12. Were readers of the reference standard blinded to the results of the biopsy?
13. Were the readers of the biopsy blinded to all other clinical information?
14. Were readers of the reference standard blinded to all other clinical information?

The domain considered to be of overriding importance for this topic was the potential for bias in the evidence base. The potential for bias was measured by the quality of the evidence as described above. The quality rating was considered to be the highest strength of evidence grade that could be achieved for each conclusion. The other domains were evaluated as either "Sufficient" or "Insufficient," and ratings of "Insufficient" for other domains caused a downgrading of the strength of evidence grade. Further details about grading the strength of evidence may be found in Appendix G.

Because of the nature of Question 3 and the sources of information used to address it, we did not draw many formal evidence-based conclusions for this question, nor, in most cases, did we attempt to rate the quality of the studies or grade the strength of the evidence. For one conclusion for Key Question 3 we considered the consistency, robustness, and strength of association between the type of biopsy and the outcome to be sufficient to support an evidence- based conclusion.

Applicability

The issue of applicability was chiefly addressed by excluding studies that enrolled patient populations that were not a general population of asymptomatic women participating in routine breast cancer screening programs. We defined this population as women at average risk of breast cancer participating in routine breast cancer screening programs (including mammography, clinical examination, and self-examination). We excluded studies that enrolled women who were referred for biopsy for the purpose of: staging of already diagnosed breast cancers; evaluation of the axillary lymph nodes; evaluation for metastatic or suspected metastatic disease; evaluation of recurrent or suspected recurrent disease; and studies that enrolled women thought to be at very high risk of breast cancer due to family history or carriers of BRCA mutations. We also excluded studies of biopsy instrumentation that are no longer commercially available on the grounds that the data reported is no longer applicable to clinical practice.

To verify that the evidence base enrolled a "typical" population we examined the prevalence of breast cancers diagnosed. The prevalence of cancers in the general population sent for breast biopsy (in the U.S.) has been reported to be around 23%.[15] If our evidence base were indeed typical for patients in the U.S., we would expect to see a similar prevalence of breast cancers.

Data Analysis and Synthesis

Several key assumptions were made: (1) the "reference standard," open surgical biopsy and/or clinical and radiologic followup for at least six months, was 100% accurate; (2) the pathologists diagnosing the open surgical biopsy results were 100% accurate in diagnosing the material submitted to them; and (3) core-needle diagnoses of malignancy (invasive or in situ) that could not be confirmed by an open surgical procedure were assumed to have been correct diagnoses where the lesion had been completely removed by the core-needle biopsy procedure.33 In addition, the majority of studies reported data on a per-lesion rather than a per-patient basis, and therefore we analyzed the data on a per-lesion basis assuming that statistical assumptions of data independence were not being violated.

We performed two primary types of analyses - a standard diagnostic accuracy analysis and an analysis of underestimation rates. For the diagnostic accuracy analysis,

- true negatives were defined as lesions diagnosed as benign on core-needle biopsy that were found to be benign by the reference standard;
- false negatives were defined as lesions diagnosed as benign on core-needle biopsy that were found to be malignant (invasive or in situ) by the reference standard;
- true positives were defined as lesions diagnosed as malignant (invasive or in situ) on core-needle biopsy as well as "high risk" lesions that were found to be malignant (invasive or in situ) on the reference standard
- false positives were defined as lesions diagnosed as "high risk"(most commonly ADH lesions) on core-needle biopsy that were found not to be malignant (invasive or in situ) by the reference standard (see Table 3).

Table 3. Definitions of diagnostic test characteristics.

		Reference standard results (open surgery or followup)	
		Malignant (invasive or in situ tumor)	**Benign**
Core-needle biopsy results	Malignant (invasive or in situ)	True positive	True positive[a]
	ADH or other "high risk" lesions type	True positive	False positive
	Benign	False negative	True negative

[a] Most authors assumed malignant diagnoses on core-needle were true positives even if no tumor was identified by surgical excision.

Sensitivity = (true positives/ (true positives + false negatives))* 100

Negative likelihood ratio = (false negatives/(true positives + false negatives)/(true negatives/false positives + true negatives)

Table 4. Definitions of underestimation rates.

		Reference standard results (open surgery or followup)		
		Malignant (invasive)	**Malignant (in situ)**	**Benign**
Core-needle biopsy results	DCIS	Underestimation	Not underestimated	Not underestimated
	ADH or other "high risk" lesion type	Underestimation	Underestimation	Not underestimated

DCIS underestimation = (number cases diagnosed as DCIS on core-needle biopsy that were found to be invasive cancer by the reference standard)/ (total number cases diagnosed as DCIS on core-needle biopsy)*100

ADH underestimation = (number cases diagnosed as ADH on core-needle biopsy that were found to be invasive or in situ cancer by the reference standard)/ (total number cases diagnosed as ADH on core-needle biopsy)*100

We meta-analyzed the data reported by the studies using a bivariate mixed-effects binomial regression model as described by Harbord et al.[34] All such analyses were computed by the STATA 10.0 statistical software package using the "midas" command.[35] The summary likelihood ratios and Bayes theorem were used to calculate the post-test probability of having a benign or malignant lesion. In cases where a bivariate binomial regression model could not be fit we meta-analyzed the data using a random-effects model and the software package Meta-Disc.36 Meta-regressions were also performed with the Meta-Disc software package.

Diagnostic tests all have a trade-off between minimizing false-negative and minimizing false-positive errors. False-positive errors that occur on core-needle biopsy are not considered to be as clinically relevant as false-negative errors. Women who experience a false-positive error will be sent for an additional biopsy procedure, and may suffer anxiety and minor temporary complications. However, women who experience a false-negative error may die from a delayed cancer diagnosis. In addition, because all "positive" diagnoses of malignancy on core-needle biopsy are assumed to be correct, the "true" false positive rate is artificially reduced towards 0%. Thus false-positive errors, and diagnostic test characteristics that evaluate the impact of false- positive errors (specificity, positive predictive value, positive likelihood ratio), are not particularly relevant for evaluating this technology.

We focused on measures that evaluate the extent of false-negative errors: sensitivity and negative likelihood ratio. A biopsy method with a very high sensitivity misses very few cancers. Negative likelihood ratios can be used along with Bayes' theorem to directly compute an individual woman's risk of having a malignancy following a "benign" diagnosis on core-needle biopsy. In general, the smaller the negative likelihood ratio the more accurate the diagnostic test is in predicting the absence of disease. However, each individual woman's post-test risk varies by her pre-test risk of malignancy. Simple nomograms are available for in-office use that allow clinicians to directly read individual patients' post-test risk off a graph without having to go through the tedium of calculations. Negative predictive value is another commonly used measure of false-negative errors; however, negative predictive values are specific to specific populations of women. They can be used to predict how many women in that particular population do not have a malignancy following a "benign" diagnosis on core-needle biopsy. Negative predictive values vary by the prevalence of disease in each specific population and should not be applied to other populations with different prevalences of disease.

The second type of analysis we performed was an analysis of underestimation rates. Lesions diagnosed as DCIS by core-needle biopsy that were found to be invasive by the reference standard were counted as underestimates. Similarly, "high risk" (most commonly ADH lesions) that were found to be malignant (in situ or invasive) by the reference standard were counted as underestimates (see Table 4). The underestimation rate was then calculated as the number of underestimates per number of DCIS (or "high risk") diagnoses and expressed as a percentage (the percentage of DCIS or ADH diagnoses that were underestimates). We meta-analyzed the underestimation rates with a random-effects model using the CMA software package.[37]

We meta-analyzed any other types of outcomes with a random-effects model using the CMA software package.[37] We did not assess the possibility of publication bias because statistical methods developed to assess the possibility of publication bias in treatment studies have not been validated for use with studies of diagnostic accuracy.[38,39]

Peer Review and Public Commentary

A draft of the completed report was sent to the peer reviewers, the representatives of the AHRQ, and the Scientific Resource Center. The draft report was posted to a Web site for public comment. In response to the comments of the peer reviewers and the public, revisions were made to the evidence report, and a summary of the comments and their disposition was submitted to AHRQ. Peer reviewer comments on a preliminary draft of this report were considered by the EPC in preparation of this final report. Synthesis of the scientific literature presented here does not necessarily represent the views of individual reviewers.

3. Results

Question 1. In Women with a Palpable or Non-Palpable Breast Abnormality What Is the Accuracy of Different Types of Core-Needle Breast Biopsy Compared with Open Biopsy for Diagnosis?

Evidence Base

Our literature searches identified 1,224 potentially relevant articles. After review of the abstracts, the full-length articles of 589 of these studies were obtained and examined in full. Of these, 107 studies met the inclusion criteria for Key Question 1. The excluded studies and primary reason for exclusion are shown in Appendix C. The studies are briefly described in Table 5. Full Full details about the included studies, the enrolled patients, the biopsy methods, and the characteristics of the breast lesions are shown in the evidence tables in Appendix E.

Thirty-five of the 107 studies were prospective in design. Forty-nine were conducted in the United States. Ninety-three were carried out in general hospitals. A total of 57,088 breast lesions were enrolled in the 107 studies. The overall quality of the entire evidence base was rated as low (median score 6.1, range 3.6 to 8.2); see Table 5 for details.

Accuracy of Open Surgical Biopsy

Obtaining information on the accuracy of open surgical biopsy was, not surprisingly, difficult. Practically all authors and experts assume that open surgical biopsy is 100% accurate. We did not identify any clinical studies of open surgical biopsy that met our inclusion criteria (see Methods section).

We identified an article by Antley et al. 1998 that reviewed the accuracy of open surgical biopsy.[40] Antley et al. reviewed the available information (published literature as well as patient charts available in the author's medical center) on the accuracy of open surgical biopsy and concluded that open surgical biopsy has been reported to miss 1 to 2% of breast cancers (a sensitivity of 98% or greater). This estimate is based upon a re-review of archived open biopsy material by a second pathologist, the charts reviewed by Antley et al., a study of cases of benign results on biopsy after a very suspicious mammogram, and expert opinion.[41-43]

We did not identify any information on estimates of underestimation rates for open surgical biopsy. However, underestimations are generally thought to be due to failure to sample all important areas of a lesion. For example, a lesion may contain a foci of carcinoma within a cluster of atypical cells. Biopsy samples collected by core-needle may fail to sample any of the carcinoma cells, leading to an underestimation. Because open surgical biopsy samples most or all of the lesion, in theory underestimations should not occur. Therefore, we have assumed that open surgical biopsy has a zero, or close to zero, underestimation rate.

Accuracy of Core-Needle Biopsy

We attempted to fit a bivariate binomial regression model to the data reported by all 107 studies but the data were too heterogeneous to allow a valid model to be fit. Due to obvious differences across studies of biopsy methods and enrolled patient populations, we did not perform further analyses on the full set of data. In the following analyses we have grouped the studies by the type of core-needle biopsy used in the study. The analyses are summarized in

Figure 1 A through Figure 4 D in the Executive Summary and in Table 6 and Table 7. Full details of the analyses and reported data are provided in Appendix F.

Freehand Core-Needle Biopsies

Five studies reported data on the accuracy of non-guided, i.e., freehand, core-needle biopsies performed with automated biopsy gun devices.[44-48] We fit a bivariate binomial model. There was very little heterogeneity in the data (I^2 = 6.95%). The summary sensitivity was 85.8% (95% CI: 75.8 to 92.1%) and the summary negative likelihood ratio was 0.143 (95% CI: 0.082 to 0.250). This ratio indicates that for a woman with a pre-test probability of malignancy of 30%, her probability of having malignancy after a negative freehand core-needle biopsy would be 5.8%. A pre-test probability of 30% was chosen because the average woman undergoing core- needle biopsy has been categorized as BI-RADS 4 before undergoing the biopsy, and such women have an approximate overall prevalence of malignancy of 30%.[15] We have used the 30% pre-test probability in the analyses that follow for the same reason. However, it is important to realize that each individual woman's pre-test probability may vary from this estimate.

None of the studies reported underestimation rates. Because there were only five studies we did not perform any sub-group or meta-regression analyses.

Cusick et al. noted that smaller lesions (less than 2 cm in diameter) were more likely to be misdiagnosed.[48] In contrast, Barreto et al. commented that neither tumor size nor patient age affected the accuracy of the procedure; however, tumors located in the right breast were much more likely to receive false-negative diagnoses, perhaps due to the fact that the persons performing the biopsy procedures were right handed.[47] Barreto et al. also noted that operator inexperience was a key factor in misdiagnoses.[47] The apparent difference in conclusions about the impact of tumor size on biopsy accuracy is probably due to the fact that the tumors in the study by Barreto et al. were all larger than 2 cm in diameter.

We graded the conclusions from this evidence as Low. The quality of the evidence base was rated as Low (median score 5.7), but quantity, consistency, and robustness were all rated as Sufficient.

Ultrasound Guided Automated Gun Core-Needle Biopsies

Sixteen studies of 7,124 biopsies used ultrasound guidance and an automated biopsy gun.[49-64] We could not fit a bivariate binomial model due to heterogeneity. The random-effects model found a summary sensitivity of 97.7% (95% CI: 97.2 to 98.2%) and a summary negative likelihood ratio of 0.030 (95% CI: 0.022 to 0.040). This ratio indicates that for a woman with a pre-test probability of malignancy of 30%, her probability of having malignancy after a negative ultrasound-guided automated gun core-needle biopsy would be 1.3%. Twelve of the sixteen studies reported data on atypia underestimation rates.[49,51-53,56-61,63,64]; the summary atypia underestimation rate was 29.2% (23.4 to 3 5.9%). Twelve studies reported data on DCIS underestimation rates.[49,51-53,55-61,64] the summary DCIS underestimation rate was 35.5% (27.1 to 45.0%). We graded the conclusions from this evidence as Low. The quality of the evidence base was rated as Low (median score 6.1), but quantity, consistency, and robustness were all rated as Sufficient.

We then proceeded to explore factors that might affect the accuracy of the biopsies by performing meta-regressions. We only performed meta-regressions if all of the studies reported information about the factor being analyzed and at least three studies were different from the rest of the studies for that factor.

Patient and Breast Lesion Factors

The studies reported insufficient information about characteristics of the lesions or the patients to explore the impact of these factors on the accuracy of the biopsies.

Biopsy Procedure Factors

Only seven of the studies reported information about patient position during the procedure, and six of these reported the patients were supine[49,51,56,60,62,63] while the seventh reported the patients were seated.[58] All but two of the studies reported using a 14G needle; one of these two studies used an 1 8G needle, and one used different sizes of needles for different patients.[59,62]

Three of the fifteen studies verified all core-needle findings with surgery[50,58,62] (the rest used a combination of surgery and patient followup), and six of the studies did not follow all patients for at least two years.[52,53,55,57,60,63] Meta-regression did not find a statistically significant impact of methods of verification of biopsy on the accuracy of the biopsies.

One study, de Lucen et al., evaluated the impact of number of cores taken on the accuracy of the procedure. The authors of the study reported that taking more than 2 cores did not improve the accuracy of the procedure.[50] However, Fishman et al. reported that taking more than 2 cores did improve the accuracy of the biopsy, with 4 cores being the optimal number.[55] Fishman et al.'s conclusion was based on one case of DCIS that would have been missed if fewer than 4 cores had been taken; the other 13 tumors identified in the study would have been correctly diagnosed if only 2 cores had been taken. de Lucen et al.'s conclusion was based on the fact that the six tumors (out of a total of 101 tumors identified in the study) that were falsely diagnosed as benign by core-needle biopsy would not have been correctly diagnosed even if up to six cores were taken.

Clinician and Facility Factors

All but one of the studies were performed in general hospitals. The studies were conducted in settings around the world; meta-regression did not find a statistically significant effect of geographic location on the accuracy of the biopsies. Most of the studies did not report data about the training or experience of the persons performing the biopsies.

Stereotactic-Guided Automated Gun Core-Needle Biopsies

Thirty-three studies of 7153 biopsies used stereotactic guidance and an automated biopsy gun.65-97 We were able to fit a bivariate binomial model. The summary sensitivity was 97.8% (95% CI: 95.8 to 98.9%) and the summary negative likelihood ratio was 0.022 (95% CI: 0.0 12 to 0.043). This ratio indicates that for a woman with a pre-test probability of malignancy of 30%, her probability of having malignancy after a negative stereotactically-guided automated gun core-needle biopsy would be 0.9%. Twenty-six of the 33 studies reported data on atypia underestimation rates.[65-69,71,73-90,94,96] and 17 reported data on DCIS underestimation rates.[65- 68,73,75,76,78-81,85,86,89-92] The atypia underestimation rate was 43.5% (95% CI: 35.7 to 51.7%) and the DCIS underestimation rate was 24.4% (95% CI: 18.0 to 32.1%). We graded the conclusions from this evidence as Low. The quality of the evidence base was rated as Low (median score 6.1), but quantity, consistency, and robustness were all rated as Sufficient.

We then proceeded to explore factors that might affect the accuracy of the biopsies by performing meta-regression. We only performed meta-regressions if all of the studies reported information about the factor being analyzed and at least three studies were different from the rest of the studies for that factor.

Patient and Breast Lesion Factors

Koskela et al. reported zero false-negatives out of 97 procedures performed on lesions detected as masses on mammography but 4 false-negatives out of 108 procedures performed on lesions with microcalcifications.[66] Walker et al. reported that the sensitivity of core-needle biopsy was much lower for microcalcifications than for any other type of lesion.[85]

The majority of the studies appeared to have enrolled patients with only non-palpable lesions but many of the studies did not report on the palpability of the lesions. The studies reported insufficient information about other characteristics of the lesions or the patients to explore the impact of these factors on the accuracy of the biopsies.

Biopsy Procedure Factors

All but three of the studies used 1 4G needles,[78,79,92] and meta-regression did not find a statistically significant impact of needle size on biopsy accuracy. Twenty-two of the studies reported that the patients were prone,[65,67,68,70,73,75,76,80,82-84,86-96] three reported the patients were seated,[66,69,72] one reported the patients were in the decubitus position,[77] one reported patients were either prone or seated,[81] but six did not report information about patient positioning.[71,74 ,78 ,79 ,85 ,97]

Eight of the studies verified all core-needle findings with surgery[68,72,73,79,94-97] (the rest used a combination of surgery and patient followup), and 22 of the studies did not follow all patients for at least two years.[66,67,69,70,74-78,80-87,89-93] Meta-regression did not find a statistically significant impact of methods of verification of biopsy on the accuracy of the biopsies.

Koskela et al. reported that more than three cores need to be taken from lesions before an accurate diagnosis can be made.[66]

Clinician and Facility Factors

Twenty-nine of the studies were conducted at a single center (the other four were multi-center studies[65,68,70,79]). Twenty-six of the studies were conducted in general hospitals,[65-69,71- 76,78,81-83,85-87,89-92,94-97] four were conducted in free-standing dedicated cancer centers,[77,80,88,93] one was conducted in a breast cancer screening clinic,[84] and one was conducted in multiple centers of different types.[70] Twenty of the studies were conducted within the United States[70,75,76,79-83,86-97] and the rest were scattered worldwide. Meta-regressions did not find that any of these factors had a statistically significant impact on biopsy accuracy.

The majority of studies reported that radiologists performed the biopsies, but many studies did not report information about the training of the operators. Very few of the studies reported the degree of experience of the operators or their caseloads.

Ultrasound-Guided Vacuum-Assisted Core-Needle Biopsies

Seven studies of 507 biopsies used ultrasound guidance and a vacuum-assisted device to perform breast biopsies.[56,98-103] There was no significant heterogeneity in the data (I^2 = 0.0%). We fit a bivariate binomial model to the data. The summary sensitivity was 96.5% (95% CI: 81.2 to 99.4%) and the summary negative likelihood ratio was 0.036 (95% CI: 0.006 to 0.212). This ratio indicates that for a woman with a pre-test probability of malignancy of 30%, her probability of having malignancy after a negative vacuum-assisted ultrasound-guided core-needle biopsy would be 1.5%. The studies reported no cases of atypia underestimation and only a single case of DCIS underestimation.[56] We graded the conclusions from this evidence as Low. The quality of the evidence base was rated as Low (median score 5.9), but quantity, consistency, and robustness were all rated as Sufficient.

Due to the lack of heterogeneity in the data, we did not perform any meta-regressions to explore the impact of factors on accuracy. The following differences between studies do not appear to affect accuracy.

Patient and Breast Lesion Factors

The studies reported very little information about the patients or lesions.

Biopsy Procedure Factors

All of the studies verified core-biopsy results by a combination of open surgery and patient followup. Only one of the seven studies followed all patients for at least two years.[98]

Five of the studies used the Mammotome device with an 11 G needle,[56,99,101 -103] one study used a VACORA device with a 10G needle,[98] and one study did not report information about the device or needle gauge.[100] Four of the studies reported the patients were supine[56,100,102,103] and the others did not report details of patient positioning.

Clinician and Facility Factors

Two of the studies were conducted in free-standing cancer centers[101,103] and the others were performed in general hospitals. The studies were conducted in many different countries worldwide. The studies generally did not report information on operator training or experience.

Stereotactic-Guided Vacuum-Assisted Core-Needle Biopsies

Twenty-two studies of 7,153 biopsies used stereotactic guidance and a vacuum-assisted device to perform core-needle biopsies.[76,80,104-123] We were able to fit a bivariate binomial model. The summary sensitivity was 99.2% (95% CI: 98.1 to 99.6%) and the summary negative likelihood ratio was 0.009 (95% CI: 0.004 to 0.02 1). This ratio indicates that for a woman with a pre-test probability of malignancy of 30%, her probability of having malignancy after a negative vacuum-assisted stereotactically-guided core-needle biopsy would be 0.4%. All of the studies reported information about atypia and DCIS underestimation rates. The summary atypia underestimation rate was 21.7% (95% CI: 17.7 to 26.4%) and the summary DCIS underestimation rate was 12.9% (95% CI: 11.1 to 15.1%). The low DCIS underestimation rate may affect treatment planning. The surgeon performing the followup open surgical procedure can be reasonably confident that a malignant tumor is not present, and therefore may plan to remove the lesion using a breast-conserving approach, and may decide to not sample the axillary lymph nodes. Some women and physicians may decide that the ADH underestimation rate is low enough to safely substitute surveillance for an open biopsy procedure after diagnosis of ADH on core-needle biopsy. We graded the conclusions from this evidence as Low. The quality of the evidence base was rated as Low (median score 6.1), but quantity, consistency, and robustness were all rated as Sufficient.

We then proceeded to explore factors that might affect the accuracy of the biopsies by performing meta-regressions. We only performed meta-regressions if all of the studies reported information about the factor being analyzed and at least three studies were different from the rest of the studies for that factor.

Patient and Breast Lesion Factors

Two studies reported that stereotactic-guided vacuum-assisted core-needle biopsy was equally accurate for lesions with microcalcifications and lesions detected as masses on mammography.[110,117]

Nine of the 21 studies reported that all of the lesions were non-palpable[76,104,108,1 10-112,114- 116] but the other studies reported no information on palpability of enrolled lesions. The studies reported insufficient information about characteristics of the lesions or the patients to explore the impact of these factors on the accuracy of the biopsies.

Biopsy Procedure Factors

All 21 studies used the Mammotome device either exclusively or in part. Seventeen of the studies used an 1 1G needle,[80,104-114,117-120,122] two used a 14G needle,[76,116] one used either a 14G or an 1 1G needle,[121] and one did not report the size of the needle.[115] All but one of the studies used a combination of open surgery and patient followup to verify the results of the biopsies, and it used open surgery on all patients.[117] Only three studies followed all patients for at least two years.[104,110,116] Meta-regression found that method of biopsy verification did not affect the accuracy of the biopsies.

The majority of the studies reported that patients were prone,[76,80,104,105,107-112,114,1 16-122] two reported that patients were seated,113,115 and one did not report information about patient positioning.[106]

Lomoschitz et al. reported that 12 cores were necessary for accurate diagnosis and taking more than 12 cores did not improve accuracy.[110]

Clinician and Facility Factors

Only two of the 21 studies were multi-center studies. Three of the studies were conducted in free-standing dedicated cancer centers,[105,106,116] one was conducted in an ambulatory surgical center,[80] and the rest were conducted in general hospitals. Six of the studies were conducted in the USA[76,80,113,114,116,118] and 12 were conducted in Europe. [104,106-112,115,117,120,121] Meta-regression did not find that the type or location of facility affected the accuracy of the biopsies.

Very few of the studies reported any information about the training or experience of the persons performing the biopsies. Pfarl et al. noted that for six of the seven false-negatives that occurred in the study, the biopsy procedure had been performed by an operator who had previously performed fewer than 15 stereotactic-guided biopsies.[117]

MRI-Guided Core-Needle Biopsies

Only one study reported data on the accuracy of MRI-guided biopsies performed with automated biopsy guns.[124]

Table 5. Studies addressing Key Questions 1 and 2.

Study	Type(s) Core Biopsy	Quality score	Type of Study	Number of Centers	Care Setting	Country Conducted in	Funded by	Number of Lesions Enrolled	Followup	% Attrition at Longest Followup
Jackman et al. 2009[123]	Stereotactic guidance vacuum-assisted 1 1G and 14G	5.4	Retrospective	1	General hospital	USA	Partially supported by Biopsys Medical, Inc., and Ethicon Endo-Surgery	1,280	2 years	10.6%
Peters et al. 2008[65]	Stereotactic guidance automated gun 14G	4.6	Retrospective	4	General hospital	Netherlands	NR	948	2 years	5%
Schueller et al. 2008[64]	US guidance automated gun 14G	5.4	Retrospective	1	General hospital	Austria	The authors reported no financial relationship to disclose	1438	2 years	6.0%
Sim and Kei et al. 2008[122]	Stereotactic guidance vacuum-assisted 1 1G	6.1	Retrospective	1	General hospital	Singapore	NR	105	2 years	12.4%
Tonegutti and Girardi 2008[104]	Stereotactic guidance vacuum-assisted 11G	6.1	Retrospective	1	General hospital	Italy	NR	268	2 years	0%
Youk et al. 2008[49]	US guidance automated gun 14G	4.6	Retrospective	1	General hospital	South Korea	NR	4,359	2 years	44%
Ciatto et al. 2007[126]	Multiple methods	4.6	Retrospective	1	Dedicated breast cancer center	Italy	Funded in part by a National Health and Medical Research Council (NHMRC) grant	4,035	1 year	26%
de Lucena et al. 2007[50]	US guidance automated gun 14G	6.8	Prospective	1	General hospital	Brazil	NR	150	Immediate surgery	0%
Vag et al. 2007[98]	US guidance vacuum- assisted 1 0G	6.1	Prospective	1	General hospital	Germany	NR	70	2 years	0%

Table 5. (Continued).

Study	Type(s) Core Biopsy	Quality score	Type of Study	Number of Centers	Care Setting	Country Conducted in	Funded by	Number of Lesions Enrolled	Followup	% Attrition at Longest Followup
Chapellier et al. 2006[106]	Stereotactic guidance vacuum-assisted 11G	6.4	Prospective	1	General cancer center	France	NR	318	Range: 4 to 16 months	0%
Cipolla et al. 2006[127]	Multiple methods	6.8	NR	1	General hospital	Italy	NR	426	1 year	0%
Dhillon et al. 2006[107]	Stereotactic guidance vacuum-assisted 1 1G	7.5	Prospective	1	General hospital	UK	NR	150	Median: 48 months	0%
Bolivar et al. 2005[51]	US guidance automated gun 14G	6.8	Prospective	1	General hospital	Spain	NR	214	2 years	5%
Crystal et al. 2005[52]	US guidance automated gun 14G	6.8	NR	1	General hospital	Israel	NR	715	Median: 39 months Range: 27 to 60 months	0%
Dillon et al. 2005[128]	Multiple methods	4.6	Retrospective	1	General hospital	Ireland	NR	2,427	Median: 24 months Range: 3 to 67 months	19%
Koskela et al. 2005[66]	Stereotactic guidance automated gun 14G	6.1	Prospective	1	General hospital	Finland	Kuopio University Hospital (the center where it was conducted)	213	Mean: 24 months Range: 6 to 39 months	4%
Sauer et al. 2005[53]	US guidance automated gun 14G	5.0	Retrospective	1	General hospital	Germany	NR	962	Mean: 22.2 months Median: 21 months Range: 8 to 36 months	13%

Study	Type(s) Core Biopsy	Quality score	Type of Study	Number of Centers	Care Setting	Country Conducted in	Funded by	Number of Lesions Enrolled	Followup	% Attrition at Longest Followup
Weber et al. 2005[108]	Stereotactic guidance vacuum-assisted 11G	7.9	Prospective	1	General hospital	Switzerland	NR	225	Median: 2.1 years Range: 0.5 to 4.4 years	15%
Wu et al. 2005[99]	US guidance vacuum- assisted 11 G	6.8	NR	1	General hospital	Taiwan	NR	113	1 year	0%
Alonso-Bartolome et al. 2004[100]	US guidance vacuum- assisted 11G	6.8	Prospective	2	General hospital	Spain	NR	102	6 to 12 months	0%
Delle and Terinde 2004[54]	US guidance automated gun 14G	6.8	NR	1	General hospital	Germany	NR	169	2 years	0%
Fajardo et al. 2004[129]	Multiple methods	8.2	Prospective	22	Academic and community practice clinical sites	USA	National Cancer Institute	2,403	2 years	30%
Kettritz et al. 2004[109]	Stereotactic guidance vacuum-assisted 11G	4.6	Prospective	5	General hospital	Germany	NR	2,893	Mean: 25 months Range: 6 to 67 months	22%
Lomoschitz et al. 2004[110]	Stereotactic guidance vacuum-assisted 11G	6.1	Prospective	1	General hospital	Austria	One author partially supported by both Ethicon Endosurgery and Biopsys Medical	100	2 years	0%
Abdsaleh et al. 2003[130]	Multiple methods	7.1	Prospective	1	General hospital	Sweden	NR	180	1 year	21%
Ambrogetti et al. 2003[111]	Stereotactic guidance vacuum-assisted 11G	4.6	Retrospective	1	General hospital	France	NR	364	Mean: 15.8 months Range: 6 to 36 months	35%

Table 5. (Continued).

Study	Type(s) Core Biopsy	Quality score	Type of Study	Number of Centers	Care Setting	Country Conducted in	Funded by	Number of Lesions Enrolled	Followup	% Attrition at Longest Followup
Fishman et al. 2003[55]	US guidance automated gun 14G	5.7	Prospective	1	General hospital	USA	NR	73	Mammo-graphic and US followup Median:21 months Range: 4 to 30 months	33%
Han et al. 2003[67]	Stereotactic guidance automated gun 14G	5.4	Retrospective	1	General hospital	Korea	NR	271	At least 6 months	27%
Kirshenbaum et al. 2003[131]	Multiple methods	5.0	Retrospective	1	General hospital	USA	NR	506	Mean: 2.1 years Range: 3 months to five years.	23%
March et al. 2003[101]	US guidance vacuum- assisted 1 1G	5.7	Prospective	2	Dedicated breast cancer center	USA	RSNA Seed Grant and the Rays of Hope charitable fund	34	6 months	9%
Pfleiderer et al. 2003[124]	MRI guidance automated gun 14G	6.4	Prospective	1	General hospital	Germany	NR	14	2 years	0%
Philpotts et al. 2003[56]	Multiple methods	4.6	Retrospective	1	General hospital	USA	NR	281	Mean: 19 months Range: 3 to 53 months for 1 4G Mean: 13 months Range: 1 to 24 for 11G	24%
Wong and Hisham 2003[44]	Freehand automated gun 14 or 16G	7.1	Prospective	1	General hospital	Malaysia	NR	150	Range: 6 to 13 months	0%

Study	Type(s) Core Biopsy	Quality score	Type of Study	Number of Centers	Care Setting	Country Conducted in	Funded by	Number of Lesions Enrolled	Followup	% Attrition at Longest Followup
Georgian-Smith et al. 2002[113]	Stereotactic guidance vacuum-assisted 11G	5.7	Retrospective	4	General hospital	USA	NR	185	Range: 6 to 12 months	21%
Jackman and Lamm 2002[132]	Multiple methods	5.4	Retrospective	1	General hospital	USA	Funded in part by Biopsys Medical	31	At least 6 months	0%
Johnson et al. 2002[102]	US guidance vacuum- assisted 11 or 8G	6.4	NR	1	General hospital	USA	Fashion Footwear of NY	101	Mean: 9.5 months	24%
Liberman et al. 2002[114]	Stereotactic guidance vacuum-assisted 1 1G	4.3	Retrospective	1	General cancer center	USA	NR	800	At least 1 year	29%
Meloni et al. 2002[115]	Stereotactic guidance vacuum-assisted	6.1	Retrospective	1	General hospital	Italy	NR	129	Mean: 18.7 months Range: 14 to 26 months	0%
Morris et al. 2002[116]	Stereotactic guidance vacuum-assisted 14G	6.4	Prospective	1	Dedicated breast cancer center	USA	NR	21	Median: 46 months Range: 40-54 months	10%
Pfarl et al. 2002[117]	Stereotactic guidance vacuum-assisted 1 1G	6.1	Retrospective	1	General hospital	Austria	NR	332	Immediate surgery	4%
Verkooijen et al. COBRA 2002[68]	Stereotactic guidance automated gun 14G	7.9	Prospective	5	General hospital	the Netherlands	Dutch National Health Insurance Fund Council	984	Immediate surgery	11%
Becker et al. 2001[69]	Stereotactic guidance automated gun 14G	5.0	Retrospective	1	General hospital	Canada	NR	232	Range: 6 to 12 months	27%
Brenner et al. 2001[70]	Stereotactic guidance automated gun 14G	6.1	Prospective	7	Cancer centers and hospitals	USA	NR	1,003	Mean:19.3 months Range: 0 to 36 months	1%

Table 5. (Continued).

Study	Type(s) Core Biopsy	Quality score	Type of Study	Number of Centers	Care Setting	Country Conducted in	Funded by	Number of Lesions Enrolled	Followup	% Attrition at Longest Followup
Cangiarella et al. 2001[118]	Stereotactic guidance vacuum-assisted 11G	6.1	NR	1	General hospital	USA	NR	160	Mean: 20.5 months Range: 6 to 35 months	38%
Dahlstrom and Jain 2001[71]	Stereotactic guidance automated gun 14G	6.8	NR	1	General hospital	Australia	NR	301	Range: 2.4 to 7.5 years	0%
Lai et al. 2001[119]	Stereotactic guidance vacuum-assisted 1 1G	6.4	NR	1	General hospital	Canada	NR	673	Mean: 6.7 months Range: 6 to 24 months	29%
Levin et al. 2001[72]	Stereotactic guidance automated gun 14G	7.1	Prospective	1	General hospital	Canada	Physician's Services Incorporated Foundation	70	Immediate surgery	0%
Margolin et al. 2001[133]	Multiple methods	5.4	Retrospective	1	General hospital	USA	NR	1,333	Mean: 14 months Range: 6 to 24 months; missing data was collected from SEER database; at the time of accession of SEER data followup ranged from 15 to 75 months.	3%
Perez-Fuentes et al. 2001[103]	US guidance vacuum- assisted 11G	4.6	NR	1	Dedicated breast cancer center	Venezuela	NR	88	Median: 11.1 months Range: 4 to 24 months.	33%

Study	Type(s) Core Biopsy	Quality score	Type of Study	Number of Centers	Care Setting	Country Conducted in	Funded by	Number of Lesions Enrolled	Followup	% Attrition at Longest Followup
Smith et al. 2001[57]	US guidance automated gun 14G	6.1	NR	1	General hospital	USA	NR	500	Mean: 22 months Median: 14 months Range: 12 to 60 months	21%
White et al. 2001 [134]	Multiple methods	4.6	Retrospective	1	General hospital	USA	NR	1,042	Median: 29 months, at least 1 year	29%
Wunderbaldinger et al. 2001[58]	US guidance automated gun 14G	6.1	Prospective	1	General hospital	Austria	author supported by Erwin Schroedinger Auslandsstipenium of the Austrian Science Fund	45	Immediate surgery	0%
Yeow et al. 2001[59]	US guidance automated gun 14 or 16G	7.1	Prospective	1	General hospital	China	NR	98	Mean: 4 years Range: 3 to 5 years	0%
Beck et al. 2000[120]	Stereotactic guidance vacuum-assisted 11G	6.8	NR	1	General hospital	Germany	NR	594	1 year	0%
Kirwan et al. 2000[73]	Stereotactic guidance automated gun 14G	5.0	Retrospective	1	General hospital	UK	NR	72	Immediate surgery	13%
Latosinsky et al. 2000[135]	Multiple methods	5.4	Retrospective	1	General hospital	USA	NIH grant	692	Median: 17.2 months Range: 2.8 to 43 months	42%

Table 5. (Continued).

Study	Type(s) Core Biopsy	Quality score	Type of Study	Number of Centers	Care Setting	Country Conducted in	Funded by	Number of Lesions Enrolled	Followup	% Attrition at Longest Followup
Makoske et al. 2000[137]	Multiple methods	5.4	Retrospective	1	General hospital	USA	NR	817	Mean: 1.7 years	30%
Ward et al. 2000[74]	Stereotactic guidance automated gun 14G	6.1	NR	1	General hospital	Canada	NR	121	Mean: 16 months Range: 4 to 36 months	7%
Welle et al. 2000[138]	Multiple methods	3.6	Retrospective	3	General hospital	USA	NR	225	Range: 6 to 24 months	20%
Helbich et al. 1999[150]	Multiple methods	6.1	Prospective	1	General hospital	Austria	Ludwig-Boltzmann Institute for Radiologic Tumor Research; one author was supported by a grant from the Max Kade Foundation	44	Immediate surgery	0%
Jackman et al. 1999[75]	Stereotactic guidance automated gun 14G	5.0	Retrospective	1	General hospital	USA	NR	483	Median: 55 months	1%
Meyer et al. 1999[139]	Multiple methods	4.6	Retrospective	1	General hospital	USA	NR	1,836	At least 1 year	25%
Puglisi et al. 1999[125]	Perforated compression grid automated gun 14G	5.4	Retrospective	1	General hospital	Italy	NR	106	At least 6 months	1%
Soo et al. 1999[76]	Multiple methods	5.0	Retrospective	1	General hospital	USA	NR	116	Mean: 16 months Range: 5 to 31 months	19%
Caruso et al. 1998[140]	Multiple methods	6.8	Prospective	1	General hospital	Italy	NR	92	Immediate surgery	13%

Study	Type(s) Core Biopsy	Quality score	Type of Study	Number of Centers	Care Setting	Country Conducted in	Funded by	Number of Lesions Enrolled	Followup	% Attrition at Longest Followup
Doyle et al. 1998[77]	Stereotactic guidance automated gun 14G	5.0	Retrospective	1	Dedicated breast cancer center	New Zealand	NR	151	Range: 6 to 36 months	11%
Fuhrman et al. 1998[141]	Multiple methods	4.6	Retrospective	1	General hospital	USA	NR	1,440	At least 6 months	18%
Heywang-Kobrunner et al. 1998[121]	Stereotactic guidance vacuum-assisted 11 or 14G	6.1	NR	1	General hospital	Germany	NR	261	6 months	31%
Ioffe et al. 1998[142]	Multiple methods	6.1	NR	1	General hospital	USA	NR	224	Range: 6 to 12 months	14%
Liberman et al. 1998[60]	US guidance automated gun 14G	6.4	NR	1	General cancer center	USA	NR	151	Median: 20 months Range: 6 to 48 months	23%
Schulz-Wendtland et al. 1998[61]	US guidance automated gun 14G	6.8	NR	1	General hospital	Germany	NR	307	2 years	0%
Vega-Bolivar et al. 1998[78]	Stereotactic guidance Surecut 15G	4.6	Retrospective	1	General hospital	Spain	NR	182	Mean: 27 months Range: 6 to 47 months	6%
Whitman et al. 1998[79]	Stereotactic guidance automated gun 16G	5.4	Retrospective	2	General hospital	USA	NR	12	Immediate surgery	0%
Zannis and Aliano 1998[80]	Multiple methods	5.7	Retrospective	1	Ambulatory surgical center	USA	NR	424	At least 6 months	31%
Bauer et al. 1997[81]	Stereotactic guidance automated gun 14G	5.7	Retrospective	NR	NR	USA	NR	799	Mean: 9 months	0%

Table 5. (Continued).

Study	Type(s) Core Biopsy	Quality score	Type of Study	Number of Centers	Care Setting	Country Conducted in	Funded by	Number of Lesions Enrolled	Followup	% Attrition at Longest Followup
Britton et al. 1997[143]	Multiple methods	6.8	NR	1	General hospital	UK	NR	202	Mean: 20.1 months Range: 5.3 to 30.8 months	2%
Helbich et al. 1997[144]	Multiple methods	7.1	Prospective	1	General hospital	Austria	NR	210	Immediate surgery	0%
Khattar et al. 1997[62]	US guidance automated gun	6.4	Prospective	1	General hospital	Denmark	NR	106	Immediate surgery	43%
Liberman et al. 1997[82]	Stereotactic guidance automated gun 14G	4.3	Retrospective	1	General cancer center	USA	NR	442	Median: 18 months Range: 6 to 46 months	34%
Pitre et al. 1997[83]	Stereotactic guidance automated gun	5.4	Retrospective	1	General hospital	USA	NR	128	1 year	8%
Stolier et al. 19971[45]	Multiple methods	5.4	Retrospective	1	General hospital	USA	NR	244	Mean: 12.8 months Range: 6 to 39 months	NR
Sutton, et al. 1997[84]	Stereotactic guidance automated gun 14G	3.6	Retrospective	1	Screening clinic	Australia	NR	206	1 year	32%
Walker et al. 1997[85]	Stereotactic guidance automated gun 14G	6.8	NR	1	General hospital	UK	NR	200	Range: 6 to 36 months	10%
Frazee et al. 1996[86]	Stereotactic guidance automated gun	7.1	Prospective	1	General hospital	USA	NR	103	At least 6 months	0%
Fuhrman et al. 1996[87]	Stereotactic guidance automated gun 14G	5.4	NR	1	General hospital	USA	NR	451	1 year	22%
Head and Haynes 1996[88]	Stereotactic guidance automated gun 18G	6.4	Prospective	1	Dedicated breast cancer center	USA	NR	115	2 years	8%

Study	Type(s) Core Biopsy	Quality score	Type of Study	Number of Centers	Care Setting	Country Conducted in	Funded by	Number of Lesions Enrolled	Followup	% Attrition at Longest Followup
Mainiero et al. 1996[89]	Stereotactic guidance automated gun 14G	6.1	Retrospective	1	General hospital	USA	NR	138	At least 6 months	14%
Meyer et al. 1996[90]	Stereotactic guidance automated gun 14G	5.4	NR	1	General hospital	USA	NR	388	1 year	30%
Nguyen et al. 1996[146]	Multiple methods	6.4	NR	1	General hospital	USA	American Cancer Society, UCLA Jonsson Comprehensive Cancer Center, and the Stein-Oppenheim Foundation	431	At least 6 months	10%
Pettine et al. 1996[91]	Stereotactic guidance automated gun 14G	6.1	Retrospective	1	General hospital	USA	NR	25	6 month repeat mammo-graphy for benign	0%
Rosenblatt et al. 1996[92]	Stereotactic guidance automated gun 14G	4.6	Retrospective	1	General hospital	USA	NR	25	1 year	16%
Scopa et al. 1996[45]	Freehand TruCut	6.8	NR	1	General hospital	Greece	NR	120	Immediate surgery	0%
Cross et al. 1995[93]	Stereotactic guidance automated gun 14G	5.0	NR	1	Dedicated breast cancer center	USA	NR	250	1 year	12%
Doyle et al. 1995[147]	Multiple methods	6.4	Prospective	1	General Hospital	USA	NR	150	Range: 6 to 24 months	3%
Hamed et al. 1995[151]	Freehand Biopty-cut	6.1	Prospective	1	General hospital	UK	NR	122	Immediate surgery	0%
Burbank et al. 1994[148]	Multiple methods	5.7	NR	1	General hospital	USA	NR	105	At least 6 months	0%
Gisvold et al. 1994[94]	Stereotactic guidance automated gun 14G	6.4	Prospective	1	General hospital	USA	NR	160	Immediate surgery	0%

Table 5. (Continued).

Study	Type(s) Core Biopsy	Quality score	Type of Study	Number of Centers	Care Setting	Country Conducted in	Funded by	Number of Lesions Enrolled	Followup	% Attrition at Longest Followup
Parker et al. 1994[149]	Multiple methods	3.9	Retrospective	20	Various hospitals, breast care centers, clinics	USA	NR	6,152	At least 6 months	39%
Smyth and Cederbom 1994[95]	Stereotactic guidance automated gun 14G	4.6	NR	1	General hospital	USA	NR	58	Immediate surgery	0%
Elvecrog et al. 1993[96]	Stereotactic guidance automated gun 14G	7.9	Prospective	1	General hospital	USA	NR	100	Immediate surgery	0%
Parker et al. 1993[63]	US guidance automated gun 14G	6.8	NR	1	Specialized imaging center	USA	NR	181	Range: 12 to 36 months	0%
McMahon et al. 1992[46]	Multiple methods	6.8	Prospective	1	General hospital	UK	NR	151	Median: 11 months Range: 1 to 24 months	0%
Barreto et al. 1991[47]	Freehand automated gun 18G	6.8	NR	1	General hospital	UK	NR	107	Immediate surgery	0%
Cusick et al. 1990[48]	Freehand	6.1	NR	1	General hospital	USA	NR	96	Immediate surgery	0%
Parker et al. 1990[97]	Stereotactic guidance automated gun	5.7	NR	1	General hospital	USA	NR	103	Immediate surgery	0%

NR = Not Reported
USA = United States of America
UK = United Kingdom

Table 6. Summary of accuracy by type of biopsy procedure.

Type of biopsy	N studies	N lesions	Prevalence of malignancy	Sensitivity (95% CI)	Negative likelihood ratio (95% CI)	Atypia underestimation rate	DCIS underestimation rate
Freehand automated gun	5	610	68.7%	85.8% (75.8 to 92.1%)	0.143 (0.082 to 0.250)	Not reported	Not reported
US guidance automated gun	16	7,124	53.9%	97.7% (97.2% to 98.2%)	0.030 (0.022 to 0.040)	0.292 (0.234 to 0.359)	0.355 (0.271 to 0.450)
Stereotactic guidance, automated gun	33	7,153	37.1%	97.8% (95.8% to 98.9%)	0.022 (0.012 to 0.043)	0.435 (0.357 to 0.517)	0.244 (0.180 to 0.321)
MRI guidance, automated gun	1	14	42.8%	83.3% (43.5% to 96.5%)	0.23 (0.05 to 0.95)	100% (1/1)	NR
Perforated compression grid automated gun	1	100	33%	91.4% (77.5% to 96.9%)	0.09 (0.03 to 0.26)	0.25 (1 out of 4)	0.286 (2 out of 7)
US guidance vacuum- assisted	7	507	15%	96.5% (81.2 to 99.4%)	0.036 (0.006 to 0.212)	None reported	Only one occurrence reported
Stereotactic guidance, vacuum- assisted	21	6,360	32.6%	99.2 % (97.9% to 99.7%)	0.009 (0.003 to 0.023)	0.217 (0.177 to 0.264)	0.130 (0.111 to 0.151)

NR = Not Reported

Table 7. Summary of the impact of factors on accuracy.

Factors	N Studies Reported Data on the Impact of the Factor on Accuracy	Conclusion
Patient age	1	Insufficient data
Breast density	1	Insufficient data
Patient co-morbidities	0	Insufficient data
Palpable vs. non-palpable	2	Insufficient data
Microcalcifications vs. masses	4	Inconsistent findings
Distortions vs. masses	1	Insufficient data
Size of lesion	2	Insufficient data
Location of lesion	1	Insufficient data
Number of cores	3	Inconsistent findings
Patient position	1	Insufficient data
Reference standard	68	Meta-regression found no impact
Use of vacuum	78	Vacuum-assistance improved accuracy
Use of image guidance	78	Image guidance improved accuracy; stereotactic guidance was more accurate than US guidance
Needle size	33	Meta-regression found no impact
Experience of operator	2	Insufficient data
Training of operator	0	Insufficient data
Facility location	68	Meta-regression found no impact
Facility type	33	Meta-regression found no impact

Perforated Compression Grid Guided Core-Needle Biopsies

Only one study reported data on the accuracy of biopsies performed with automated biopsy guns guided by a perforated compression grid.[125]

Multiple Core-Needle Methods

There were an additional 24 studies that used multiple core-needle biopsy methods in their studies and did not report the data for different biopsy methods separately.[126-149] Some of these studies reported information relevant to this topic as discussed below.

Patient and Breast Lesion Factors

Abdasaleh et al. reported that technical failures were more likely to occur with women with very dense breast tissue.[130]

The authors of Ciatto et al., who used multiple methods of performing core-needle biopsy, reported the percentage of procedures that gave false-negative results by lesion type: 2.7% palpable lesions, 2.2% nonpalpable lesions, 2.3% masses on mammography, 1.4% distortions on mammography, and 2.5% of microcalcifications.[126] Cipolla et al. reported that correspondence between core-needle biopsy and surgical biopsy results was 100% for palpable lesions but only 88% for nonpalpable lesions.[127] Fajardo reported that the sensitivity of core- needle biopsies for nonpalpable lesions and lesions with microcalcifications was 90.7%, much lower than the 97.4% sensitivity of core-needle biopsy for masses detected on mammography.[129]

Biopsy Procedure Factors

Abdasaleh et al. reported that taking two cores instead of one increased the accuracy of the procedure.[130]

Helbich et al. randomly assigned patients to be biopsied in different positions - seated upright, supine, or prone. The accuracy data were not reported separately for each group, but the authors did comment that patient position did not affect the biopsy procedure.[144]

Clinician and Facility Factors

Ciatto et al. reported that sensitivity of core-needle biopsies improved as the operators (radiologists) gained experience, from 88% in the first year of the study to 96% in the last year (eight years overall) of the study.[126]

Question 2. In women with a palpable or non-palpable breast abnormality, what are the harms associated with core-needle breast biopsy compared to the open biopsy technique in the diagnosis of breast cancer?

The evidence for Key Question 1, 107 studies of overall low quality, was used to address Key Question 2. Fifty of the 107 included studies did not report any harms (see Appendix F); whether this was because no harms occurred is unclear. Five studies only reported that no severe complications or harms occurred. Tonegutti and Giradi reported that (unspecified) complications only occurred during the first year of performing stereotactically-guided vacuum-assisted biopsies.[104]

Very few of the included studies reported information about complications occurring in association with open surgical biopsy procedures. We consulted a narrative review published in 2007 to obtain further information about complications of open surgical biopsy procedures.

In this review, Vitug and Newman report that 2 to 10% of breast surgeries are complicated by hematoma formation, and that 3.8% are complicated by infections.[152] Rissanen et al. reviewed a series of 425 wire-localized open biopsy procedures and reported that 10.2% were complicated by vasovagal reactions.[153]

Use of Pain Medications

Four studies reported information on the use of pain medications.[80,101,102,124]These studies reported that 100% of patients were sent home with narcotics after an open biopsy procedure, and only one patient (0.17%) required narcotics after a core-needle procedure.[102] Twenty (3.5%) patients were reported to have required acetaminophen after a core-needle procedure.[101] Note that being sent home with a medication may not necessarily mean the patients required or used the medication.

Bruising, Bleeding, and Hematomas

Twenty-four studies of 17,585 core-needle biopsy procedures reported that only 0.085% were complicated by hematomas that required treatment.[56,57,59,66,81,90,94,96,100-102,104,106,109,1 12- 115,120,138,139,143,146,149] These studies reported that 3.85% of vacuum-assisted procedures were complicated by hematoma formation, and only 0.14% of vacuum-assisted procedures were complicated by hematomas that required treatment. In comparison, only 0.24% of non-vacuumassisted procedures were reported to be complicated by hematoma formation, and only 0.035% of non-vacuum-assisted procedures were complicated by hematomas that required treatment. Due to inconsistency in reporting, these percentages should be used with caution; however, vacuum-assisted procedures do appear to have a higher rate of hematoma formation than other core-needle biopsy methods, although overall, hematomas rarely complicate core-needle procedures.

Twenty-four studies of 8,474 core-needle biopsy procedures reported that 1.4% were complicated by bleeding, but only 0.3% were complicated by bleeding that required treatment.[44,46,53,56,69,80,85,97,98,100,102-104,109,1 12-115,121,130-132,135,138] Of the vacuum-assisted procedures, 0.94% were reported to be complicated by bleeding, but only 0.34% of vacuum-assisted procedures were complicated by bleeding that required treatment or termination of the procedure. In comparison, 0.55% of non-vacuum-assisted procedures were reported to be complicated by bleeding, and only 0.20% of non-vacuum-assisted procedures were reported to be complicated by bleeding that required treatment. Due to inconsistency in reporting these percentages should be viewed with caution; however, vacuum-assisted procedures do appear to be complicated by bleeding more often than non-vacuum-assisted procedures, although bleeding is a rare complication of core-needle procedures.

Nine studies reported that bruising occurred after core-needle biopsy procedures.[46,57,59,85,90,99,101,108,141] Three of the nine reported that bruising was a common event,46,85,141 two reported that approximately 50% of patients had bruising,[90,101] and four studies reported that 45 out of 976 patients (4.6%) had severe bruising.[57,59,99,108] These nine studies used a variety of core-needle procedures.

Infections

March et al. reported that 2.1% of open biopsy procedures were complicated by the development of an abscess, but zero abscesses complicated 234 ultrasound-guided vacuum-assisted core-needle procedures.[101] Tonegutti and Girardi reported that one abscess that required surgical treatment occurred in a series of 268 stereotactically-guided vacuum-assisted procedures.[104] None of the other studies reported the occurrence of abscesses.

Twenty studies of 16,407 core-needle procedures reported that only 0.15% of the procedures were complicated by infections.[44,53,57,59,66,77,81,85,93,94,97,98,102,106, 108,109,133,135,139,149] Zannis and Aliano reported that 6.3% of open surgical biopsies were complicated by infections.[80]

Pain

Three vacuum-assisted biopsy procedures (out of over 6000 performed) were reported to have been terminated after patients complained of severe pain.[76,108,114] No other types of biopsy procedures were reported to have been terminated due to patient complaints of pain. Seventeen studies of a wide variety of biopsy methods reported information about patient pain during the procedure, and overall only 1.7% of patients were reported to have experienced severe pain.[44,46,76,84-86,93,94,96,100,101,108,112,114,121,146]

Frazee et al. reported the mean pain score (10-point VAS scale) was 2.5 for open biopsy procedures and 2.8 for stereotactically-guided automated gun core-needle biopsies (the difference was not statistically significant).[86]

Wong and Hisham reported no difference in the amount of pain experienced by patients undergoing a 14G core-needle procedure vs. a 16G core-needle procedure.[44] McMahon et al. reported that patients undergoing 18G core-needle procedures had significantly less pain than patients undergoing 14G core-needle procedures, but there was no significant difference in pain between 14G and 16G procedures.[46]

Vasovagal Reactions

Twenty-two studies of 7,526 core-needle procedures reported that 1% were complicated by vasovagal reactions (fainting or near-fainting).[58,66,69,72,77-79,85,94,97,98, 104,109,113-115,125,131,138,139,143,144] More than 40% of the vasovagal reactions occurred in patients who were reported to have been positioned sitting upright for the biopsy procedure (many of the studies did not report patient position so the other 60% of vasovagal reactions could have occurred in patients positioned in a variety of positions, or could have occurred primarily in seated patients).

Kirshenbaum et al. commented that the majority of vasovagal reactions occurred when inexperienced operators performed the biopsy procedures.[131]

Time to Recovery

One study, Frazee et al., reported information about time to recovery, measured by asking patients how long it had taken for them to return to their normal activities after the biopsy procedure. This study reported that the average time of recovery was 3.5 days for open biopsy procedures and 1.5 days for stereotactically-guided automated gun core-needle biopsy procedures.[86]

Impact of Biopsy Procedure on Usual Activities

One study, March et al., reported that ultrasound-guided vacuum-assisted procedures did not impact the usual activities of 47% of the women at all.[101]

Impact of Biopsy Procedure on Subsequent Mammographic Procedures

Three studies reported information about the impact of core-needle biopsies on subsequent mammographic examinations.[109,120,121] All three studies performed stereotacticguided vacuum-assisted core-needle procedures. These three studies enrolled 3,748 patients of whom 3,345 (89.2%) were reported to have no mammographically visible scarring after the biopsy procedures. Only seven of the patients (0.19%) were reported to have scars that were potentially diagnostically confusing on subsequent mammographic procedures.

Miscellaneous Reported Harms

Four studies of 2,600 patients reported that four cases of pneumothorax, none of which required treatment, had occurred.[104,109,113,120] None of these four studies used the same method of performing the core-needle biopsies.

Two studies reported that one patient per study (out of 3,487 patients) had suffered a seizure during a stereotactic-guided vacuum-assisted procedure.[109,120]

One study of 268 patients undergoing stereotactic-guided vacuum-assisted biopsies reported that three patients developed acute inflammation at the biopsy site after the procedure.[104]

Table 8. Dissemination of Cancerous Cells During Biopsy Procedures.

Type of study	Number of studies	Number of patients	Summary of findings
Histopathological demonstration of dissemination of cells	3 case reports[155-157] 1 retrospective study[163] 6 prospective studies[154,158-162]	786	The percentage of needle tracks reported to contain displaced cancerous cells ranged from 0% to 65%. Factors reported to increase the risk of finding displaced cancerous cells include: duration of the biopsy procedure,[158] multiple passes of the needle,[159] and a short interval between core-needle procedure and surgical excision.[154] Factors reported to decrease the risk of finding displaced cancerous cells include: diagnosis of invasive lobular carcinoma,[159] and use of vacuum-assisted core-needle biopsy.[154]
Tumor recurrence at the biopsy site	3 case reports[155,161, 164]	6	6 cases of tumor recurrence at the biopsy site were presented. All were treated with skin-sparing mastectomy following core-needle biopsy , and three were reported to have not received radiation treatment.[155,161] It was not reported whether the other 3 cases received radiation treatment.[164]
Risk of tumor recurrence following biopsy	4 retrospective studies[165-168]	1,879	Three of the four studies reported that women treated with open excisional biopsies had a higher rate of tumor recurrence than women who received pre-operative core-needle biopsies;[165-167]the fourth study reported opposite findings.[168] The majority of women in all four studies were treated with breast-conserving surgery and radiation therapy.
Risk of metastasis to the lymph nodes following biopsy	3 retrospective studies[169-171]	3,103	Two studies reported that the method of biopsy did not correlate with the rate of metastases to the sentinel lymph nodes;[169, 171] one study reported that the rate of metastases to the sentinel lymph nodes was higher in women who underwent some type of pre-operative needle biopsy than in women who underwent open excisional biopsy. [170]

One study of 185 stereotactic-guided vacuum-assisted procedures reported that one patient vomited during the procedure.[113]

Dissemination of Cancerous Cells During the Biopsy Procedure

To address this possible harm of a breast biopsy we did not use formal inclusion criteria; any clinical study that addressed the topic was included for discussion. Full details of the studies are shown in Appendix E. The results of the studies are summarized in Table 8.

We identified ten studies that used histopathology to demonstrate dissemination of cancerous cells by core-needle biopsy procedures.[154-163] The percentage of needle tracks reported to contain displaced cancerous cells ranged from 0% to 65%. Diaz et al. demonstrated that the time elapsed between core-needle biopsy and examination of the needle track strongly influenced the findings, with fewer and fewer displaced cancerous cells observed the longer the interval, suggesting that the majority of displaced cancerous cells die off over time.[154] However, we also identified six case reports of patients developing tumor recurrences at the site of prior core- needle biopsies, indicating that not all displaced cancerous cells are non-viable.[155,161,164] Three of these six women were reported not to have received radiation therapy for the primary tumor; for the other three women it was not reported whether or not they had received radiation therapy.

Table 9. Summary of Harms Complicating Core-Needle Biopsies.

Harms	N Studies Reported	N Lesions	N Occurrences	% Affected
Did not report	50	28,280	NR	NR
Reported no complications occurred	5	3,954	0	0%
Negative impact on quality of life	0	0	NR	NR
Patients dissatisfied with the procedure	2	328	2	0.61%
Hematomas requiring treatment	24	17,585	15	0.09%
Bleeding, severe	24	8,474	61	0.72%
Infections	20	16,407	24	0.15%
Pneumothorax	4	2,600	4	0.15%
Usual activities significantly affected by the biopsy procedure	1	34	4	11.80%
Time to recovery	1	103	1.5 days on average	NA
Bruising	9	3,256	Reported to be "common"	NR
Required pain medications	4	573	21	3.70%
Diagnostically confusing scars subsequent to the procedure	3	3,748	7	0.18%
Vasovagal reactions	22	7,631	77	1.00%
Severe pain during the biopsy procedure	17	3,128	52	1.70%

NR = Not Reported
NA = Not Applicable

The risk of tumor recurrence following biopsy was explored by four retrospective studies of 1,879 women.[165-168] Three of these four studies reported that women who did not have a preoperative needle biopsy had a higher rate of tumor recurrence than women who did receive a preoperative needle biopsy;[165-167] the fourth study reported the opposite.[168] The majority of the women in these four studies were treated with breast-conserving surgery and radiation therapy.

The risk of seeding the lymph nodes with cancerous cells by biopsy procedures was examined in three retrospective studies of 3,[103] patients. [169-171] Two of the three studies reported that the method of biopsy did not affect the rate of positive sentinel lymph nodes;[169,171] the third study reported that the rate of metastases to the sentinel lymph node was higher in women who underwent some form of pre-operative biopsy.[170]

Table 10. Summary of the Impact of Factors on Harms.

Factors	N Studies Reported Data on the Impact of the Factor on Harms	Conclusion
Patient age	0	Insufficient data
Breast density	0	Insufficient data
Patient co-morbidities	0	Insufficient data
Palpable vs. non-palpable	0	Insufficient data
Microcalcifications vs. masses	0	Insufficient data
Distortions vs. masses	0	Insufficient data
Size of lesion	0	Insufficient data
Location of lesion	0	Insufficient data
Number of cores	0	Insufficient data
Patient position	22	Vasovagal reactions occur more often in patients seated upright
Reference standard	0	Insufficient data
Use of vacuum	24	Use of vacuum increased the percentage of procedures complicated by severe bleeding and hematoma formation
Use of image guidance	0	Insufficient data
Needle size	1	Insufficient data
Experience of operator	0	Insufficient data
Training of operator	0	Insufficient data
Facility location	0	Insufficient data
Facility type	0	Insufficient data

In 2006 Bleiweiss et al. reported 25 cases of false-positive sentinel lymph nodes.[172] All 25 cases appeared to be caused by displacement of benign epithelial cells during a prior biopsy procedure. Twelve of the false-positive cases had undergone core-needle biopsy prior to the sentinel lymph procedure, 12 had undergone wire-localization open biopsy procedures, and one had undergone a fine-needle aspiration procedure. Although these cases are not, strictly speaking, cases of seeding lymph nodes with cancerous cells, this study is of clinical importance. False-positive sentinel lymph node procedures are likely to lead to over-treatment of patients, thus causing harm. These false-positive cases had stained positively for the presence of cytokeratins due to the presence of benign breast epithelial cells in the lymph nodes. Fifteen of the false-positives occurred in women with pure DCIS, and the remainder had DCIS plus invasive carcinoma. Twenty-two of the 25 cases had intraductal papilloma, (a not uncommon breast lesion) at the biopsy site and showed signs of displacement of benign cells at the biopsy site. The authors of this series of case reports suggest using caution when interpreting sentinel lymph node histopathology in cases where intraductal papilloma was noted during the initial biopsy procedure.

Question 3. How do open biopsy and various core-needle techniques differ in terms of patient preference, availability, costs, availability of qualified pathologist interpretations, and other factors that may influence choice of a particular technique?

We did not use formal inclusion criteria to select literature that addressed Key Question 3 due to the nature of the question. Data addressing this question were collected and are shown in Appendix E. The data are summarized in Table 13, Table 14, and Table 15, and are discussed outcome-by-outcome below. Economic factors that may influence the choice of a particular technique are discussed first, followed by factors highly important to patients, followed by other factors such as availability of equipment. Because of the nature of the question and the sources of information used to address it, we did not draw many formal evidence-based conclusions for this question, nor, in most cases, did we attempt to rate the quality of the studies or grade the strength of the evidence.

Relative Costs

Articles identified by our searches that analyzed the costs of open and various core-needle biopsy techniques in the U.S. health care system within the last five years (published in or after 2004) are summarized in Table 11. The relative costs of open surgical biopsy and various core-needle biopsy techniques have been evaluated by six studies. Some of the studies developed models, while others prospectively followed a patient population. When evaluating the costs of these techniques and procedures, the studies have reviewed factors such as the initial purchase price of the devices used, the costs of staffing, the costs of processing and analyzing the biopsy samples, the patient volume where the device will be utilized, if the device is used as a complementary procedure, and what mammography results determine the use of a core-needle biopsy technique.

According to the literature reviewed, the costs of open surgical biopsy are substantially higher than core-needle techniques. A study by Hatmaker et al. in 2007 found that the average total cost of an open surgical biopsy performed in the operating room was $4,368 (presumably 2003-2005 U.S. dollars) with a median cost of $3,479 and the average total cost of image-guided core-needle biopsy was $1,267 with a median cost of $1,239.[173]

The results of a mammogram help surgeons and radiologists decide which core-needle technique, if any, would be beneficial and ultimately cost-effective for the patient and facility. Soo et al. used a decision analysis model to compare the costs of a 14-gauge core-needle biopsy to a 14-gauge and 11-gauge vacuum-assisted biopsy for noncalcified lesions. They found that the 14-gauge CNB is less costly for noncalcified lesions, which is not surprising since vacuum- assisted equipment is more expensive.[174] Golub et al. prepared a cost-minimization model and found that image-guided core-needle biopsy was favored (cost the least) over open biopsy for low suspicion lesions, calcifications, and masses, primarily due to savings from reducing the overall number of surgeries performed.[175]

The cost to purchase a core-needle biopsy system is another factor of interest to facilities. In an article published in 2003, Kirshenbaum et al. reported that the average list price for a breast imaging center to make an existing mammography unit biopsy ready (i.e add-on unit) was $90,000 and the average list price for a dedicated prone biopsy table was $226,000.[131] Current quoted prices (not list prices) are about $170,000 (2008 U.S. dollars) for a dedicated table (which also requires a large dedicated room) and about $100,000 for an add-on unit.[176] Unlike a dedicated prone biopsy table, a mammography unit with an add-on device can be used for general mammography purposes when not being used for a biopsy procedure. However, add-on units have limitations, including limited access angles, limited ability to restrict patient movement, and less patient comfort than dedicated units.[176]

Ultrasound-guided core-needle biopsies do not require special equipment and can be performed with a standard multi-purpose US device. Vacuum-assisted core-needle devices currently cost around $37,000 (2008 U.S. dollars) to purchase a console, and require $270 single- use probes.[176] MRI-guidance is the most expensive method of performing core-needle biopsies, requiring expensive specialized equipment as well as access to an MRI facility.[176]

Spared Surgical Procedures

We identified 31 studies that reported information on how the use of core-needle biopsy spares women additional surgical procedures (see Table 12; also see Appendix E for further details). Women who undergo open biopsy with positive findings often undergo additional surgical procedures to ensure the entire lesion has been removed and to sample the lymph nodes. Women who undergo a core-needle biopsy procedure with positive findings may be able to undergo a single surgical procedure that simultaneously confirms the diagnosis and removes the entire lesion, and samples the lymph nodes if necessary, thus being spared additional surgical procedures. Women who undergo a core-needle biopsy with negative findings may be able to avoid surgical procedures altogether. Liberman et al. reported that, before the introduction of core-needle biopsy, 29% of women diagnosed with cancer had only one surgical procedure, but after the introduction of core-needle biopsy that number rose to 84%.[177] The studies consistently reported that approximately 75% of women who underwent a core-needle biopsy procedure were spared further procedures, with a mean of approximately 1.2 procedures per woman compared to 1.5 to 2.0 procedures per woman who was initially evaluated with open surgical biopsy.

Seven of the studies reported information about the percentage of women who, after being diagnosed with breast cancer by either core-needle or open biopsy, were able to be treated for their cancer with a single surgical procedure. We combined the data reported by these studies in a meta-analysis. The data were consistent (I2 = 2.2%). The summary odds ratio is 13.7 (95% CI: 5.6 to 34.6), an extremely large magnitude of effect. We felt that the strength of association between the type of biopsy and being able to treat the breast cancer with only one surgical procedure was strong enough to support an evidence-based conclusion. Although the internal validity (study quality) was low, the evidence was robust, consistent, and had an extremely large magnitude of effect. We therefore graded the strength of evidence supporting the conclusion as Moderate.

Procedure Preference

We identified 20 studies that reported data on patient preferences (see Table 12; also see Appendix E for further details). Ten of the 20 studied vacuum-assisted methods. The majority of the studies did not directly compare different biopsy procedures and instead reported information such as that the patients tolerated the procedure well or would recommend it to others in the future. One study reported that patients preferred the decubitus position to the prone position.138 Two studies reported that vacuum-assisted procedures were more comfortable than other types of core-needle biopsies.[178,179] Two authors reported that patients lost less time to core-needle procedures than to open procedures.[100,180] The majority of the studies concluded that core-needle biopsies were preferable to open biopsies, but one study reported that a survey of patients found that 90% were satisfied with their open surgical biopsy compared to only 80% satisfied with a vacuum-assisted core-needle biopsy.[181]

Cosmetic Results

We identified ten studies that reported information on cosmetic results (see Table 12; also see Appendix E for further details). The studies all used vacuum-assisted core-needle biopsy methods. The authors of the studies reported information on how patients felt about the cosmetic results post-procedure. Overall, patients were reported to have been satisfied with the cosmetic results. Only one of the ten studies, Chun et al., compared a group of patients undergoing core- needle biopsy to a group of patients undergoing open biopsy.[181] Chun et al. compared cosmetic results of patients undergoing wire-localized open biopsy to patients undergoing vacuum-assisted 11-gauge core-needle biopsy two years post-procedure. Ninety-five percent of the core-needle biopsy group and only 25% of the open biopsy group were very satisfied with the appearance of their breast. None of the core-needle biopsy group said the cosmetic results were unacceptable compared to 20% of the open biopsy group who found the results unacceptable.

Although all of the studies reporting on cosmetic results used vacuum-assisted methods, it is likely the results apply to most forms of core-needle biopsy. Regardless of the needle gauge or method used, the actual incision cut in the skin for core-needle procedures is always approximately 1/4" long.[176]

Physician Experience

We identified ten studies that reported information concerning physician experience (see Table 12; for further details see Appendix E). Authors of some of the studies commented that certain devices were easier for inexperienced physicians to use. In general, however, the authors of the studies concluded that greater experience with particular devices improved the accuracy of the biopsy procedures, shortened procedure duration times, and led to a decrease in the number of open biopsies that were performed.

Availability of a Qualified Pathologist

We identified two studies that discussed pathologist qualifications and availability (see Table 12; for further details see Appendix E). One reported that whether a specimen was read by a local or central pathologist made little difference because concordance between readings was 96.1% ($\kappa = 0.90$) for core needle biopsy and 92.6% ($\kappa = 0.93$) for open surgical biopsy. However, there was greater disagreement with respect to ADH and ALH for both biopsy types, with underestimation of the lesion by local pathologists in comparison to the central pathology laboratory (for CNB, ADH agreement 63% and ALH agreement 53%; for open, ADH agreement 45% and ALH agreement 73%).[182] The authors of the other study speculated that lack of an experienced pathologist was the cause of the low accuracy of the core-needle biopsies performed during the course of their study.[183]

Availability of Equipment

We identified three studies that talked about the impact of equipment availability (see Table 12; for further details see Appendix E). One reported that vacuum-assisted devices were more commonly available in the U.S. than in Europe.[184] One reported that wait times for access to core-needle procedures were significantly shorter than wait times for access to open surgical procedures.[185] The authors of the third study reported that wait times for access to a dedicated prone biopsy table were longer than wait times for other types of core-needle biopsy.[186]

Resource Usage

We identified two studies that talked about resource usage (see Table 12; for further details see Appendix E). The authors of one study reported that vacuum-assisted procedures required more physician and room time than free-hand ultrasound-guided procedures.[187] The other study reported that dedicated prone tables use four times as much space as non-prone units.[188]

Table 11. Economic considerations.

Reference	Source of Cost Data	Methods or Models of Analysis	Primary Conclusions
Hatmaker et al. 2006[173]	The Massachusetts Utilization Multiprogramming System and the Decision Support System software packages were used to track costs of procedures, by Current Procedure Terminology (CPT) code and date of service.	Data were analyzed and described using the R statistical computing environment. Costs for all service related to each procedure were linked through billing procedures by the date of service and classified as related to radiology costs, to pathology or laboratory costs, or to procedural costs	"The average total cost to evaluate a patient with a breast mass or mammographic abnormality through an OSB in the operating room was $4,368 (SD: $2,586) with a median cost of $3,479. The average total cost for a CNB was $1,267 (SD: $536) with a median cost of $1,239. For VA hospitals with available resources, the option of CNB is a cost-effective and more preferable alternative to OSB." (US currency year not specified; data collected between 2003-2005)
Orel et al. 2006[190]	NR	NR	"The total Medicare allowance for one MR-guided vacuum-assisted CNB procedure is approximately $500." (presumed to be 2005 US dollars) "Additional investigation is needed to develop more cost-efficient systems. In addition, the cost of the needles will probably decrease as the use of them increases"
Shin et al. 2006[191]	NR	NR	"If the surgeon chooses to perform a diagnostic core biopsy and then excise the lesion for definitive treatment, the overall cost would be between $12,000 and $15,000, depending on the initial modality used for biopsy. Extrapolating this to our small pilot study of 156 patients, the observation arm would cost $619,000 for ultrasound-guided CNB and $1,028,820 for stereotactic-guided CNB. OSB for diagnosis and treatment with routine screening follow-up would cost $1,454,544 at our institution." The costs appear to be charges ("costs billed at our institution). Currency year not specified but the data were collected between 2000 –

Reference	Source of Cost Data	Methods or Models of Analysis	Primary Conclusions
Soo et al. 2005[174]	Cost & probability variables were estimated from the authors'institution over a three-year period. Ratios were used representing the relative dollar values of the estimated costs	Decision Analysis Model was used to compare costs of 14-gauge CNB to 14-gauge and 11-gauge vacuum-assisted CNB for stereotactic biopsy of noncalcified breast lesions	2003, and the study was presented in 2005.) The 14-G vacuum-assisted CNB was 1.19 times as expensive as the multipass automated gun CNB method, and the 1 1-G vacuum-assisted CNB was 1.22 times as expensive as the multi pass automated gun CNB. The 14-G CNB is less costly for stereotactic biopsy of non-calcified lesions over a wide range of cost estimates
Golub et al. 2004[175]	Patient billing records at the Lynn Sage Breast Center	A decision analytic model of the outcomes of all biopsy patients seen at the Lynn Sage Breast Center during a 2 year period was constructed. Costs were analyzed by considering only patients receiving breast-conserving surgery (lumpectomy alone), and subgroup based on degree of suspicion and on radiographic abnormality type. The sum of the mean costs determined from the patient billing records was used as the base-line outcome measures in the decision tree. Costs were measured from a societal perspective. Only direct costs related to inpatient care were considered, and they included CNB, OSB, lumpectomy with or without reexcision, lumpectomy with or without lymph node dissection, mastectomy with or without lymph node dissection, and lymph node dissection alone. Costs were derived by application of the institution's cost-to-charge multiplier	"The total cost of diagnosis and surgical treatment was $1,849 for CNB versus $2,775 for OSB. When the probabilities were biased to favor OSB, the cost was $2,297 for CNB and $2,458 for OSB. CNB was favored for low suspicion lesions, calcifications, and masses. OSB was favored for high suspicion lesionsand architectural distortion. Total costs were $926 less for the CNB group. CNB can be cost-saving compared with OSB, particularly when mammographic abnormality is classified as low suspicion or consists of calcifications or masses." (Currency year not specified, but costs were in U.S. dollars and data were collected in 1996-1998.)

Table 11 (Continued).

Reference	Source of Cost Data	Methods or Models of Analysis	Primary Conclusions
Kirshenbaum et al. 2003[131]	NR	NR	"A breast imaging center need spend only approximately $90,000 (average list price of add-on device) to make an existing mammography unit biopsy-ready. For a dedicated prone biopsy table, a center would need to spend $226,000 (average listprice). If one includes the addit-ional cost of purchasing a mammo-graphy machine (average $80,000) that might be required because the add-on unit is incompatible with the existing machine, the cost differe-ntial is substantially reduced. When not being used for biopsies, add-on units can be used for general scree-ning and diagnostic work, whereas prone units can only be used for biopsies." (U.S. Currency year not specified; manuscript submitted in 2002)

Procedure Duration Time

We identified 40 studies that reported information about the duration of different biopsy procedures (see Table 12; for further details see Appendix E). The studies reported a wide range of times, from 10 minutes to 128 minutes. The wide range of times may be in part due to different definitions of when exactly the procedure was defined as starting and ending: for example, does the procedure start when the patient enters the room? When the incision is made? Does it end when the sample is collected or when the patient is released to go home? In general, study authors did not define what exactly they meant by procedure duration time.

The reported mean or median time to perform core-needle biopsies under ultrasound guidance ranged from 10 to 60 minutes; the mean or median time to perform core-needle biopsies under stereotactic guidance ranged from 19 to 70 minutes; and the mean or median time to perform core-needle biopsies under MRI guidance ranged from 31 to 70 minutes. Vacuum- assisted core-needle biopsies were reported to have a mean or median duration of 10 to 70 minutes. Open surgical biopsies were generally reported to have longer duration times than core- needle procedures, but only two studies reported estimated duration times of open biopsy—40 to 45 minutes.[51,189]

Wait Time for Test Results

We identified two studies that reported mean or median times to get a diagnosis following a breast biopsy (see Table 12; for further details see Appendix E). The authors reported that wait times after a core-needle procedure were 7 to 10 days shorter than after an open excisional biopsy.[183,185]

Table 12. Key Question 3: other Outcomes.

Outcome	Number of Studies	Number of Patients	Summary of Findings
Cosmetic results	5 prospective studies[101, 103,192- 194] and 5 retrospective studies[108,120,181,195,196]	4,732	In eight of the ten studies, the authors reported how all included study patients felt about their scar appearance at some point in time from one week to six months post-procedure. Overall, patients were satisfied with the cosmetic outcome. In two of the ten studies, the authors made direct comparisons between two types of biopsy procedures. Weber et al. compared the cosmetic results of the Mammotome with an 11-gauge needle to those of the ABBI.[108] They found the ABBI group was less satisfied with the appearance of the biopsy site than those in the Mammotome group. Chun et al. compared patients having either an ABBI or the Mammotome with an 11-gauge needle to those undergoing a wire localized biopsy.[181] These authors found that many patients in the wire localized group were unhappy with their cosmetic result, while all of the patients having Mammotome or ABBI found the scar appearance to be acceptable or excellent.
Physician experience	5 prospective studies[46,58,97,178,197] and 5 retrospective studies[198-202]	23,332	Eight of the ten included studies described the study physicians' level of experience and how that may have impacted the studies' results. In two of these cases (Schneider et al.[197] and Wunderbaldinger et al.[58]), the study investigators were testing a new CNB device and concluded that the device is suitable for physicians without a great deal of experience performing biopsies. The other two articles described how the availability of highly experienced biopsy operators has led to a decrease in the use of diagnostic excisional biopsies (Holloway et al.[198] and Hoffman et al.[199]).
Procedure time	23 prospective Studies[51,58,78,96,97,100,103, 106,112,12, 4,144,158,178,179, 187,194,197, 203-208] and [17] retrospective Studies[69,77,79,108,120,138,189, 190,196, 200,201,209-214]	6,121	A total of 40 studies reported procedure times for the various breast biopsy procedures. There was great variation in reported procedure times by study, with a range of between 10 and [128] minutes. Some studies indicated that changing from a conventional to an add-on unit and increased operator experience tended to decrease procedure times, while other studies suggested that cases in which benign epithelial cells were disseminated or where ABBI and wire localized procedures were used procedure times tended to be increased.

Table 12. (Continued).

Outcome	Number of Studies	Number of Patients	Summary of Findings
Spared procedure rates	8 prospective Studies[51,103,106,112,185,186, 215,216] and [23] retrospective Studies[60,69,84,114,136,177,214, 217-230]	8,407	31 studies reported how diagnostic CNB spared patients a surgical procedure as compared with a diagnostic excisional biopsy. CNB appears to spare a majority of patients additional surgical procedures. One particularly important finding was that women diagnosed with breast cancer by core-needle biopsy were usually able to have their cancer treated with a single surgical procedure, but women diagnosed with breast cancer by open surgical biopsy often required more than one surgical procedure to treat their cancer (odds ratio 13.7, 95% CI: 5.5 to 34.6).
Availability of a qualified pathologist	1 prospective study[183] and 1 retrospective study[182]	2,112	Two studies addressed the availability of a qualified pathologist for interpreting biopsy specimens. The first, Collins et al., found that whether a specimen was read by a local or central pathologist made very little difference.1 82 Agreement rates between the two were very high for both CNB and open biopsy, although agreement rates were somewhat lower for open biopsy specimens. The second study, Gukas et al, evaluated the accuracy of TruCut versus excisional biopsy in Nigeria.[183] The pathologist used in their study did not have a lot of experience with the TruCut device, and the authors concluded that his lack of experience explains TruCut's poor performance compared with excisional biopsy.
Availability of equip-ment	2 prospective studies[185,186] and 1 retrospective study[184]	5,921	Three studies addressed the availability of various breast biopsy devices. One, Deurloo et al., explained that while vacuum-assisted CNB is on the rise in the United States, in Europe automated gun CNB is the preferred technique, suggesting that European women are much less likely to have access to a vacuum-assisted procedure than are women in this country.[184] Verkooijen et al. report that median wait times, from initial physician referral to first diagnostic procedure, were shorter for patients having a CNB than those requiring an open biopsy (4 vs. 13 days, respectively), while Williams et al. found a longer wait list for prone CNB patients than for a historical cohort in the pre-prone table days.[185,186]
Resource usage	2 prospective studies[187,188]	393	Two studies addressed how the various breast biopsy techniques impact resource usage. Mainiero et al. compared the amount of physician time and room time utilized by vacuum-assisted CNB compared to freehand ultrasound- guided CNB.[187] They found the vacuum-assisted method required more physician and room time. Wunderbaldinger et al. reported that prone devices use four times the amount of hospital/office space as non-prone units.[188]

Outcome	Number of Studies	Number of Patients	Summary of Findings
Procedure preference	12 prospective Studies[100,101,106,178-180,183, 192-194,231,232] and [8] retrospective studies[77,108,120,138,181, 196, 222,233]	5,001	Twenty studies collected data on patient preferences for breast biopsy procedures. Overall, these studies reported that patients tolerated the CNB procedure well and that a good percentage indicated they would recommend the procedure to others.
Wait time for test results	2 prospective studies[183,185]	272	Two studies reported how long it may take patients to receive a diagnosis following either a CNB or open biopsy procedure. In both studies, wait times were shorter for the CNB (7.3 days less and 9 vs. 19 days, respectively).

Table 13. Summary of economic aspects of core-needle biopsy.

Aspect	N Studies	Conclusions and Comments
Relative costs open biopsy vs. core-needle biopsy	8	All report that core-needle biopsy costs less than open biopsy procedures.
Relative costs of different types of core-needle biopsy	3	Insufficient data. All three studies reported information on different comparisons.
Resource usage	2	Insufficient data. Both studies reported information on different topics.

Table 14. Summary of Patient Perspectives on Choice of Biopsy Method.

Aspect	N Studies	Conclusions and Comments
Procedure preference	20	The majority of the studies concluded that patients preferred core-needle procedures over open procedures
Spared surgical procedures	31	Approximately 75% of women who underwent a core-needle procedure were spared further procedures, with a mean of 1.2 procedures per woman compared to 1.5 to 2.0 procedures per woman who went straight to open biopsy.
Cosmetic results	10	Overall patients were satisfied with the cosmetic results of a vacuum-assisted core-needle procedure.
Procedure duration time	40	US-guided core-needle procedures took 10 to 60 minutes, stereotactically-guided core-needle procedures took 19 to 70 minutes, vacuum-assisted core-needle biopsies took 10 to 70 minutes. Open biopsy procedures were estimated to take 40 to 45 minutes.
Wait time for test result	2	Insufficient data

Table 15. Summary of clinician and facility factors related to core-needle biopsy.

Aspect	N Studies	Conclusions and Comments
Clinician experience	10	Greater experience with particular devices improved accuracy. Some types of devices were easier for inexperienced clinicians to use than others.
Availability of Equipment	3	Insufficient data
Availability of qualified pathologists	2	Insufficient data

Previously Published Systematic Reviews

Our searches identified two previously published systematic reviews. Verkooijen et al. reviewed the literature published prior to 1999 on core-needle biopsy of non-palpable lesions.[234] Fahrbach et al. reviewed the literature published from 1996 to 2004 on core-needle biopsy of patients referred for biopsy after screening mammography.[235]

We assessed the quality of each systematic review using the 'assessment of multiple systematic reviews' (AMSTAR) measurement tool.[236] The AMSTAR consists of 11 items, which have been tested for face and content validity. The items assess whether or not a systematic review includes important elements, such as a comprehensive literature search, assessment of study quality, appropriate methods to combine study findings, and assessment of publication bias. Responses to each item are checked as 'Yes' if the review includes that item, 'No' if it does not, 'Can't tell' if the item cannot be answered by the information provided in the review, or Not applicable' if the item is not applicable. The AMSTAR does not provide a method for rating the quality of a review. To rate the quality of the reviews, we applied the following criteria: a rating of 'High' if the review received mostly 'yes' responses (at least 8), a rating of 'Low' if the review received mostly 'no' responses (at least 8), and a rating of 'Moderate' if the review received mixed responses. Both systematic reviews were rated as Moderate quality. The reviews were not rated as High quality because neither systematic review stated conflicts of interest or incorporated ratings of the quality of the literature into their conclusions. See Appendix E for details about the quality rating.

Verkooijen et al. included only five cohort studies in their review. Their inclusion criteria were studies of non-palpable lesions, either surgical biopsy or at least two years of followup to verify the true diagnosis, and a minimum of five cores taken per lesion. All included studies happened to have used stereotactic guidance. The authors assumed core-needle biopsy had no false-positives (i.e., malignant diagnoses on core needle that were not found on open surgery were assumed to have been completely removed by the core-needle procedure). Their analyses found that the DCIS underestimation rate was 15% (95% CI: 8.0 to 26.0%), the ADH underestimation rate was 40% (95% CI: 26.0 to 56.0%), and the overall sensitivity of core- needle biopsy for non-palpable lesions was 97.0% (95% CI: 95.0% to 99.0%). Only two complications were reported, one hematoma and one case of infection.[234]

Fahrbach et al. included 12 studies of stereotactically-guided vacuum-assisted core-needle biopsy and compared them to 25 studies of stereotactically-guided automated gun core- needle biopsy. One of their inclusion criterion was that the study must have been conducted in a western-style health care system (North America, Europe, Australia, or New Zealand). Their analyses found the false-negative rate of vacuum-assisted biopsy was 1.2%, the DCIS underestimation rate was 13.7%, and the ADH underestimation rate was 2 9.2%. Automated gun core-needle biopsy had a false-negative rate of 2%, a DCIS underestimation rate of 27.1%, and an ADH underestimation rate of 47.4%. Further, the authors performed analyses of possible factors that may have affected the results. Study location was a significant predictor of the false- negative rate, but type of reference standard and patient position had no significant impact on the results.

The authors of both systematic reviews concluded that core-needle biopsy rarely misdiagnosed malignant lesions as benign. Fahrbach et al. concluded that vacuum-assisted biopsy may provide lower miss and underestimation rates than automated gun core-needle biopsy.[235]

4. Discussion

Open surgical biopsy is the "gold standard" method of evaluating a suspicious breast lesion. However, it is a surgical procedure that, like all surgeries, places the patient at risk of experiencing morbidities and, in rare cases, mortality. The majority of women who undergo breast biopsy procedures do not have cancer. Exposing large numbers of women to invasive surgical procedures when the majority of these women do not benefit from the procedure may be considered an unacceptable medical practice. A less invasive method would be preferable if it were sufficiently accurate.

Open surgical biopsy has been reported to miss 1 to 2% of breast cancers.40 Our analysis found that stereotactically-guided vacuum-assisted core-needle biopsy is almost as accurate as open surgical biopsy with a much lower complication rate. US-guided automated gun core-needle biopsy may be almost as accurate as stereotactically-guided vacuum-assisted biopsy, and may have a slightly lower complication rate than vacuum-assisted biopsy. Both US-guided automated gun biopsy and stereotactically-guided vacuum-assisted biopsy meet the criteria of being sufficiently accurate and safer than open surgical biopsy, and therefore under most clinical conditions are preferable to open surgical biopsy. It is possible that US-guided vacuum-assisted biopsy and stereotactically guided automated gun also meet the criteria of being sufficiently accurate and safer than open surgical biopsy, but the confidence intervals around the point estimates of accuracy are too wide to be certain.

Diagnoses of "pure" DCIS determined on the basis of core-needle biopsy may be incorrect due to the inability of needle biopsy to sample all parts of the tumor. Rakha and Ellis reviewed the literature in 2007 and reported that 15 to 20% of cases diagnosed as "pure" DCIS by core-needle biopsy were subsequently found to contain associated invasive carcinoma upon excision. 16 Our analyses found that DCIS underestimation rates ranged from 13% to 36%, justifying current clinical practice of referring all DCIS diagnoses for open surgery.

The management of "high risk" lesions such as ADH is somewhat controversial. Our analysis found that at least 20% of ADH diagnoses on core-needle biopsy are actually malignant, suggesting that some patients diagnosed with atypia on core needle may benefit from open surgery as well.

In Figure 5E, in the Executive Summary, we present a simple model of what might happen if the same cohort of 1000 women underwent various types of breast biopsy. The cohort of women includes 300 women with malignant tumors, and 700 women with benign lesions. The model is based on the point estimates of accuracy from our analyses and do not incorporate estimates of uncertainty in the point estimates. Refer to Figure 1 A through Figure 4 D in the Executive Summary for a visual representation of the degree of uncertainty in the point estimates.

Limitations of the Evidence Base

The evidence base is very large but of generally low quality. The majority of the available studies are poorly reported retrospective chart reviews. Most of the studies included all patients who underwent core-needle biopsy at a particular center or centers during a certain time period and had no other inclusion criteria for enrollment. Very few studies reported any characteristics of their patients; some did not even report how many patients were enrolled. Details of operator training and experience were often omitted, as were details about the training and experience of the pathologists reading the biopsy material. Many studies combined results for multiple core-needle biopsy methods. Others changed biopsy methodology in mid-study. Descriptions of biopsy methods were often inadequate. Characteristics of the breast lesions being biopsied were often omitted. Biopsy diagnoses were often collapsed into "benign" and "malignant" categories, instead of being presented in a more granular form by type of lesion. Sources of funding for the studies were usually not mentioned. Presentation of results was often haphazard and confusing. Many patients diagnosed as "benign" on core-needle biopsy had inadequate followup data. Poor reporting of biopsy methodology, patient characteristics, and details of lesions precluded answering the majority of the sub-questions about factors affecting the accuracy and harms of core-needle biopsy.

Applicability

We used inclusion criteria intended to restrict the evidence base to only those studies that included the population of interest: women of average risk undergoing breast biopsy after discovery of a suspicious lesion on routine screening. However, our analysis found that the prevalence of cancers in the study populations tended to be slightly higher than expected. The prevalence of cancers in the general population sent for breast biopsy (in the USA) has been reported to be around 23%.[15] The studies in our analysis generally reported prevalence in the thirties to forties, and up to 55% for freehand biopsies. This may be due to the fact that many of the studies were conducted in non-USA locations, where the prevalence of cancers in populations sent for biopsy has been reported to be 60 to 70%.[234] It may also be an artifact caused by attrition. Many of the studies had fairly high rates of attrition, and most of the lost patients had been diagnosed as benign on core-needle biopsy. The lost patients were of necessity removed from the analysis, and this may have artificially elevated the prevalence of disease. Interestingly, the studies of US-guided vacuum-assisted biopsy reported an overall prevalence of disease of only 15%, suggesting that lesions selected for this method may have a low probability of being malignant. Lesions selected for US-guided procedures generally do not contain microcalcifications and must be clearly visible on US.

Possible Impact of Key Assumptions on the Conclusions

Several key assumptions were made: (1) the "reference standard", a combination of open surgery and followup for at least six months, was 100% accurate; (2) the pathologists examining the open surgical biopsy results were 100% accurate; and (3) core-needle diagnoses of malignancy (invasive or in situ) that could not be confirmed by open surgery were assumed to have been correct diagnoses where the lesion had been completely removed by the core-needle biopsy procedure. In addition, the majority of studies reported data on a per-lesion rather than a per-patient basis, and therefore we analyzed the data on a per-lesion basis.

Key assumption #1, that the reference standard was 100% accurate, is almost certainly not true. Open surgical biopsy has been reported to have a false-negative rate of 1 to 2% when two years of patient followup was used as the reference standard.40 If a small percentage of the surgical biopsies were false-negatives then our estimates of the accuracy of core-needle biopsy are slightly lower than the actual "true" accuracy of core-needle biopsy. If a small percentage of the patients declared "benign" on six-month patient followup actually had cancers then our estimates of the accuracy of core-needle biopsy are higher than the actual "true" accuracy of core-needle biopsy. Logically one would expect short-term patient followup to be more prone to error than open surgical biopsy; thus it seems likely that our estimates of core-needle biopsy accuracy are slightly higher than the actual "true" accuracy. However, some of the studies did follow all patients for at least two years, and other studies did perform open biopsy on all patients. We performed meta-regressions and found no statistically significant impact of the type of reference standard used or length of followup on the reported accuracy of the core-needle biopsies.

Key assumptions #2 and #3 are inter-related and both depend on pathologists being 100% accurate in reading open surgical biopsy material. The errors that pathologists make when examining core-needle biopsy specimens are incorporated into our conclusions about the accuracy of core-needle biopsy: causes of misdiagnosis include errors of sampling as well as errors of pathologists examining the core-needle specimens. The literature reports pathology errors in general as being rare, affecting 0.08 to 1.2% of specimens examined.[237] The fact that open surgical biopsy has a false-negative rate of less than 2% also suggests that open surgical biopsy pathology errors are quite rare; this low false-negative rate includes errors of surgery as well as errors of pathologists. A 2006 review of medical malpractice suits filed against pathologists for breast biopsy misdiagnoses reported that about half the suits involved false- negative errors and about half involved false-positive errors.[237] Even if a very small percentage of patients declared "true positive" in our analysis were actually false-positives and a very small percentage of patients declared "true negatives" were actually false-negatives, it seems unlikely that our estimates of core-needle biopsy accuracy can be significantly different than the actual true accuracy. The clinical impact of pathology errors, however, is not insignificant, since it can lead to over- and under- treatment.

Key assumption #4, that analyzing the data on a per-lesion rather than a per-patient basis would not violate statistical assumptions of independence, was unavoidable. Very few of the studies reported data on a per-patient basis. The percentage of patients with more than one lesion was, in most studies, quite low. Each lesion was subjected to an independent core-needle biopsy. A patient diagnosed with multiple benign lesions would have all lesions managed by followup, but a patient with one malignant lesion and a benign lesion may have had the benign lesion surgically biopsied at the same time as the malignant lesion was biopsied. Thus the independence of data at the per-lesion level is not quite complete. The impact of this minor lack of independence on the results of our analyses is most likely insignificant.

Correlation with Findings from Prior Systematic Reviews

As discussed previously, two prior systematic reviews of core-needle biopsy have been published.[234,235] Both prior reviews and our review calculated very similar false-negative rates for stereotactically-guided automated gun core-needle biopsy: 2.2%, 3.0%, and 2.0%. Both prior reviews and our review calculated very similar rates of ADH underestimation for stereotactically-guided automated gun core-needle biopsy: 40%, 43.5%, and 47.4%. The DCIS underestimation rate reported by Verkooijen et al. for stereotactically-guided core-needle biopsy was much lower (only 15.0%) than the DCIS underestimation rates reported by Fahrbach et al. and our review (24.4%, 27.1%, respectively). This difference may be related to the fact that our review and Fahrbrach et al. included both palpable and non-palpable lesions in the analysis whereas Verkooijen et al. restricted their analysis to non-palpable lesions.

Table 16. Unanswered Questions.

Unanswered questions about accuracy
What is the accuracy of MRI-guided core-needle biopsy?
What impact does patient age have on the accuracy of different methods of performing breast biopsy?
What impact does breast density have on the accuracy of different methods of performing breast biopsy?
What impact do patient co-morbidities have on the accuracy of different methods of performing breast biopsy?
Do different methods of breast biopsy have different accuracies for palpable vs. non-palpable lesions, microcalcifications vs. masses, distortions vs. masses?
What impact does the size of the lesion have on the accuracy of different methods of performing breast biopsy?
What impact does the location of the lesion have on the accuracy of different methods of performing breast biopsy?
What impact does the number of cores taken have on the accuracy of different methods of performing breast biopsy?
What impact does patient positioning have on the accuracy of different methods of performing breast biopsy?
What impact does experience of the operator have on the accuracy of different methods of performing breast biopsy?
What impact does the training of the operator have on the accuracy of different methods of performing breast biopsy?
Unanswered questions about harms
What impact does the type of image guidance (none, MRI, stereotactic, or US) have on adverse events of breast biopsy?
What impact does patient age have on adverse events related to breast biopsy?
What impact does breast density have on adverse events of breast biopsy?
What impact do patient co-morbidities have on adverse events of breast biopsy?
Does the type of lesion- palpable vs. non-palpable lesions, microcalcifications vs. masses, distortions vs. masses- have an impact on adverse events of breast biopsy?

What impact does the size of the lesion have on adverse events of breast biopsy?
What impact does the location of the lesion have on adverse events of breast biopsy?
What impact does the number of cores taken have on adverse events of breast biopsy?
Unanswered questions about accuracy
What impact does the needle size have on adverse events of breast biopsy?
What impact does experience of the operator have on adverse events of breast biopsy?
What impact does the training of the operator have on adverse events of breast biopsy?
What impact does the facility location or type of facility have on adverse events of breast biopsy?
Unanswbered questions about economic aspects
What impact does the cost of different types of core-needle breast biopsy have on the choice to perform a particular type of breast biopsy?
What impact does the availability of equipment and resources have on the choice to perform a particular type of breast biopsy?
What impact does the availability of a qualified pathologist have on the choice to perform a particular type of breast biopsy?

Verkooijen et al. did not study stereotactically-guided vacuum-assisted core-needle biopsy. Our review and Fahrbach et al. found very similar accuracy figures for stereotacticallyguided vacuum-assisted core-needle biopsy: false negative rate, 1.2% and 0.8%; ADH underestimation rate, 29.2% and 21.9%; DCIS underestimation rate, 13.7% and 13.0%.

Fahrbach et al. found that study location was a significant predictor of the false-negative rate, but type of reference standard and patient position had no significant impact on the results. We also found that the type of reference standard had no impact on the results, but we found no impact of study location on the results. The reason for this apparent discrepancy may be that we included studies conducted worldwide, whereas Fahrbach et al. included only studies conducted in North America, Europe, Australia, or New Zealand.

Future Research Needed

For many interventions, randomized controlled trials that measure patient-oriented outcomes are necessary in order to justify the routine use of the intervention. However, it is generally believed that early diagnosis and treatment of breast tumors leads to improved survival rates and quality of life. Women found to have benign lesions on biopsy are able to avoid unnecessary treatment and receive reassurance that they do not have breast cancer. There is no need to conduct randomized controlled trials reporting patient-oriented outcomes of breast biopsy procedures. Establishing that a type of breast biopsy is safer than open surgical biopsy while being as or almost as accurate as open surgical biopsy is sufficient to justify its routine use. Our systematic review has found that both stereotactically guided vacuum-assisted and US- guided automated gun core-needle biopsy are safer than open surgical biopsy and are almost as accurate as open surgical biopsy, justifying their routine use.

However, well-reported retrospective chart reviews, retrospective database analyses, or prospective diagnostic accuracy studies are needed to address the as-yet-unanswered questions as to what factors affect the accuracy and harms of core-needle breast biopsy. We have listed the most important as-yet unanswered questions in Table 16. Answers to such questions are important for both patients and clinicians when faced with the decision of what type of breast biopsy is best for each individual patient. The unanswered questions can be addressed by a prospective or retrospective diagnostic cohort study that reports relevant information in a format that allows each unanswered question to be directly addressed. It is possible that many of the studies included in the current systematic review collected information that addressed some of the unanswered questions but did not report it.

In addition, our conclusions are often rated as being supported by a low strength of evidence. The low rating is almost entirely due to the fact that the evidence base, while large, consists of universally poorly reported studies. The studies omitted important details about patients, methods, and results. The studies presented results in an often confusing and haphazard manner. The poor reporting made it difficult to determine whether the studies were likely to be unaffected by bias, and therefore we rated the evidence base as being of low quality. Publication of better-reported diagnostic accuracy studies would permit verification that our conclusions are accurate and not influenced by biases in the studies included in this technology assessment.

References and Included Studies

(Note: There is a separate set of references at the end of Appendix G whose reference numbers are different from those in the text of the report.)

[1] American Cancer Society (ACS). Cancer facts and figures 2003. Atlanta, GA: American Cancer Society (ACS); 2003. Available at: http://www.cancer p.

[2] American Cancer Society (ACS). Cancer facts & figures 2009. Atlanta, GA: American Cancer Society (ACS); 2009. Available at: http://www.cancer 09web.pdf.

[3] National Cancer Institute. Surveillance Epidemiology and End Results. SEER stat fact sheets—cancer of the breast. Available at: http://seer.cancer.gov/statfacts/html/breast_p rint.html. *Accessed February*, 5, 2007.

[4] Feuer, EJ; Wun, LM. DEVCAN: probability of developing or dying of cancer software, version 4.1. Available at: http://canques.seer.cancer.gov/cgi- bin/cq_submit?dir-devcan1 999&db=1 &rpt=TAB&sel=. Accessed May, 28, 2002.

[5] Levine, P; Simsir, A; Cangiarella, J. Management issues in breast lesions diagnosed by fine-needle aspiration and percutaneous core breast biopsy. *Am J Clin Pathol,*, 2006, Jun;125 Suppl:S124-S134. PMID: 16830962.

[6] American Cancer Society (ACS). Cancer facts & figures 2008. Atlanta, GA: American Cancer Society (ACS); 2008. Available at: http://www.cancer. U.S. Preventive Services Task Force (USPSTF). Screening for breast cancer: recommendations and rationale. Washington, DC: Agency for Healthcare Research and Quality, February 2002. AHRQ Publication No. 02-507A. Available at: http://www.ahrq.gov/clinic/3rduspstf/breastc ancer.

[7] U.S. Preventive Services Task Force (USPSTF). Screening for breast cancer: recommendations and rationale. Washington, DC: Agency for Healthcare Research and

Quality, February 2002. AHRQ Publication No. 02-507A. Available at: http://www.ahrq.gov/clinic/3rduspstf/breastcancer.

[8] Humphrey, LL; Helfand, M; Chan, BK; et al. Breast cancer screening: a summary of the evidence for the U.S. Preventive Services Task Force. Ann Intern Med 2002, Sep 3, 137(5 Part 1), 347-367. PMID: 12204020.

[9] Rosato, FE; Rosato, EL. Examination techniques: roles of the physician and patient in evaluating breast diseases. In: Bland KI; Copeland 3rd EM; eds. The breast: comprehensive management of benign and malignant diseases. 2nd ed. Vol. 1. Philadelphia, PA: WB. *Saunders Company*; 1998, 615-623.

[10] U.S. Preventive Services Task Force. Screening for breast cancer: U.S. Preventive Services Task Force recommendation statement. Ann Intern Med 2009, Nov 17, 151(10), 716-726, W236. PMID: 19920272.

[11] Liberman, L; Menell, JH. Breast imaging reporting and data system (BI-RADS). *Radiol Clin North Am*, 2002, May, 40(3), 409- 430. PMID, 12117184.

[12] Diagnostic and Interventional Radiology Department. Mammography. Omaha, NE: Creighton University School of Medicine. Available at: http://radiology.creighton.edu/mammo.html.

[13] Obenauer, S; Hermann, KP; Grabbe, E. Applications and literature review of the BI-RADS classification. *Eur Radiol*, 2005, May, 15(5), 1027-1036. PMID: 15856253.

[14] Wallis, M; Tardivon, A; Helbich, T; et al. Guidelines from the European Society of Breast Imaging for diagnostic interventional breast procedures. *Eur Radiol*, 2007, Feb, 17(2), 581-588. PMID: 17013595.

[15] Lacquement, MA; Mitchell, D; Hollingsworth, AB. Positive predictive value of the Breast Imaging Reporting and Data System. *J Am Coll Surg*, 1999, Jul;189(1), 34-40. PMID: 10401738.

[16] Rakha, EA; Ellis, IO. An overview of assessment of prognostic and predictive factors in breast cancer needle core biopsy specimens. *J Clin Pathol*, 2007, Dec, 60(12), 1300-1306. PMID: 17630399.

[17] American Cancer Society (ACS). Detailed guide: breast cancer. How is breast cancer staged? Available at: http://www.cancer.org/docroot/CRI/content/ CRI_2_4_3X_How_is_breast_cancer_stage d_5.asp. Accessed May 25, 2007.

[18] NCCN clinical practice guidelines in oncology: breast cancer V.2.2007. Jenkintown, PA: National Comprehensive Cancer Network (NCCN); 2007, Mar 28.

[19] Fryback, DG; Thornbury, JR. The efficacy of diagnostic imaging. Med Decis Making 1991 Apr-Jun, 11(2), 88-94. PMID: 1907710.

[20] Deeks, JJ. Systematic reviews of evaluations of diagnostic and screening tests. In: M; Egger, GD; Smith, DG; Altman, eds. Systematic reviews in health care: meta-analysis in context. 2nd ed. London, England: BMJ Books; 2001, 248-282.

[21] Lijmer, JG; Mol, BW; Heisterkamp, S; et al. Empirical evidence of design-related bias in studies of diagnostic tests. *JAMA*, 1999, Sep 15, 282(11), 1061-1066. PMID: 10493205.

[22] Moher, D; Pham, B; Klassen, TP; et al. What contributions do languages other than English make on the results of meta- analyses? *J Clin Epidemiol*, 2000, Sep, 53(9), 964-972. PMID: 11004423.

[23] Juni, P; Holenstein, F; Sterne, J; et al. Direction and impact of language bias in meta-analyses of controlled trials: empirical study. *Int J Epidemiol*, 2002, Feb;31(1), 1 15-123. PMID: 11914306.

[24] Chalmers, I; Adams, M; Dickersin, K; et al. A cohort study of summary reports of controlled trials. JAMA 1990, Mar 9, 263(10), 1401-1405. PMID: 2304219.

[25] Neinstein, LS. A review of Society for Adolescent Medicine abstracts and Journal of Adolescent Health Care articles. *J Adolesc Health Care,* 1987 Mar;8(2), 198- 203. PMID: 3818406.

[26] Dundar, Y; Dodd, S; Williamson, P; et al. Case study of the comparison of data from conference abstracts and full-text articles in health technology assessment of rapidly evolving technologies: does it make a difference? *Int J Technol Assess Health Care,* 2006, Jul;22(3), 288-294.

[27] De Bellefeuille, C; Morrison, CA; Tannock, IF. The fate of abstracts submitted to a cancer meeting: factors which influence presentation and subsequent publication. *Ann Oncol,* 1992, Mar;3(3), 187-191. PMID: 1586615.

[28] Scherer, RW; Langenberg, P. Full publication of results initially presented in abstracts. In: Cochrane Library [Cochrane methodology review]. Issue 2. Oxford: Update Software; 2001. Available at: http://www.cochrane.org/index.htm. *Accessed April*, 23, 2001.

[29] Marx, WF; Cloft, HJ; Do, HM; et al. The fate of neuroradiologic abstracts presented at national meetings in 1993, rate of subsequent publication in peer-reviewed, indexed journals. *AJNR Am J Neuroradiol,* 1999, Jun-Jul;20(6), 1173-1177. PMID: 10445467.

[30] Yentis, SM; Campbell, FA; Lerman, J. Publication of abstracts presented at anaesthesia meetings. *Can J Anaesth*, 1993, Jul, 40(7), 632-634. PMID: 8403137.

[31] Whiting, P; Rutjes, AW; Reitsma, JB; et al. The development of QUADAS: a tool for the quality assessment of studies of diagnostic accuracy included in systematic reviews. BMC *Med Res Methodol*, 2003, Nov 10, 3(1), 25. PMID: 14606960.

[32] Treadwell, JR; Tregear, SJ; Reston, JT; et al. A system for rating the stability and strength of medical evidence. *BMC Med Res Methodol*, 2006, 6, 52. PMID: 17052350.

[33] Rakha, EA; El-Sayed, ME; Reed, J; et al. Screen-detected breast lesions with malignant needle core biopsy diagnoses and no malignancy identified in subsequent surgical excision specimens (potential false- positive diagnosis). *Eur J Cancer*, 2009, May;45(7), 1162-1167. PMID: 19121932.

[34] Harbord, RM; Deeks, JJ; Egger, M; et al. A unification of models for meta-analysis of diagnostic accuracy studies. *Biostatistics,* 2007, Apr;8(2), 239-25 1. PMID: 16698768.

[35] STATA statistics/data analysis. MP parallel edition. College Station (TX), StataCorp; 1984-2007. Single user Stata for Windows. Available at: http://www.stata.com.

[36] Zamora, J; Abraira, V; Muriel, A; et al. MetaDiSc: a software for meta-analysis of test accuracy data. *BMC Med Res Methodol*, 2006, 6, 31. PMID: 16836745.

[37] Borenstein, M; Hedges, L; Higgins, J; et al. Comprehensive meta-analysis. Version 2. Englewood (NJ), Biostat; 2005. Available at: http://www.metaanalysis.com/pages/about_us.html.

[38] Deeks, J; Macaskill, P; Irwig, L. Detecting publication bias in systematic reviews of diagnostic test accuracy [abstract O-009]. In: Cochrane Collaboration [database online]. Oxford (UK), Cochrane Collaboration; 2004. Available at: http://www.cochrane.org/colloquia/abstracts /ottawa/O-009.htm. Accessed May 25, 2005.

[39] Deeks, J; Macaskill, P; Irwig, L. By how much does publication bias affect the results of systematic reviews of diagnostic test accuracy? (abstract O-010). In: Cochrane Collaboration [database online]. Oxford (UK), Cochrane Collaboration; 2004. Available at: http://www.cochrane.org/colloquia/abstracts /ottawa/O-010.htm. Accessed May 25, 2005.

[40] Antley, CM; Mooney, EE; Layfield, LJ. A comparison of accuracy rates between open biopsy, cutting-needle biopsy, and fine- needle aspiration biopsy of the breast: A 3-year experience. *Breast J*, 1998, 4(1), 3-8.

[41] Meyer, JE; Kopans, DB. Analysis of mammographically obvious carcinomas of the breast with benign results upon initial biopsy. Surg Gynecol Obstet 1981 Oct; 1 53(4), 570-572. PMID: 6269239.

[42] Patchefsky, AS; Potok, J; Hoch, WS; et al. Increased detection of occult breast carcinoma after more thorough histologic examination of breast biopsies. *Am J Clin Pathol,* 1973, Dec, 60(6), 799-804. PMID: 4357121.

[43] Grady, D; Hodgkins, ML; Goodson 3rd, WH. The lumpy breast. *West J Med*, 1988, Aug;149(2), 226-229. PMID: 3073579

[44] Wong, TE; Hisham, AN. Core needle biopsy of palpable breast lump: the influence of needle size. *Med J Malaysia*, 2003, Aug; 58(3), 399-404. PMID: 14750380.

[45] Scopa, CD; Koukouras, D; Spiliotis, J; et al. Comparison of fine needle aspiration and Tru-Cut biopsy of palpable mammary lesions. *Cancer Detect Prev*, 1996, 20(6), 620-624. PMID: 8939348.

[46] McMahon, AJ; Lutfy, AM; Matthew, A; et al. Needle core biopsy of the breast with a spring-loaded device. *Br J Surg*, 1992, Oct;79(10), 1042-1045. PMID: 1422715.

[47] Barreto, V; Hamed, H; Griffiths, AB; et al. Automatic needle biopsy in the diagnosis of early breast cancer. *Eur J Surg Oncol*, 1991, Jun, 17(3), 237-239. PMID: 2044776.

[48] Cusick, JD; Dotan, J; Jaecks, RD; et al. The role of Tru-Cut needle biopsy in the diagnosis of carcinoma of the breast. Surg Gynecol Obstet 1990 May;170(5), 407-410. PMID: 2183373.

[49] Youk, JH; Kim, EK; Kim, MJ; et al. Sonographically guided 14-gauge core needle biopsy of breast masses: a review of 2,420 cases with long-term follow-up. *AJR Am J Roentgenol,*, 2008, Jan;190(1), 202-207. PMID: 18094312.

[50] de Lucena, CE; Dos Santos Junior, JL; de Lima Resende, CA; et al. Ultrasound-guided core needle biopsy of breast masses: How many cores are necessary to diagnose cancer? *J Clin Ultrasound*, 2007, Sep, 35(7), 363-366. PMID: 17663457.

[51] Bolivar, AV; Alonso-Bartolome, P; Garcia, EO; et al. Ultrasound-guided core needle biopsy of non-palpable breast lesions: a prospective analysis in 204 cases. *Acta Radiol*, 2005, Nov;46(7), 690-695. PMID: 16372687.

[52] Crystal, P; Koretz, M; Shcharynsky, S; et al. Accuracy of sonographically guided 14-gauge core-needle biopsy: Results of 715 consecutive breast biopsies with at least two-year follow-up of benign lesions. *J Clin Ultrasound,* 2005, Feb, 33(2), 47-52. PMID: 15674836.

[53] Sauer, G; Deissler, H; Strunz, K; et al. Ultrasound-guided large-core needle biopsies of breast lesions: Analysis of 962 cases to determine the number of samples for reliable tumour classification. *Br J Cancer*, 2005, Jan 31, 92(2), 23 1-235. PMID: 15611793.

[54] Delle Chiaie, L; Terinde, R. Three- dimensional ultrasound-validated large-core needle biopsy: is it a reliable method for the histological assessment of breast lesions. *Ultrasound Obstet Gynecol*, 2004, Apr, 23(4), 393-397. PMID: 15065192.

[55] Fishman, JE; Milikowski, C; Ramsinghani, R; et al. US-guided core-needle biopsy of the breast: How many specimens are necessary? *Radiology*, 2003, Mar 1, 226(3), 779-782. PMID: 12601206.

[56] Philpotts, LE; Hooley, RJ; Lee, CH. Comparison of automated versus vacuum- assisted biopsy methods for sonographically guided core biopsy of the breast. *AJR Am J Roentgenol,*, 2003, Feb; 1 80(2), 347-35 1. PMID: 12540431.

[57] Smith, DN; Rosenfield Darling, ML; et al. The utility of ultrasonographically guided large-core needle biopsy: results from 500 consecutive breast biopsies. *J Ultrasound Med*, 2001, Jan;20(1), 43-49. PMID: 11149527.

[58] Wunderbaldinger, P; Helbich, TH; Partik, B; et al. First experience with a new dedicated ultrasound system for computer-guided large-core breast biopsy. *Eur Radiol,* 2001, 11(12), 2460-2464. PMID: 11734940.

[59] Yeow, KM; Lo, YF; Wang, CS; et al. Ultrasound-guided core needle biopsy as an initial diagnostic test for palpable breast masses. *J Vasc Interv Radiol*, 2001, Nov;12(11), 1313-1317. PMID: 11698631.

[60] Liberman, L; Feng, TL; Dershaw, DD; et al. US-guided core breast biopsy: use and cost- effectiveness. *Radiology*, 1998, Sep, 208(3), 717-723. PMID: 9722851.

[61] Schulz-Wendtland, R; Kramer, S; Lang, N; et al. Ultrasonic guided microbiopsy in mammary diagnosis: indications, technique and results. *Anticancer Res*, 1998, May-Jun; 18(3C), 2 145-2146. PMID: 9703772.

[62] Khattar, SC; Torp-Pedersen, S; Horn, T; et al. Ultrasound-guided biopsy of palpable breast masses. *Eur J Ultrasound*, 1997, 6(1), 1-7.

[63] Parker, SH; Jobe, WE; Dennis, MA; et al. US- guided automated large-core breast biopsy. *Radiology*, 1993, May; 187(2), 507-511. PMID: 8475299.

[64] Schueller, G; Jaromi, S; Ponhold, L; et al. US- guided 14-gauge core-needle breast biopsy: results of a validation study in 1352 cases. *Radiology*, 2008, Aug, 248(2), 406-413. PMID, 18641246.

[65] Peters, N; Hoorntje, L; Mali, W; et al. Diagnostic performance of stereotactic large core needle biopsy for nonpalpable breast lesions in routine clinical practice. *Int J Cancer,* 2008, Jan 15, 122(2), 468-47 1. PMID: 17935136.

[66] Koskela, AK; Sudan, M; Berg, MH; et al. Add-on device for stereotactic core-needle breast biopsy: How many biopsy specimens are needed for a reliable diagnosis? *Radiology*, 2005, Sep, 236(3), 801-809. PMID: 16020555.

[67] Han, BK; Choe, YH; Ko, YH; et al. Stereotactic core-needle biopsy of non-mass calcifications: outcome and accuracy at long-term follow-up. *Korean J Radiol*, 2003, Oct-Dec;4(4), 2 17-223. PMID: 14726638.

[68] Verkooijen, HM; Core Biopsy After Radiological Localisation (COBRA) Study Group. Diagnostic accuracy of stereotactic large-core needle biopsy for nonpalpable breast disease: results of a multicenter prospective study with 95% surgical confirmation. *Int J Cancer,* 2002, Jun 20, 99(6), 853-859. PMID: 12115488.

[69] Becker, L; Taves, D; McCurdy, L; et al. Stereotactic core biopsy of breast microcalcifications: comparison of film versus digital mammography, both using an add-on unit. *AJR Am J Roentgenol,*, 2001, Dec, 177(6), 1451-1457. PMID: 11717106.

[70] Brenner, RJ; Bassett, LW; Fajardo, LL; et al. Stereotactic core-needle breast biopsy: a multi-institutional prospective trial. *Radiology*, 2001, Mar;2 18(3), 866-872. PMID: 11230668.

[71] Dahlstrom, JE; Jain, S. Histological correlation of mammographically detected microcalcifications in stereotactic core biopsies. *Pathology*, 2001, 33(4), 444-448. PMID: 11827410.

[72] Levin, MF; Papoff, WJ; Doan, L; et al. Stereotaxic percutaneous core biopsy versus surgical biopsy of nonpalpable breast lesions using a standard mammographic table with an add-on device. *Can Assoc Radiol J,* 2001, 52(1), 29-32. PMID: 11247262.

[73] Kirwan, SE; Denton, ER; Nash, RM; et al. Multiple 14G stereotactic core biopsies in the diagnosis of mammographically detected stellate lesions of the breast. *Clin Radiol,* 2000, Oct;55(10), 763-766. PMID: 11052877.

[74] Ward, SE; Taves, DH; McCurdy, LI. Stereotaxic core needle biopsy of breast microcalcifications obtained using a standard mammography table with an add- on unit. *Can Assoc Radiol J,* 2000, Feb, 51(1), 10-15. PMID: 10711288.

[75] Jackman, RJ; Nowels, KW; Rodriguez-Soto, J; et al. Stereotactic, automated, large-core needle biopsy of nonpalpable breast lesions: false-negative and histologic underestimation rates after long-term follow-up. *Radiology*, 1999, Mar;2 10(3), 799-805. PMID: 10207484.

[76] Soo, MS; Ghate, S; Delong, D. Stereotactic biopsy of noncalcified breast lesions: utility of vacuum-assisted technique compared to multipass automated gun technique. *Clin Imaging*, 1999, Nov-Dec;23(6), 347-352. PMID: 10899415.

[77] Doyle, AJ; Collins, JP; Forkert, CD. Decubitus stereotactic core biopsy of the breast: technique and experience. *AJR Am J Roentgenol,,* 1999, Mar; 1 72(3), 688-690. PMID: 10063861

[78] Vega Bolivar, A; Ortega Garcia, E; Garijo Ayensa, F. Stereotaxic core needle aspiration biopsy with multiple passes in nonpalpable breast lesions. *Acta Radiol*, 1998, Jul;39(4), 389-394. PMID: 9685825.

[79] Whitman, GJ; Kopans, DB; McCarthy, KA; et al. Coaxial core needle biopsy under mammographic guidance: indications and applications. *AJR Am J Roentgenol,,* 1998, 171(1), 67-70. PMID: 9648766.

[80] Zannis, VJ; Aliano, KM. The evolving practice pattern of the breast surgeon with disappearance of open biopsy for nonpalpable lesions. *Am J Surg*, 1998, Dec, 176(6), 525-528. PMID: 9926783.

[81] Bauer, RL, Sung, J; Eckhert Jr, KH; et al. Comparison of histologic diagnosis between stereotactic core needle biopsy and open surgical biopsy. *Ann Surg Oncol*, 1997, Jun;4(4), 316-320. PMID: 9181231.

[82] Liberman, L; Dershaw, DD; Glassman, JR; et al. Analysis of cancers not diagnosed at stereotactic core breast biopsy. *Radiology*, 1997, Apr, 203(1), 151-157. PMID: 9122384

[83] Pitre, B; Baron, PL; Baron, LF; et al. Stereotactic core biopsy of the breast: Results of one-year follow-up of 101 patients. *Am Surg*, 1997, 63(12), 1124-1 127. PMID: 9393264.

[84] Sutton, S; Dahlstrom, JE; Jain, S. Stereotactic large-gauge core biopsy: its role in the diagnosis of non-palpable mammographic abnormalities presenting to a screening service. *Australas Radiol*, 1997, May, 41(2), 103-108. PMID: 9153803.

[85] Walker, TM. Impalpable breast lesions: Stereotactic core biopsy with an 'add-on' unit. *Breast*, 1997 Jun;6(3), 126-131.

[86] Frazee, RC; Roberts, JW; Symmonds, RE; et al. Open versus stereotactic breast biopsy. *Am J Surg*, 1996, Nov, 172(5), 491-493, 494-495. PMID: 8942551.

[87] Fuhrman, G; Cederbom, G; Champagne, J; et al. Stereotactic core needle breast biopsy is an accurate diagnostic technique to assess nonpalpable mammographic abnormalities. *J La State Med Soc*, 1996, Apr, 148(4), 167-170. PMID: 8935619.

[88] Head, JF; Haynes, AE; Elliott, MC; et al. Stereotaxic localization and core needle biopsy of nonpalpable breast lesions: two- year follow-up of a prospective study. *Am Surg,* 1996, Dec, 62(12), 1018-1023. PMID: 8955240.

[89] Mainiero, MB; Philpotts, LE; Lee, CH; et al. Stereotaxic core needle biopsy of breast microcalcifications: correlation of target accuracy and diagnosis with lesion size. *Radiology*, 1996, Mar, 198(3), 665-669. PMID: 8628852.

[90] Meyer, JE; Christian, RL; Lester, SC; et al. Evaluation of nonpalpable solid breast masses with stereotaxic large- needle core biopsy using a dedicated unit. *AJR Am J Roentgenol,*, 1996, 167(1), 179-1 82.

[91] Pettine, S; Place, R; Babu, S; et al. Stereotactic breast biopsy is accurate, minimally invasive, and cost effective. *Am J Surg,* 1996, May, 171(5), 474-476. PMID: 8651388.

[92] Rosenblatt, R; Fineberg, SA; Sparano, JA; et al. Stereotactic core needle biopsy of multiple sites in the breast: efficacy and effect on patient care. *Radiology*, 1996, Oct;201(1), 67-70. PMID: 8816522.

[93] Cross, MJ; Evans, WP; Peters, GN; et al. Stereotactic breast biopsy as an alternative to open excisional biopsy. *Ann Surg Oncol*, 1995, May, 2(3), 195-200. PMID: 7641014.

[94] Gisvold, JJ; Goellner, JR; Grant, CS; et al. Breast biopsy: a comparative study of stereotaxically guided core and excisional techniques. *AJR Am J Roentgenol,*, 1994, Apr; 162(4), 8 15-820. PMID: 8140997.

[95] Smyth, AT; Cederbom, GJ. Core biopsy of breast lesions. J La State Med Soc 1994 Nov;146(1 1), 499-501. PMID: 7806950.

[96] Elvecrog, EL; Lechner, MC; Nelson, MT. Nonpalpable breast lesions: correlation of stereotaxic large-core needle biopsy and surgical biopsy results. *Radiology*, 1993, Aug;188(2), 453-455. PMID: 8327696.

[97] Parker, SH; Lovin, JD; Jobe, WE; et al. Stereotactic breast biopsy with a biopsy gun. *Radiology*, 1990, Sep;176(3), 741-747. PMID: 2167501.

[98] Vag, T; Pfleiderer, SO; Bottcher, J; et al. Ultrasound-guided breast biopsy using a 10-gauge self-contained vacuum-assisted device. *Eur Radiol,* 2007, Dec;17(12), 3 100-3, 102. PMID: 17639409.

[99] Wu, YK; Huang, YM; Chou, AS; et al. Management of breast fibroadenomas by ultrasound-guided vacuum-assisted biopsy - Three years experience. *Tzu Chi Med J*, 2005, Dec, 17(6), 405-408, 52.

[100] Alonso-Bartolome, P; Vega-Bolivar, A; Torres-Tabanera, M; et al. Sonographically guided 11 -G directional vacuum-assisted breast biopsy as an alternative to surgical excision: utility and cost study in probably benign lesions. *Acta Radiol*, 2004, Jul;45(4), 390-396. PMID: 15323390.

[101] March, DE; Coughlin, BF; Barham, RB; et al. Breast masses: Removal of all US evidence during biopsy by using a handheld vacuum- assisted device— Initial experience. *Radiology*, 2003, May 1;227(2), 549-555. PMID: 12676972.

[102] Johnson, AT; Henry-Tillman, RS; Smith, LF; et al. Percutaneous excisional breast biopsy. *Am J Surg,* 2002, Dec;184(6), 550-554; discussion 554. PMID: 12488164.

[103] Perez-Fuentes, JA; Longobardi, IR; Acosta, VF; et al. Sonographically guided directional vacuum-assisted breast biopsy: preliminary experience in Venezuela. AJR *Am J Roentgenol*, 2001, Dec, 177(6), 1459-1463. PMID: 11717107.

[104] Tonegutti, M; Girardi, V. Stereotactic vacuum-assisted breast biopsy in 268 nonpalpable lesions. *Radiol Med,* 2008, Feb;113(1), 65-75. PMID: 18338128.

[105] Uematsu, T; Yuen, S; Kasami, M; et al. Dynamic contrast-enhanced MR imaging in screening detected microcalcification lesions of the breast: is there any value? Breast *Cancer Res Treat*, 2007, Jul;103(3), 269-281. PMID: 17063274.

[106] Chapellier, C; Balu-Maestro, C; Amoretti, N; et al. Vacuum-assisted breast biopsies: Experience at the Antoine Lacassagne Cancer Center (Nice, France). *Clin Imaging*, 2006, Mar, 30(2), 99-1 07. PMID: 16500540.

[107] Dhillon, MS; Bradley, SA; England, DW. Mammotome biopsy: Impact on preoperative diagnosis rate. *Clin Radiol*, 2006, Mar;61(3), 276-281. PMID: 16488210.

[108] Weber, WP; Zanetti, R; Langer, I; et al. Mammotome: Less invasive than ABBI with similar accuracy for early breast cancer detection. World J Surg 2005, Apr;29(4), 495-499. PMID: 15770379.

[109] Kubota, K; Gomi, N; Wakita, T; et al. Magnetic resonance imaging of the metal clip in a breast: safety and its availability as a negative marker. Breast Cancer 2004;11(1), 55-59. PMID: 14718794.

[110] Lomoschitz, FM; Helbich, TH; Rudas, M; et al. Stereotactic 11-gauge vacuum-assisted breast biopsy: influence of number of specimens on diagnostic accuracy. Radiology 2004, Sep;232(3), 897-903. PMID: 15273332.

[111] Ambrogetti, D; Bianchi, S; Ciatto, S. Accuracy of percutaneous core biopsy of isolated breast microcalcifications identified by mammography. Experience with a vacuum-assisted large-core biopsy device. *Radiol Med,* 2003, Oct; 1 06(4), 3 13-319. PMID: 14612823.

[112] Apesteguia, L; Mellado, M; Saenz, J; et al. Vacuum-assisted breast biopsy on digital stereotaxic table of nonpalpable lesions non- recognisable by ultrasonography. *Eur Radiol*, 2002, Mar;12(3), 638-645. PMID: 11870480.

[113] Georgian-Smith, D; D'Orsi, C; Morris, E; et al. Stereotactic biopsy of the breast using an upright unit, a vacuum-suction needle, and a lateral arm-support system. *AJR Am J Roentgenol,* 2002, Apr;178(4), 1017-1024. Available at: http://www.ajronline.org. PMID: 11906893.

[114] Liberman, L; Kaplan JB; Morris EA; et al. To excise or to sample the mammographic target: what is the goal of stereotactic 11- gauge vacuum-assisted breast biopsy. *AJR Am J Roentgenol,* 2002, Sep;179(3), 679-683. PMID: 12185043

[115] Meloni, GB; Becchere, MP; Soro, D; et al. Percutaneous vacuum-assisted core breast biopsy with upright stereotactic equipment. Indications, limitations and results. *Acta Radiol,* 2002, Nov, 43(6), 575-578. PMID: 12485254.

[116] Morris, EA; Liberman, L; Trevisan, SG; et al. Histologic heterogeneity of masses at percutaneous breast biopsy. *Breast J*, 2002, Jul-Aug, 8(4), 187-191. PMID: 12100109.

[117] Pfarl, G; Helbich, TH; Riedl, CC; et al. Stereotactic 11-gauge vacuum-assisted breast biopsy: a validation study. *AJR Am J Roentgenol,* 2002, Dec; 179(6), 1503-1507. PMID: 12438044.

[118] Cangiarella, J; Waisman, J; Symmans, WF; et al. Mammotome core biopsy for mammary microcalcification: analysis of 160 biopsies from 142 women with surgical and radiologic followup. *Cancer*, 2001, Jan 1, 91(1), 173-177. PMID: 11148574.

[119] Lai, JT; Burrowes, P; MacGregor, JH. Diagnostic accuracy of a stereotaxically guided vacuum-assisted large-core breast biopsy program in Canada. *Can Assoc Radiol J*, 2001, Aug;52(4), 223-227. PMID: 11512293.

[120] Beck, RM; Gotz, L; Heywang-Kobrunner, SH. Stereotaxic vacuum core breast biopsy—experience of 560 patients. *Swiss Surg*, 2000, 6(3), 108-110. PMID: 10894010.

[121] Heywang-Kobrunner, SH; Schaumloffel, U; Viehweg, P; et al. Minimally invasive stereotaxic vacuum core breast biopsy. *Eur Radiol*, 1998, 8(3), 377-385. PMID: 9510569.

[122] Sim, LS; Kei, PL. Upright stereotactic vacuum-assisted needle biopsy of suspicious breast microcalcifications. *J Med Imaging Radiat Oncol*, 2008, Aug, 52(4), 358-364. PMID: 18811759.

[123] Jackman, RJ; Marzoni, Jr FA; Rosenberg, J. False-negative diagnoses at stereotactic vacuum-assisted needle breast biopsy: longterm follow-up of 1,280 lesions and review of the literature. *AJR Am J Roentgenol,* 2009, Feb, 192(2), 341-351. PMID: 19155393.

[124] Pfleiderer, SOR; Reichenbach, JR; Azhari, T; et al. A manipulator system for 14-gauge large core breast biopsies inside a high-field whole-body MR scanner. *J Magn Reson Imaging*, 2003, Apr 1, 17(4), 493-498.

[125] Puglisi, F; Pertoldi, B; Ramello, M; et al. Diagnostic accuracy of perforated compression grid approach for mammographically guided core needle biopsy of breast lesions. *Cancer Lett*, 1999, Nov 15, 146(2), 181-188. PMID: 10656624.

[126] Ciatto, S; Houssami, N; Ambrogetti, D; et al. Accuracy and underestimation of malignancy of breast core needle biopsy: the Florence experience of over 4000 consecutive biopsies. *Breast Cancer Res Treat*, 2007, Mar; 101(3), 291 -297. PMID: 16823506.

[127] Cipolla, C; Fricano, S; Vieni, S; et al. Validity of needle core biopsy in the histological characterisation of mammary lesions. *Breast*, 2006, Feb; 15(1), 76-80. PMID: 16473738.

[128] Dillon, MF; Hill, AD; Quinn, CM; et al. The accuracy of ultrasound, stereotactic, and clinical core biopsies in the diagnosis of breast cancer, with an analysis of false-negative cases. *Ann Surg*, 2005, Nov, 242(5), 701-707. PMID: 16244544.

[129] Fajardo, LL; Pisano, ED; Caudry, DJ; et al. Radiologist Investigators of the Radiologic Diagnostic Oncology Group V. Stereotactic and sonographic large-core biopsy of nonpalpable breast lesions: results of the Radiologic Diagnostic Oncology Group V study. *Acad Radiol*, 2004, Mar; 11(3), 293- 308. PMID: 15035520.

[130] Abdsaleh, S; Azavedo, E; Lindgren, PG. Semiautomatic core biopsy. A modified biopsy technique in breast diseases. *Acta Radiol*, 2003, Jan, 44(1), 47-5 1. PMID: 12630998.

[131] Kirshenbaum, KJ; Voruganti, T; Overbeeke, C; et al. Stereotactic core needle biopsy of nonpalpable breast lesions using a conventional mammography unit with an add-on device. *AJR Am J Roentgenol,* 2003, Aug;181(2), 527-331. PMID: 12876040.

[132] Jackman, RJ; Lamm, RL. Stereotactic histologic biopsy in breasts with implants. *Radiology*, 2002, Jan, 222(1), 157-164. PMID, 11756720.

[133] Margolin, FR; Leung, JW; Jacobs, RP; et al. Percutaneous imaging-guided core breast biopsy: 5 years' experience in a community hospital. *AJR Am J Roentgenol,* 2001, Sep;177(3), 559-564. PMID: 11517047.

[134] White, RR; Halperin, TJ; Olson, Jr JA; et al. Impact of core-needle breast biopsy on the surgical management of mammographic abnormalities. *Ann Surg*, 2001, Jun, 233(6), 769-777. PMID: 11371735.

[135] Latosinsky, S; Cornell, D; Bear, HD; et al. Evaluation of stereotactic core needle biopsy (SCNB) of the breast at a single institution. *Breast Cancer Res Treat*, 2000, Apr;60(3), 277-283. PMID: 10930116.

[136] Liberman, L; Ernberg, LA; Heerdt, A; et al. Palpable breast masses: is there a role for percutaneous imaging-guided core biopsy. *AJR Am J Roentgenol,* 2000, Sep; 175(3), 779-787. PMID: 10954467.

[137] Makoske, T; Preletz, R; Riley, L; et al. Longterm outcomes of stereotactic breast biopsies. *Am Surg*, 2000, 66(12), 1104-1109.

[138] Welle, GJ; Clark, M; Loos, S; et al. Stereotactic breast biopsy: recumbent biopsy using add-on upright equipment. *AJR Am J Roentgenol,* 2000, Jul; 175(1), 59-63. PMID: 10882246.

[139] Meyer, JE; Smith, DN; Lester, SC; et al. Large-core needle biopsy of nonpalpable breast lesions. *JAMA*, 1999, May, 5, 281(17), 1638-1641. PMID: 10235159.

[140] Caruso, ML; Gabrieli, G; Marzullo, G; et al. Core Biopsy as Alternative to Fine-Needle Aspiration Biopsy in Diagnosis of Breast Tumors. *Oncologist*, 1998, 3(1), 45-49. PMID: 10388083.

[141] Fuhrman, GM; Cederbom, GJ; Bolton, JS; et al. Image-guided core-needle breast biopsy is an accurate technique to evaluate patients with nonpalpable imaging abnormalities. *Ann Surg*, 1998, Jun, 227(6), 932-939. PMID: 9637557.

[142] Ioffe, OB; Berg, WA; Silverberg, SG; et al. Mammographic-histopathologic correlation of large-core needle biopsies of the breast. *Mod Pathol*, 1998, Aug; 11(8), 72 1-727. PMID: 9720499.

[143] Britton, PD; Flower, CD; Freeman, AH; et al. Changing to core biopsy in an NHS breast screening unit. *Clin Radiol*, 1997, Oct, 52(10), 764-767. PMID: 9366536.

[144] Helbich, TH; Mayr, W; Schick, S; et al. Coaxial technique: approach to breast core biopsies. Radiology 1997 Jun;203(3), 684-690. PMID: 9169689.

[145] Stolier, AJ. Stereotactic breast biopsy: A surgical series. J Am Coll Surg 1997;185(3), 224-228. PMID: 9291397.

[146] Nguyen, M; McCombs, MM; Ghandehari, S; et al. An update on core needle biopsy for radiologically detected breast lesions. *Cancer*, 1996, Dec 1, 78(11), 2340-2345. PMID: 8941004.

[147] Doyle, AJ; Murray, KA; Nelson, EW; et al. Selective use of image-guided large-core needle biopsy of the breast: accuracy and cost-effectiveness. *AJR Am J Roentgenol,* 1995, Aug; 165(2), 281-284. PMID: 7618540.

[148] Burbank, F; Kaye, K; Belville, J; et al. Image- guided automated core biopsies of the breast, chest, abdomen, and pelvis. *Radiology*, 1994, Apr; 191(1), 165-171. PMID: 8134564.

[149] Parker, SH; Burbank, F; Jackman, RJ; et al. Percutaneous large-core breast biopsy: a multi-institutional study. *Radiology*, 1994, Nov;193(2), 359-364. PMID: 7972743.

[150] Helbich, TH; Rudas, M; Bohm, G; et al. Randomized in vitro and in vivo evaluation of different biopsy needles and devices for breast biopsy. *Clin Radiol*, 1999, 54(1), 56-62. PMID: 9915512.

[151] Hamed, H; De Freitas, Jr R; Rasbridge, S; et al. A prospective randomized study of two gauges of biopty-cut needle in diagnosis of early breast cancer. *Breast*, 1995, 4(2), 135-136.

[152] Vitug, AF; Newman, LA. Complications in breast surgery. *Surg Clin North Am*, 2007, Apr, 87(2), 431-451. PMID: 17498536.

[153] Rissanen, TJ; Makarainen, HP; Mattila, SI; et al. Wire localized biopsy of breast lesions: a review of 425 cases found in screening or clinical mammography. *Clin Radiol*, 1993, Jan, 47(1), 14-22. PMID: 8428412.

[154] Diaz, LK; Wiley, EL; Venta, LA. Are malignant cells displaced by large-gauge needle core biopsy of the breast. *AJR Am J Roentgenol,* 1999, Nov, 173(5), 1303-1313. PMID: 10541110.

[155] Chao, C; Torosian, MH; Boraas, MC; et al. Local recurrence of breast cancer in the stereotactic core needle biopsy site: case reports and review of the literature. Breast J 2001, Mar-Apr, 7(2), 124-127. PMID: 11328321.

[156] Youngson, BJ; Cranor, M; Rosen, PP. Epithelial displacement in surgical breast specimens following needling procedures. *Am J Surg Pathol*, 1994, Sep, 18(9), 896-903. PMID: 8067510.

[157] Harter, LP; Curtis, JS; Ponto, G; et al. Malignant seeding of the needle track during stereotaxic core needle breast biopsy. *Radiology*, 1992, Dec, 185(3), 713-714. PMID: 1343569.

[158] Michalopoulos, NV; Zagouri, F; Sergentanis, TN;et al. Needle tract seeding after vacuum- assisted breast biopsy. *Acta Radiol*, 2008, Apr;49(3), 267-270. PMID: 18365811.

[159] Uematsu, T; Kasami, M. Risk of needle tract seeding of breast cancer: cytological results derived from core wash material. *Breast Cancer Res Treat*, 2008, Jul, 110(1), 51-55. PMID: 17674195.

[160] Hoorntje, LE; Schipper, MEI; Kaya, A; et al. Tumour cell displacement after 14G breast biopsy. *Eur J Surg Oncol*, 2004, Jun, 30(5), 520-525.

[161] Stolier, A; Skinner, J; Levine, EA. A prospective study of seeding of the skin after core biopsy of the breast. *Am J Surg*, 2000, Aug;180(2), 104-107. PMID: 11044522.

[162] Liberman, L; Vuolo, M; Dershaw, DD; et al. Epithelial displacement after stereotactic 11- gauge directional vacuum-assisted breast biopsy. *AJR Am J Roentgenol,* 1999, Mar; 1 72(3), 677-68 1. PMID: 10063859.

[163] Youngson, BJ; Liberman, L; Rosen, PP. Displacement of carcinomatous epithelium in surgical breast specimens following stereotaxic core biopsy. *Am J Clin Pathol,* 1995, May, 103(5), 598-602. PMID: 7741106.

[164] Uriburu, JL; Vuoto, HD; Cogorno, L; et al. Local recurrence of breast cancer after skin-sparing mastectomy following core needle biopsy: Case reports and review of the literature. *Breast J*, 2006, May, 12(3), 194-198. PMID: 16684314.

[165] Fitzal, F; Sporn, EP; Draxler, W; et al. Preoperative core needle biopsy does not increase local recurrence rate in breast cancer patients. *Breast Cancer Res Treat*, 2006, May;97(1), 9-15. PMID: 16502019.

[166] Chen, AM; Haffty, BG; Lee, CH. Local recurrence of breast cancer after breast conservation therapy in patients examined by means of stereotactic core-needle biopsy. *Radiology*, 2002, Dec, 225(3), 707-7 12. PMID: 12461249.

[167] Knight, R; Horiuchi, K; Parker, SH; et al. Risk of needle-track seeding after diagnostic image-guided core needle biopsy in breast cancer. *J Soc Laparoendosc Surg*, 2002, Jul-Sep;6(3), 207-209. PMID: 12166757.

[168] King, TA; Hayes, DH; Cederbom, GJ; et al. Biopsy technique has no impact on local recurrence after breast-conserving therapy. *Breast J*, 2001, Jan-Feb, 7(1), 19-24. PMID: 11348411.

[169] Newman, EL; Kahn, A; Diehl, KM; et al. Does the method of biopsy affect the incidence of sentinel lymph node metastases? *Breast J*, 2006, Jan, 12(1), 53-57. PMID: 16409587.

[170] Hansen, NM; Ye, X; Grube, BJ; et al. Manipulation of the primary breast tumor and the incidence of sentinel node metastases from invasive breast cancer. *Arch Surg*, 2004, Jun;139(6), 634-640.

[171] Peters-Engl, C; Konstantiniuk, P; Tausch, C; et al. The impact of preoperative breast biopsy on the risk of sentinel lymph node metastases: Analysis of 2502 cases from the Austrian sentinel node biopsy study group. *Br J Cancer*, 2004, Nov 15, 91(10), 1782-1786.

[172] Bleiweiss, IJ; Nagi, CS; Jaffer, S. Axillary sentinel lymph nodes can be falsely positive due to iatrogenic displacement and transport of benign epithelial cells in patients with breast carcinoma. *J Clin Oncol*, 2006, May 1, 24(13), 2013-2018.

[173] Hatmaker, AR; Donahue, RM; Tarpley, JL; et al. Cost-effective use of breast biopsy techniques in a Veterans health care system. *Am J Surg*, 2006, Nov, 192(5), e37-e41. PMID: 17071179.

[174] Soo, MS; Kliewer, MA; Ghate, S; et al. Stereotactic breast biopsy of noncalcified lesions: A cost-minimization analysis comparing 14-gauge multipass automated core biopsy to 14- and 11-gauge vacuum- assisted biopsy. *Clin Imaging*, 2005, Jan, 29(1), 26-33.

[175] Golub, RM; Bennett, CL; Stinson, T; et al. Cost minimization study of image-guided core biopsy versus surgical excisional biopsy for women with abnormal mammograms. *J Clin Oncol,* 2004, 22(12), 2430-2437.

[176] Launders, JH. (ECRI Institute, Plymouth Meeting, PA). CER Breast Biopsy Project. August 12, 2008.

[177] Liberman, L; Latrenta, LR; Dershaw, DD; et al. Impact of core biopsy on the surgical management of impalpable breast cancer. *AJR Am J Roentgenol,* 1997, 168(2), 495-499.

[178] Duchesne, N; Parker, SH; Lechner, MC; et al. Multicenter evaluation of a new ultrasound- guided biopsy device: Improved ergonomics, sampling and rebiopsy rates. *Breast J*, 2007, Jan-Feb, 13(1), 36-43. PMID: 17214791.

[179] Hui, JY; Chan, LK; Chan, RL; et al. Prone table stereotactic breast biopsy. *Hong Kong Med J*, 2002, Dec;8(6), 447-451. PMID: 12459602.

[180] Geller, BM; Oppenheimer, RG; Mickey, RM; et al. Patient perceptions of breast biopsy procedures for screen-detected lesions. *Am J Obstet Gynecol,* 2004, Apr; 190(4), 1063-1069. PMID: 15118643.

[181] Chun, K; Velanovich, V. Patient-perceived cosmesis and satisfaction after breast biopsy: Comparison of stereotactic incisional, excisional, and wire-localized biopsy techniques. *Surgery*, 2002, 131(5), 497-501. PMID: 12019401.

[182] Collins, LC; Connolly, JL; Page, DL; et al. Diagnostic agreement in the evaluation of image-guided breast core needle biopsies: results from a randomized clinical trial. *Am J Surg Pathol*, 2004, Jan, 28(1), 126-131. PMID: 14707874.

[183] Gukas, ID; Nwana, EJ; Ihezue, CH; et al. Trucut biopsy of palpable breast lesions: a practical option for pre-operative diagnosis in developing countries. *Cent Afr J Med,* 2000, May;46(5), 127-130. PMID: 11210334

[184] Deurloo, EE; Gilhuijs, KGA; Schultze Kool, LJ; et al. Displacement of breast tissue and needle deviations during stereotactic procedures. *Invest Radiol*, 2001, 36(6), 347-353.

[185] Verkooijen, HM; Borel Rinkes, IH; Peeters, PH; et al. Impact of stereotactic large-core needle biopsy on diagnosis and surgical treatment of non-palpable breast cancer. *Eur J Surg Oncol,* 2001, 27(3), 244-249.

[186] Williams, AB; Roberts, JV; Michell, MJ; et al. Prone stereotactic breast core biopsy: The impact on surgical management of nonpalpable breast cancers. *Breast*, 1999, Feb, 8(1), 12-15.

[187] Mainiero, MB; Gareen, IF; Bird, CE; et al. Preferential use of sonographically guided biopsy to minimize patient discomfort and procedure time in a percutaneous image-guided breast biopsy program. *J Ultrasound Med,* 2002, Nov;21(1 1), 1221-1226. PMID: 12418763.

[188] Wunderbaldinger, P; Wolf, G; Turetschek, K; et al. Comparison of sitting versus prone position for stereotactic large-core breast biopsy in surgically proven lesions. *AJR Am J Roentgenol,* 2002, 178(5), 1221-1225. PMID: 11959735.

[189] Chen, SC; Yang, HR; Hwang, TL; et al. Intraoperative ultrasonographically guided excisional biopsy or vacuum-assisted core needle biopsy for nonpalpable breast lesions. *Ann Surg*, 2003, Nov, 238(5), 738-742. PMID: 14578737.

[190] Orel, SG; Rosen, M; Mies, C; et al. MR imaging-guided 9-gauge vacuum-assisted core-neddle breast biopsy: Initial experience. *Radiology*, 2006, Jan, 238(1), 54-61. PMID: 16304093.

[191] Shin, S; Schneider, HB; Cole, Jr FJ; et al. Follow-up recommendations for benign breast biopsies. *Breast J*, 2006, Sep; 12(5), 41 3-417.

[192] Fine, RE; Whitworth, PW; Kim, JA; et al. Low-risk palpable breast masses removed using a vacuum-assisted hand-held device. *Am J Surg*, 2003, Oct, 186(4), 362-367. PMID: 14553851.

[193] Krainick-Strobel, U; Huber, B; Majer, I; et al. Complete extirpation of benign breast lesions with an ultrasound-guided vacuum biopsy system. *Ultrasound Obstet Gynecol*, 2007, Mar;29(3), 342-346.

[194] Wong, TT; Cheung, PS; Ma, MK; et al. Experience of stereotactic breast biopsy using the vacuum-assisted core needle biopsy device and the advanced breast biopsy instrumentation system in Hong Kong women. *Asian J Surg*, 2005, Jan, 28(1), 18-23.

[195] Kettritz, U; Rotter, K; Schreer, I; et al. Stereotactic vacuum-assisted breast biopsy in 2874 patients: a nmlticenter study. *Cancer*, 2004, Jan, 15, 100(2), 245-251. PMID: 14716757.

[196] Mariotti, C; Feliciotti, F; Baldarelli, M; et al. Digital stereotactic biopsies for nonpalpable breast lesion. *Surg Endosc*, 2003, Jun, 17(6), 911-917. PMID: 12632135.

[197] Schneider, E; Rohling, KW; Schnall, MD; et al. An apparatus for MR-guided breast lesion localization and core biopsy: Design and preliminary results. *J Magn Reson Imaging,* 2001, 14(3), 243-253.

[198] Holloway, CMB; Saskin R; Brackstone M; et al. Variation in the use of percutaneous biopsy for diagnosis of breast abnormalities in Ontario. *Ann Surg Oncol*, 2007, Oct; 14(10), 2932-2939.

[199] Hoffmann, J. Analysis of surgical and diagnostic quality at a specialist breast unit. *Breast*, 2006, Aug; 15(4), 490-497.

[200] Lehman, CD; DePeri, ER; Peacock, S; et al. Clinical experience with MRI-guided vacuum-assisted breast biopsy. *AJR Am J Roentgenol,* 2005, Jun; 184(6), 1782-1787. PMID: 15908530.

[201] Liberman, L; Holland, AE; Marjan, D; et al. Underestimation of atypical ductal hyperplasia at MRI-guided 9-gauge vacuum- assisted breast biopsy. *AJR Am J Roentgenol,* 2007, Mar; 188(3), 684-690. PMID: 17312054.

[202] Popiela, TJ; Tabor, J; Nowak, W;et al. Detectability of pre-clinical breast pathologies in own experience. *Pol Przegl Chir*, 2002, 74(1), 36-43.

[203] Liberman, L; Morris, EA; Dershaw, DD; et al. Fast MRI-guided vacuum-assisted breast biopsy: initial experience. *AJR Am J Roentgenol,* 2003, Nov, 1 81(5), 1283-1293. PMID: 14573421.

[204] Perlet, C; Heywang-Kobrunner SH; Heinig, A; et al. Magnetic resonance-guided, vacuum-assisted breast biopsy: Results from a European multicenter study of 538 lesions. *Cancer*, 2006, Mar 1, 106(5), 982-990. PMID: 16456807.

[205] Diebold, T; Hahn, T; Solbach, C; et al. Evaluation of the stereotactic 8G vacuum-assisted breast biopsy in the histologic evaluation of suspicious mammography findings (BI-RADS IV). *Invest Radiol*, 2005, Jul, 40(7), 465-47 1. PMID: 15973139.

[206] Bloomston, M; D'Angelo, P; Galliano, D; et al. One hundred consecutive advanced breast biopsy instrumentation procedures: complications, costs, and outcome. *Ann Surg Oncol*, 1999, Mar, 6(2), 195-199. PMID: 10082046.

[207] Rotenberg, L; Verhille, R; Schulz-Wendtland, R; et al. Multicenter clinical experience with large core soft tissue biopsy without vacuum assistance. *Eur J Cancer Prev,* 2004, Dec;13(6), 491-498. PMID: 15548942.

[208] Janes, RH; Bouton, MS. Initial 300 consecutive stereotactic core-needle breast biopsies by a surgical group. *Am J Surg,* 1994 Dec; 1 68(6), 533-536; discussion 536-537. PMID: 7977991.

[209] Uematsu, T; Kasami, M; Uchida, Y, et al. Ultrasonographically guided 18-gauge automated core needle breast biopsy with post-fire needle position verification (PNPV). *Breast Cancer*, 2007, 14(2), 2 19-228. PMID: 17485909.

[210] Viehweg, P; Bernerth, T; Kiechle, M; et al. MR-guided intervention in women with a family history of breast cancer. *Eur J Radiol*, 2006, Jan, 57(1), 81-89. PMID: 16364583

[211] Florentine, BD; Cobb, CJ; Frankel, K; et al. Core needle biopsy: A useful adjunct to fine-needle aspiration in select patients with palpable breast lesions. *Cancer*, 1997, Feb 25, 81 (1), 33-39.

[212] Howisey, RL; Acheson, MB; Rowbotham, RK; et al. A comparison of Medicare reimbursement and results for various imaging- guided breast biopsy techniques. *Am J Surg,* 1997 May;173(5), 395-398. PMID: 9168074.

[213] Burbank, F. Stereotactic breast biopsy of atypical ductal hyperplasia and ductal carcinoma in situ lesions: Improved accuracy with directional; vacuum- assisted biopsy. *Radiology*, 1997, Mar, 202(3), 843- 847.

[214] Yim, JH; Barton, P; Weber, B; et al. Mammographically detected breast cancer. Benefits of stereotactic core versus wire localization biopsy. *Ann Surg*, 1996, Jun, 223(6), 688-697; discussion 697-670. PMID: 8645042.

[215] Strong, JW; Worsham, GF; Austin, RM; et al. Stereotactic core biopsy of nonpalpable breast lesions. *J S C Med Assoc*, 1995, Dec;91(12), 489-496. PMID: 8587312.

[216] Morrow, M; Venta, L; Stinson, T; et al. Prospective comparison of stereotactic core biopsy and surgical excision as diagnostic procedures for breast cancer patients. *Ann Surg*, 2001, Apr;233(4), 537-541. PMID: 11303136.

[217] Liberman, L; Gougoutas, CA; Zakowski MF; et al. Calcifications highly suggestive of malignancy: comparison of breast biopsy methods. *AJR Am J Roentgenol,* 2001, Jul;177(1), 165-172. PMID: 11418420.

[218] Altomare, V; Guerriero, G; Giacomelli, L; et al. Management of nonpalpable breast lesions in a modern functional breast unit. *Breast Cancer Res Treat*, 2005, Sep, 93(1), 85- 89. PMID: 16184463.

[219] Carmon, M; Rivkin, L; Abu-Dalo, R; et al. Increased mammographic screening and use of percutaneous image-guided core biopsy in non-palpable breast cancer: Impact on surgical treatment. *Isr Med Assoc J*, 2004, Jun, 6(6), 326-328. PMID: 15214456.

[220] Lind, DS; Minter, R; Steinbach, B; et al. Stereotactic core biopsy reduces the reexcision rate and the cost of mammographically detected cancer. *J Surg Res*, 1998, Jul, 15, 78(1), 23-26.

[221] Smith, DN; Christian, R; Meyer, JE. Large- core needle biopsy of nonpalpable breast cancers. The impact on subsequent surgical excisions. *Arch Surg*, 1997, Mar, 132(3), 256- 259; discussion 260. PMID: 9125023.

[222] Elliott, RL; Haynes, AE; Bolin, JA; et al. Stereotaxic needle localization and biopsy of occult breast lesions: first year's experience. *Am Surg*, 1992, Feb, 58(2), 126-131. PMID: 1550304.

[223] Liberman, L; Dershaw, DD; Rosen, PP; et al. Stereotaxic core biopsy of impalpable spiculated breast masses. *AJR Am J Roentgenol,* 1995, 165(3), 551-554.

[224] Pijnappel, RM; Peeters, PH; van den Donk, M; et al. Diagnostic strategies in non-palpable breast lesions. *Eur J Cancer*, 2002, Mar, 38(4), 550-555. PMID: 11872348.

[225] Al-Sobhi, SS; Helvie, MA; Pass, HA; et al. Extent of lumpectomy for breast cancer after diagnosis by stereotactic core versus wire localization biopsy. *Ann Surg Oncol,* 1999, Jun, 6(4), 330-335.

[226] Johnson, JM; Dalton, RR; Landercasper, J; et al. Image-guided or needle-localized open biopsy of mammographic malignant- appearing microcalcifications? *J Am Coll Surg,* 1998, 1 87(6), 604-609. PMID: 9849733.

[227] Kaufman, CS; Delbecq, R; Jacobson, L. Excising the reexcision: stereotactic core-needle biopsy decreases need for reexcision of breast cancer. *World J Surg,* 1998, Oct;22(10), 1023-1027. PMID: 9747160.

[228] Fenoglio, ME; Gallagher, JQ; Joy, N; et al. Stereotactic core breast biopsy versus needle localization breast biopsy—The effect of initial diagnostic modality on surgical therapy in patients with breast cancer. Minim Invasive *Ther Allied Technol*, 1997, Jun, 6(3), 225-227.

[229] Whitten, TM; Wallace, TW; Bird, RE; et al. Image-guided core biopsy has advantages over needle localization biopsy for the diagnosis of nonpalpable breast cancer. *Am Surg,* 1997 Dec;63(12), 1072-1077; discussion 1077-1078. PMID: 9393255.

[230] Friese, CR; Neville, BA; Edge, SB; et al. Breast biopsy patterns and outcomes in Surveillance, Epidemiology, and End Results-Medicare data. *Cancer*, 2009, Feb 15, 115(4), 716-724. PMID: 19152430.

[231] Handy, RB; Fajardo, LL; Innis, CA; et al. Patient perceptions of stereotaxic large-core breast biopsy. *Acad Radiol*, 1996, Dec, 3(12), 1007-1011. PMID: 9017015.

[232] Helbich, TH, Rudas, M; Haitel, A; et al. Evaluation of needle size for breast biopsy: Comparison of 14-, 16-, and 18-gauge biopsy needles. *AJR Am J Roentgenol,* 1998, Jul;171(1), 59-63. PMID: 9648764.

[233] Killebrew, LK; Oneson, RH. Comparison of the diagnostic accuracy of a vacuum-assisted percutaneous intact specimen sampling device to a vacuum-assisted core needle sampling device for breast biopsy: Initial experience. *Breast J*, 2006, Jul;12(4), 302-308. PMID: 16848839.

[234] Verkooijen, HM; Peeters, PH; Buskens, E; et al. Diagnostic accuracy of large-core needle biopsy for nonpalpable breast disease: a meta-analysis. *Br J Cancer*, 2000, Mar;82(5), 1017-1021. PMID: 10737383.

[235] Fahrbach, K; Sledge, I; Cella, C; et al. A comparison of the accuracy of two minimally invasive breast biopsy methods: a systematic literature review and meta- analysis. *Arch Gynecol Obstet*, 2006, May, 274(2), 63-73. PMID: 16598478.

[236] Shea, BJ; Grimshaw, JM; Wells, GA; et al. Development of AMSTAR: a measurement tool to assess the methodological quality of systematic reviews. *BMC Med Res Methodol*, 2007, 7, 10. PMID: 17302989.

[237] Troxel, DB. Medicolegal aspects of error in pathology. *Arch Pathol Lab Med*, 2006, May, 130(5), 617-619. PMID: 16683874.

List of Acronyms/Abbreviations

ADH	Atypical Ductal Hyperplasia
AHRQ	Agency for Healthcare Research and Quality
ALH	Atypical Lobular Hyperplasia
BI-RADS®	Breast Imaging Reporting and Data System
CI	Confidence Interval
DCIS	Ductal Carcinoma In Situ
FN	False Negative
FP	False Positive
G	Gauge
LCIS	Lobular Carcinoma In Situ
MRI	Magnetic Resonance Imaging
NA	Not Applicable
NR	Not Reported
TN	True Negative
TP	True Positive

UK	United Kingdom
US	Ultrasound
USA	United States of America

Glossary of Selected Terms

Atypical ductal hyperplasia (ADH). A condition in which the cells that line the milk ducts of the breast experience abnormal growth. The lesion itself is not malignant but may sometimes contain foci of malignant cells and women with ADH have an elevated risk of developing a malignant lesion.

Automated biopsy gun. A device used to obtain core-needle samples. The device is pressed against the tissue at the appropriate location and angle and then the needle is "fired" into the tissue. After confirming the core-needle has sampled the appropriate tissue the needle is withdrawn and the tissue sample ejected from the needle into a sampling container. Some units use a coaxial needle. With a coaxial needle, a cannula (hollow tube) is advanced into the tissue until in contact with the area to be sampled, and then the sampling needle is "fired" through the cannula and into the lesion.

Ductal carcinoma in situ (DCIS). A carcinoma of the milk ducts of the breast that is confined within the duct.

High-risk lesion. Any of a number of different types of non-cancerous lesions of the breast that have been observed to sometimes contain foci of malignant cells, and women diagnosed with these types of lesions have an elevated risk of developing a malignant lesion. Some common types of high-risk lesions include atypical ductal hyperplasia (ADH), radial scars, papillary lesions, atypical lobular hyperplasia (ALH), and lobular carcinoma in situ (LCIS).

Microcalcification. A tiny deposit of calcium visible as a bright spot on a mammogram. Tight clusters of microcalcifications may be a sign of a malignant lesion.

Negative likelihood ratio. A measure of the ability of the diagnostic test to accurately "rule out" disease. The smaller the negative likelihood ratio is, the more accurate the test is.

Palpable lesion. A breast lesion that can be felt by manual manipulation.

Sensitivity. Sensitivity is the proportion of people with the disease who have a positive test for the disease. A test with high sensitivity will rarely misclassify people with the disease as not having the disease (the test has a low rate of false-negatives).

Stereotactic guidance. X-rays are taken from multiple locations in order to accurately identify the exact location of the lesion to be sampled. After using the images to determine where to sample, the needle is inserted. Further x-ray images are usually taken to confirm the needle has penetrated the lesion.

Ultrasound guidance. High-frequency sound waves are used to visualize the exact location of the lesion to be sampled. After using the images to determine where to sample, the needle is inserted. Images can be taken continuously during needle insertion to guide and confirm the needle has penetrated the lesion.

Vacuum-assisted. After insertion of a hollow biopsy needle a vacuum can be applied to pull tissue into the needle.

Underestimation rate. The percentage of lesions that were diagnosed on core-needle biopsy as lesion types of lesser concern than the final diagnosis. For example, a lesion diagnosed as ADH on core-needle biopsy that is diagnosed as malignant on open biopsy was "underestimated" by the core-needle biopsy.

End Notes

[a] Formula:((raw score +14)/28)*10

In: Effectiveness of Core-Needle and Open Surgical Biopsy... ISBN: 978-1-61209-799-2
Editor: Leslie D. Schmidt

Chapter 2

Comparative Effectiveness of Core-Needle and Open Surgical Biopsy for the Diagnosis of Breast Lesions Appendix

Agency for Healthcare Research and Quality

Appendix A. Technical Experts and Peer Reviewers

Table A1. Technical Expert Panel.

Name	Title	Specialty	Organization
Wendie Berg, MD, PhD	American Radiology Services Johns Hopkins at Greenspring Lutherville, Maryland	Radiology	American College of Radiology representative
R. James Brenner, MD, JD, FACR, FCLM	Professor, Clinical Radiology and Chief, Breast Imaging, UCSF	Radiology	UCSF
Patty Carney, PhD	Professor of Family Medicine, and Associate Director for Population Studies at the OHSU Cancer Institute	Family Medicine	OHSU
Joanne Elmore, MD, MPH	Section Head, Division of General Internal Medicine Professor of Medicine Adjunct Associate Professor of Epidemiology Associate Director UW Robert Wood Johnson Clinical Scholars Program	Internal Medicine/ Epidemiology	University of Washington
Richard E. Fine, MD, FACS	Director Advanced Breast Care of Georgia	Surgery	Surgeon-Oncology

Table A1. (Continued).

Name	Title	Specialty	Organization
Carol Lee, MD	Yale University School of Medicine Chair of the American College of Radiology Breast Commission	Radiology	Yale University School of Medicine
Bev Parker, PhD	Research Analyst	Consumer	Y-ME National Breast Cancer Organiation
Elizabeth Steiner, MD	Assistant Professor of Family Medicine	Family Medicine	OHSU
Maria Wetzel, BS	Clinical Laboratory Scientist	Consumer	National Breast Cancer Coalition
Pamela Wilcox	Assistant Exec. Dir. of ACR	Radiology	American College of Radiology representative
Bonnie Yankaskas, PhD, MPH	Professor of Radiology, Adjunct Professor of Epidemiology, Principal Investigator for the Carolina Mammography Registry (CMR)	Radiology	University of North Carolina

Appendix B. Methods of Identifying the Literature

Electronic Database Searches

The following databases have been searched for relevant information:

Name	Date Limits	Platform/Provider
CINAHL (Cumulative Index to Nursing and Allied Health Literature)	1990 through October 30, 2008	OVID
The Cochrane Central Register of Controlled Trials (CENTRAL)	Through 2008, Issue 2	www.thecochranelibrary.com
The Cochrane Database of Methodology Reviews (Methodology Reviews)	Through 2008, Issue 2	www.thecochranelibrary.com
The Cochrane Database of Systematic Reviews (Cochrane Reviews)	Through 2008, Issue 2	www.thecochranelibrary.com
Database of Abstracts of Reviews of Effects (DARE)	Through 2008, Issue 2	www.thecochranelibrary.com
ECRI Institute Library Catalog	Through May 2008	ECRI Institute
EMBASE (Excerpta Medica)	1990 through September 11, 2009	OVID
Health Technology Assessment Database (HTA)	Through 2008, Issue 2	www.thecochranelibrary.com
Healthcare Standards	1990 through May 2008	ECRI
International Health Technology Assessment (IHTA)	Through May 2008	ECRI
MEDLINE	1990 through September 11, 2009	OVID
PreMEDLINE	Searched October 30, 2008	OVID
U.K. National Health Service Economic Evaluation Database (NHS EED)	Through 2008, Issue 2	www.thecochranelibrary.com
U.S. National Guideline ClearinghouseTM (NGC)	Searched May 2008	www.ngc.gov

Hand Searches of Journal and Nonjournal Literature

Journals and supplements maintained in ECRI Institute's collections were routinely reviewed. Nonjournal publications and conference proceedings from professional organizations, private agencies, and government agencies were also screened. Other mechanisms used to retrieve additional relevant information included review of bibliographies/reference lists from peer-reviewed and gray literature.

Search Strategies

The search strategies employed combinations of freetext keywords as well as controlled vocabulary terms including (but not limited to) the following concepts. The strategy below is presented in OVID syntax; the search was simultaneously conducted across EMBASE, MEDLINE, and PsycINFO. A parallel strategy was used to search the databases comprising the Cochrane Library.

Medical Subject Headings (MeSH), EMTREE, PsycINFO and Keywords

Conventions

OVID

$	=	truncation character (wildcard)
exp	=	"explodes" controlled vocabulary term (e.g., expands search to all more specific related terms in the vocabulary's hierarchy)
de.	=	limit controlled vocabulary heading
fs.	=	floating subheading
hw.	=	limit to heading word
md.	=	type of methodology (PsycINFO)
mp.	=	combined search fields (default if no fields are specified)
pt.	=	publication type
ti.	=	limit to title
tw.	=	limit to title and abstract fields

PubMed

[mh]	=	MeSH heading
[majr]	=	MeSH heading designated as major topic
[pt]	=	Publication Type
[sb]	=	Subset of PubMed database (PreMEDLINE, Systematic, OldMEDLINE)
[sh]	=	MeSH subheading (qualifiers used in conjunction with MeSH headings)
[tiab]	=	keyword in title or abstract
[tw]	=	Text word

Topic-Specific Search Terms.

Concept	Controlled Vocabulary	Keywords
Adverse events	Ae.fs. Co.fs. Cross infection Drainage Surgical wound infection	
Breast and breast diseases	Breast Breast cancer/di exp Breast disease/di exp Breast diseases/di Breast neoplasms/di	Breast$ Calcification$ Calcinosis Cancer Carcinoma$ Lesion$ Lump$ Mammar$ Papilloma Tum?or$
Breast biopsy	Biopsy Biopsy needle Breast biopsy Directional vaccum assisted biopsy Needle biopsy Percutaneous biopsy Stereotactic breast biopsy Tumor biopsy	Large core Mammatome Mammotome Needle Vacuum
Open biopsy	Breast/su Breast tumor/su Su.fs.	Excision$ Incision$ Open Surgical
Patient Satisfaction/QOL	Pain assessment Pain measurement Patient satisfaction Quality of life Visual analog scale	Preference$ QOL Satisf$
Seeding		seeding

CINAHL/Embase/Medline

English Language, Human.

Set N	Concept	Search statement
1	Breast biopsy	(breast biopsy or stereotactic breast biopsy or directional vacuum assisted biopsy).de.
2	Breast	Breast
3	Breast diseases	Exp breast cancer/di or exp breast neoplasms/di or exp breast disease/di or exp breast diseases/di
4		(breast or mammar$) and (Papilloma or calcification$ or calcinosis

Set N	Concept	Search statement
		or tum?or$ or lesion$ or cancer or carcinoma$ or lump$)
5	Combine sets	or/2-4
6	Biopsy	5 and ((Biopsy or tumor biopsy).de. or biops$)
7	Large core needle biopsy	6 and ((needle biopsy or biopsy needle or percutaneous biopsy).de. or (large core or needle or mammotome or mammatome or vacuum))
8	Open biopsy	6 and (breast/su or breast tumor/su)
9		6 and (su.fs. or open or excision$ or incision$ or surgical)
10	Combine sets	8 or 9
11	Combine sets	or/1,7,10
12	Limit by publication type	11 not ((letter or editorial or news or comment or case reports or note or conference paper).de. or (letter or editorial or news or comment or case reports).pt.)
13	Diagnostics filter	12 and (exp prediction and forecasting/ or (predictive value of tests or receiver operating characteristic or ROC curve or sensitivity and specificity or accuracy or diagnostic accuracy or precision or likelihood).de. or ((false or true) adj (positive or negative)))
14	Clinical trials filter	13 and ((Randomized controlled trials or random allocation or double-blind method or single-blind method or placebos or cross-over studies or crossover procedure or double blind procedure or single blind procedure or placebos or latin square design or crossover design or double-blind studies or single-blind studies or triple-blind studies or random assignment or exp controlled study/ or exp clinical trial/ or exp comparative study/ or cohort analysis or follow-up studies.de. or intermethod comparison or parallel design or control group or prospective study or retrospective study or case control study or major clinical study).de. or Case control studies/ or Cohort/ or Longitudinal studies/ or Evaluation studies/ or Follow-up studies/ or Prospective studies/ or Retrospective studies/ or Case control study/ or Cohort analysis/ or Longitudinal study/ or Follow up/ or Cohort analysis/ or Followup studies/ or random$.hw. or random$.ti. or placebo$.mp. or ((singl$ or doubl$ or tripl$ or trebl$) and (dummy or blind or sham or mask)).mp. or latin square.mp. or (time adj series) or (case adj (study or studies) or ISRCTN$.mp. or ACTRN$.mp. or (NCT$ not nctc$)))
15	Combine sets	13 or 14
16	Eliminate overlap	
17	Seeding	12 and seeding.ti,ab.
18	Patient satisfaction/Q OL	12 and ((patient satisfaction or pain measurement or pain assessment or visual analog scale or quality of life).de. or satisf$ or QOL or preference$)
19	Adverse events	12 and ((ae or co).fs. or (cross infection or drainage or surgical wound infection).de.)
20	Disfiguration	12 and (disfigur$ or deform$)
21	Combine sets	or/1 6-20

Appendix C. Excluded Studies

Table C2. Studies that did not meet the inclusion criteria for Key Questions 1 and 2.

Study	Primary Reason for Exclusion
Bukhari et al. 2009 [1]	Patients were selected for core-needle biopsy on the basis of prior fine-needle aspiration results
Eliahou et al. 2009[2]	Enrolled a high-risk population
Peters et al. 2009[3]	Enrolled a high-risk population
Salem et al. 2009[4]	Enrolled a high-risk population
Tozaki et al. 2009[5]	Enrolled a high-risk population
Bernik et al. 2008[6]	Retrospective case study
Brem et al. 2008[7]	Retrospective case study
Carder et al. 2008[8]	Retrospective case study
Cheung et al. 2008[9]	Did not address Key Question 1
Choo et al. 2008[10]	Did not verify core-needle diagnoses
Doren et al. 2008[11]	Retrospective case study
Eby et al. 2008[12]	Retrospective case study
Eun et al. 2008[13]	Enrolled only patients with benign masses
Forgeard et al. 2008[14]	Retrospective case study
Hahn et al. 2008[15]	Enrolled only patients with benign masses
Hauth et al. 2008[16]	Enrolled a high-risk population
He et al. 2008[17]	Enrolled a high-risk population
Herti et al. 2008[18]	Did not address Key Question 1
Hemmer et al. 2008[19]	Did not address Key Question 1
Hukkinen et al. 2008[20]	Enrolled only patients with malignant masses
Hwang et al. 2008[21]	Retrospective case study
Jang et al. 2008[22]	Retrospective case study
Ji et al. 2008[23]	Duplicate report of Youk et al. 200824
Kil et al. 2008[25]	Retrospective case study
Kim et al. 2008[26]	Did not verify benign diagnoses
Kim et al. 2008[27]	Retrospective case study
Kumaroswamay et al. 2008[28]	Did not verify benign diagnoses
Lee et al. 2008[29]	Did not verify benign diagnoses
Londero et al. 2008[30]	Retrospective case study
Mahoney et al. 2008[31]	Enrolled patients with a prior diagnosis of breast cancer
Menon et al. 2008[32]	Retrospective case study
Michalopoulos et al. 2008[33]	Did not address Key Question 1
Perretta et al. 2008[34]	Enrolled a high-risk population
Peter et al. 2008[35]	Fewer than 50% of enrolled patients completed the study
Resetkova et al. 2008[36]	Retrospective case study
Rizzo et al. 2008[37]	Retrospective case study

Study	Primary Reason for Exclusion
Salem et al. 2008[38]	Did not address Key Question 1
Shin et al. 2008[39]	Retrospective case study
Sigal-Zafrani et al. 2008[40]	Fewer than 50% of enrolled patients completed the study
Skandarajah et al. 2008[41]	Retrospective case study
Smetherman et al. 2008[42]	Retrospective case study
Sohn et al. 2008[43]	Retrospective case study
Somerville et al. 2008[44]	Did not address Key Question 1
Tagaya et al. 2008[45]	Enrolled only patients with benign masses
Taourel et al. 2008[46]	Did not verify benign diagnoses
Tozaki et al. 2008[47]	Enrolled a high-risk population
Tseng et al. 2008[48]	Retrospective case study
Zagouri et al. 2008[49]	Did not address Key Question 1
Zografos et al. 2008[50]	Enrolled a high-risk population
Zografos et al. 2008[51]	Did not verify benign diagnoses
Zografos et al. 2008[52]	Did not verify any core-needle diagnoses
Andreu et al. 2007[53]	Fewer than 50% of enrolled patients completed the study
Arora et al. 2007[54]	Retrospective case study
Ashkenazi et al. 2007[55]	Retrospective case study
Bode et al. 2007[56]	Retrospective case study
Cassano et al. 2007[57]	Patients were selected for core-needle biopsy on the basis of prior fine-needle aspiration results
Ciatto et al. 2007[58]	Enrolled a high-risk population
Dillon et al. 2007[59]	Retrospective case study
Douglas-Jones et al. 2007[60]	Retrospective case study
Duchesne et al. 2007[61]	Fewer than 50% of enrolled patients completed the study
Duijm et al. 2007[62]	Fewer than 50% of enrolled patients completed the study
Easley et al. 2007[63]	Fewer than 50% of enrolled patients completed the study
Esserman et al. 2007[64]	Retrospective case study
Foxcroft et al. 2007[65]	Retrospective case study
Garg et al. 2007[66]	Patients were selected for core-needle biopsy on the basis of prior fine-needle aspiration results
Hollloway et al. 2007[67]	Did not verify benign diagnoses
Houssami et al. 2007[68]	Retrospective case study
Karabakhtsian et al. 2007[69]	Retrospective case study
Kikuchi et al. 2007[70]	Did not verify benign diagnoses
Kim et al. 2007[71]	Fewer than 50% of enrolled patients completed the study
Ko et al. 2007[72]	Retrospective case study
Krainick-Strobel et al. 2007[73]	Enrolled only patients with benign masses
Kumaraswamy and Carder 2007[74]	Fewer than 50% of enrolled patients completed the study
u and Kleer 2007[75]	Retrospective case study

Appendix C (Continued)

Study	Primary Reason for Exclusion
Lavoue et al. 2007[76]	Retrospective case study
Lee et al. 2007[77]	Enrolled a high-risk population
Lee et al. 2007[78]	Enrolled a high-risk population
Leikola et al. 2007[79]	Retrospective case study
Liberman et al. 2007[80]	Enrolled a high-risk population
Londero et al. 2007[81]	Retrospective case study
Lourenco et al. 2007[82]	Retrospective case study
Luczynska et al. 2007[83]	Did not verify benign diagnoses
Martel et al. 2007[84]	Retrospective case study
Mathew et al. 2007[85]	Enrolled only patients with benign masses
Mendel et al. 2007[86]	Fewer than 10 patients enrolled
Murta De Lucena et al. 2007[87]	Did not verify benign diagnoses
Nakano et al. 2007[88]	Patients were selected for core-needle biopsy on the basis of prior fine-needle aspiration results
Popiela et al. 2007[89]	Enrolled a high-risk population
Povoski and Jimenez 2007[90]	Did not report sufficient data to address Key Question 1
Rustein et al. 2007[91]	Retrospective case study
Schaefer et al. 2007[92]	Did not address any of the Key Questions
Smitt and Horst 2007[93]	Enrolled only patients with malignant masses
Sohn et al. 2007[94]	Retrospective case study
Sydnor et al. 2007[95]	Retrospective case study
Uematsu and Kasami 2007[96]	Did not address Key Question 1
Uematsu et al. 2007[97]	Did not verify benign diagnoses
Usami et al. 2007[98]	Enrolled only patients with malignant masses
Zagouri et al. 2007[99]	Retrospective case study
Zografos et al. 2007[100]	Did not verify benign diagnoses
Zuiani et al. 2007[101]	Enrolled a high-risk population
Al-Attar et al. 2006[102]	Did not address Key Question 1
Becker et al. 2006[103]	Retrospective case study
Bedei et al. 2006[104]	Retrospective case study
Chrzan et al. 2006[105]	Retrospective case study
Cox et al. 2006[106]	Retrospective case study
Dillon et al. 2006[107]	Retrospective case study
Dillon et al. 2006[108]	Retrospective case study
Fine and Staren 2006[109]	Enrolled only patients with benign masses
Fitzal et al. 2006[110]	Did not address Key Question 1
Gebauer et al. 2006[111]	Less than 50% of enrolled patients completed the study
Ghate et al. 2006[112]	Did not verify benign diagnoses
Govindarajulu et al. 2006[113]	Enrolled only patients with malignant masses
Hanley and Kessaram 2006[114]	Enrolled only patients with malignant masses

Study	Primary Reason for Exclusion
Hoffmann 2006[115]	Did not address Key Question 1
Huo et al. 2006[116]	Retrospective case study
Jackman and Rodriguez-Soto 2006[117]	Did not address Key Question 1
Jensen et al. 2006[118]	Fine-needle aspiration results were used in decisions about verification of results
Kamer et al. 2006[119]	Fewer than 10 patients enrolled
Killebrew and Oneson 2006[120]	Did not verify benign diagnoses
Koskela et al. 2006[121]	Did not report sufficient data to address Key Question 1
Lam et al. 2006[122]	Retrospective case study
Lannin et al. 2006[123]	Did not address Key Question 1
Liberman et al. 2006[124]	Retrospective case study
Lieske et al. 2006[125]	Fine-needle aspiration results were used in decisions about verification of results
Lim et al. 2006[126]	Retrospective case study
Lopez-Medina et al. 2006[127]	Retrospective case study
Margenthaler et al. 2006[128]	Enrolled a high-risk population
Mercado et al. 2006[129]	Retrospective case study
Newman et al. 2006[130]	Enrolled only patients with malignant masses
Orel et al. 2006[131]	Enrolled a high-risk population
Perlet et al. 2006[132]	Enrolled a high-risk population
Popiela et al. 2006[133]	Less than 50% of enrolled patients completed the study
Renshaw et al. 2006[134]	Retrospective case study
Renshaw et al. 2006[135]	Retrospective case study
Senn et al. 2006[136]	Did not verify benign diagnoses
Shin et al. 2006[137]	Did not address Key Question 1
Sie et al. 2006[138]	Retrospective case study
Uriburu et al. 2006[139]	Did not address Key Question 1
Valdes et al. 2006[140]	Retrospective case study
Vargas et al. 2006[141])	Did not address Key Question 1
Viehweg et al. 2006]142]	Enrolled a high-risk population
Wu et al. 2006[143]	Less than 50% of enrolled patients completed the study
Yazici et al. 2006[144]	Did not address Key Question 1
Altomare et al. 2005[145]	Did not verify benign diagnoses
Badoual et al. 2005[146]	Enrolled only patients with malignant masses
Bonifacino et al. 2005[147]	Fine-needle aspiration results were used in decisions about verification of results
Brem et al. 2005[148]	Retrospective case study
Caines et al. 2005[149]	Did not address Key Question 1
Cho et al. 2005[150]	Unresolvable multiple discrepancies in reported data
Costantini et al. 2005[151]	Did not verify benign diagnoses

Appendix C. (Continued).

Study	Primary Reason for Exclusion
Diebold et al. 2005[152]	Did not report sufficient data to address Key Question 1
Doridot et al. 2005[153]	Used a core-needle instrument that is no longer commercially available
Doyle et al. 2005[154]	Did not address Key Question 1
Elsheikh et al. 2005[155]	Retrospective case study
Gambos et al. 2005[156]	Retrospective case study
Grady et al. 2005[157]	Retrospective case study
Hanna et al. 2005[158]	Used a core-needle instrument that is no longer commercially available
Homesh et al. 2005[159]	Fine-needle aspiration results were used in decisions about verification of results
Lehman et al. 2005[160]	Did not verify benign diagnoses
Monticciolo 2005[161]	Enrolled only patients with malignant masses
Pilgrim and Ravichandran 2005[162]	Fine-needle aspiration results were used in decisions about verification of results
Qazi and Mohayuddin 2005[163]	Fine-needle aspiration results were used in decisions about verification of results
Riedl et al. 2005[164]	Did not address Key Question 1
Rulli et al. 2005[165]	Used a core-needle instrument that is no longer commercially available
Satchithananda et al. 2005[166]	Did not address Key Question 1
Schneider et al. 2005[167]	Used a core-needle instrument that is no longer commercially available
Soo et al. 2005[168]	Did not address Key Question 1
Wahner-Roedler et al. 2005[169]	Fewer than 10 patients enrolled
Wiratkapun et al. 2005[170]	Retrospective case study
Wong et al. 2005[171]	Did not verify benign diagnoses
You et al. 2005[172]	Retrospective case study
Zuiani et al. 2005[173]	Retrospective case study
Agoff et al. 2004[174]	Retrospective case study
Arpino et al. 2004[175]	Retrospective case study
Carmon et al. 2004[176]	Did not address Key Question 1
Chagpar et al. 2004[177]	Enrolled only patients with malignant masses
Chen et al. 2004[178]	Did not verify benign diagnoses
Collins et al. 2004[179]	Did not address Key Question 1
Docktor et al. 2004[180]	Did not address Key Question 1
Foster et al. 2004[181]	Retrospective case study
Gan et al. 2004[182]	Did not address Key Question 1
Geller et al. 2004[183]	Did not address Key Question 1
Gendler et al. 2004[184]	Retrospective case study

Study	Primary Reason for Exclusion
Georgina-Smith et al. 2004[185]	Retrospective case study
Golshan et al. 2004[186]	Enrolled only patients with malignant masses
Golub et al. 2004[187]	Did not address Key Question 1
Hansen et al. 2004[188]	Did not address Key Question 1
Hoorntje et al. 2004[189]	Did not address Key Question 1
Hoorntje et al. 2004[190]	Did not address Key Question 1
Ivan et al. 2004[191]	Retrospective case study
Margolin et al. 2004[192]	Did not address Key Question 1
Mendez et al. 2004[193]	Did not confirm benign diagnoses
O'Leary et al. 2004[194]	Did not address Key Question 1
Peters-Engl et al. 2004[195]	Enrolled only patients with malignant masses
Piana et al. 2004[196]	Enrolled only patients with malignant masses
Pijnappel et al. 2004[197]	Enrolled a high-risk population
Renshaw 2004[198]	Did not address Key Question 1
Renshaw et al. 2004[199]	Retrospective case study
Rotenberg et al. 2004[200]	Did not confirm benign diagnoses
Agarwal et al. 2003[201]	Enrolled only patients with malignant masses
Baez et al. 2003[202]	Enrolled only patients with benign masses
Bauer et al. 2003[203]	Retrospective case study
Berg et al. 2003[204]	Retrospective case study
Bonnett et al. 2003[205]	Retrospective case study
Brenner et al. 2003[206]	Retrospective case study
Carder and Liston 2003[207]	Enrolled patients with a benign mass
Cawson et al. 2003[208]	Retrospective case study
Charles et al. 2003 [209]	Enrolled patients with a malignant mass
Chen et al. 2003 [210]	Did not report sufficient data to address Key Question 1
Corn 2003 [211]	Used a core-needle instrument that is no longer commercially available
Crisi et al. 2003 [212]	Retrospective case study
Crowe et al. 2003 [213]	Did not verify benign diagnoses
Dennison et al. 2003 [214]	Fine-needle aspiration results were used in decisions about verification of results
Dmytrasz et al. 2003 [215]	Retrospective case study
Farshid and Rush 2003 [216]	Fine-needle aspiration results were used in decisions about verification of results
Fine et al. 2003 [217]	Enrolled only patients with benign masses
Fures et al. 2003 [218]	Did not verify benign diagnoses
Harris et al. 2003 [219]	Enrolled patients with a malignant mass
Hoorntje et al. 2003 [220]	Retrospective case study
Jackman and Marzoni 2003 [221]	Did not address Key Question 1

Appendix C. (Continued).

Study	Primary Reason for Exclusion
Kneeshaw et al. 2003 [222]	Retrospective case study
Komenaka et al. 2003 [223]	Retrospective case study
Lee et al. 2003 [224]	Enrolled only patients with malignant masses
Leifland et al. 2003 [225]	Fine-needle aspiration results were used in decisions about verification of results
Leifland et al. 2003 [226]	Fine-needle aspiration results were used in decisions about verification of results
Liberman et al. 2003 [227]	Enrolled a high-risk population
Mariotti et al. 2003 [228]	Did not verify benign diagnoses
Masood et al. 2003 [229]	Retrospective case study
Middleton et al. 2003 [230]	Retrospective case study
Miller et al. 2003 [231]	Retrospective case study
Puglisi et al. 2003 [232]	Retrospective case study
Shah et al. 2003 [233]	Retrospective case study
Sneige et al. 2003 [234]	Retrospective case study
Sperber et al. 2003 [235]	Enrolled only patients with benign masses
Tsang et al. 2003 [236]	Used a core-needle instrument that is no longer commercially available
Verkooijen et al. 2003 [237]	Did not address Key Question 1
Winchester et al. 2003 [238]	Retrospective case study
Witt et al. 2003 [239]	Did not address Key Question 1
Yeh et al. 2003 [240]	Retrospective case study
Zhao et al. 2003 [241]	Retrospective case study
Acheson et al. 2002 [242]	Retrospective case study
Bonnett et al. 2002 [243]	Retrospective case study
Chen et al. 2002 [244]	Enrolled patients with recurrent breast cancer
Chun and Velanovich et al. 2002 [245]	Did not address Key Question 1
Fine et al. 2002 [246]	Enrolled only patients with benign masses
Gal-Gombos et al. 2002 [247]	Retrospective case study
Giardina et al. 2002 [248]	Did not verify benign diagnoses
Haj et al. 2002 [249]	Used a core-needle instrument that is no longer commercially available
Harvey et al. 2002 [250]	Retrospective case study
Hoorntje et al. 2002 [251]	Did not verify benign diagnoses
Hui et al. 2002 [252]	Did not address Key Question 1
Insausti et al. 2002 [253]	Used a core-needle instrument that is no longer commercially available
Jackman et al. 2002 [254]	Retrospective case study
Jan et al. 2002 [255]	Fine-needle aspiration results were used in decisions about verification of results
Knight et al. 2002 [256]	Did not address Key Question 1
Liberman et al. 2002 [257]	Did not address Key Question 1

Study	Primary Reason for Exclusion
Lifrange et al. 2002 [258]	Used a core-needle instrument that is no longer commercially available
Mainiero et al. 2002 [259]	Did not address Key Question 1
McKee et al. 2002 [260]	Did not address Key Question 1
Perlet et al. 2002 [261]	Not published in English
Pijnappel et al. 2002 [262]	Enrolled a high-risk population
Popiela et al. 2002 [263]	Did not verify benign diagnoses
Rao et al. 2002 [264]	Retrospective case study
Renshaw 2002 [265]	Retrospective case study
Renshaw et al. 2002 [266]	Retrospective case study
Rosen et al. 2002 [267]	Retrospective case study
Schneider et al. 2002 [268]	Enrolled a high-risk population
Shin and Rosen 2002 [269]	Retrospective case study
Smyczek-Gargya et al. 2002 [270]	Did not verify benign diagnoses
Soo et al. 2002 [271]	Did not verify benign diagnoses
Tan et al. 2002 [272]	Fine-needle aspiration results were used in decisions about verification of results
Tse et al. 2002 [273]	Retrospective case study
Verkooijen and Peeters 2002 [274]	Enrolled a high-risk population
Verkooijen et al. 2002 [275]	Did not address Key Question 1
Watermann et al. 2002 [276]	Used a core-needle instrument that is no longer commercially available
Wunderbaldinger et al. 2002 [277]	Enrolled only patients with malignant masses
Bagnall et al. 2001 [278]	Enrolled only patients with malignant masses
Berg et al. 2001 [279]	Enrolled a high-risk population
Berg et al. 2001 [280]	Retrospective case study
Brem et al. 2001 [281]	Did not verify benign diagnoses
Chao et al. 2001 [282]	Not published in English
Clarke et al. 2001 [283]	Fine-needle aspiration results were used in decisions about verification of results
Daniel et al. 2001 [284]	Did not verify benign diagnoses
Deurloo et al. 2001 [285]	Did not address Key Question 1
Ely et al. 2001 [286]	Retrospective case study
Fine et al. 2001 [287]	Did not address Key Question 1
Grimes et al. 2001 [288]	Did not address Key Question 1
Hung et al. 2001 [289]	Fine-needle aspiration results were used in decisions about verification of results
Ibrahim et al. 2001 [290]	Fine-needle aspiration results were used in decisions about verification of results
Jackman et al. 2001 [291]	Retrospective case study

Appendix C. (Continued).

Study	Primary Reason for Exclusion
Jacobs et al. 2001 [292]	Core-needle biopsies were performed with a device no longer commercially available
Joshi et al. 2001 [293]	Did not verify benign diagnoses
Kaufman et al. 2001 [294]	Did not address Key Question 1
King et al. 2001 [295]	Did not address Key Question 1
Kuhl et al. 2001 [296]	Enrolled high-risk patients
Liberman et al. 2001 [297]	Did not address Key Question 1
Liberman et al. 2001 [298]	Did not address Key Question 1
Lifrange et al. 2001 [299]	Used a core-needle instrument that is no longer commercially available
Maganini et al. 2001 [300]	Retrospective case study
Marti et al. 2001 [301]	Used a core-needle instrument that is no longer commercially available
Meloni et al. 2001 [302]	Fine-needle aspiration results were used in decisions about verification of results
Mendez et al. 2001 [303]	Retrospective case study
Mercado et al. 2001 [304]	Retrospective case study
Morrow et al. 2001 [305]	Did not address Key Question 1
O'Driscoll et al. 2001 [306]	Fewer than 10 patients enrolled
Parker et al. 2001 [307]	Less than 50% of enrolled patients completed the study
Parker et al. 2001 [308]	Did not address Key Question 1
Renshaw 2001 [309]	Retrospective case study
Renshaw et al. 2001 [310]	Retrospective case study
Saarenmaa et al. 2001 [311]	Enrolled only patients with malignant masses
Schneider et al. 2001 [312]	Did not verify benign diagnoses
Schoonjans and Brem 2001 [313]	Less than 50% of enrolled patients completed the study
Shannon et al. 2001 [314]	Fine-needle aspiration results were used in decisions about verification of results
Sklair-Levy et al. 2001 [315]	Retrospective case study
Smith et al. 2001 [316]	Enrolled patients at high risk
Sun et al. 2001 [317]	Fine-needle aspiration results were used in decisions about verification of results
Verkooijen et al. 2001 [318]	Did not address Key Question 1
Westenend et al. 2001 [319]	Fine-needle aspiration results were used in decisions about verification of results
Adrales et al. 2000 [320]	Did not verify benign diagnoses
Bagnall et al. 2000 [321]	Enrolled only patients with malignant masses
Burns et al. 2000 [322]	Did not verify benign diagnoses
Darling et al. 2000 [323]	Retrospective case study
Cangiarella et al. 2000 [324]	Fine-needle aspiration results were used in decisions about verification of results
Cangiarella et al. 2000 [325]	Did not address Key Question 1

Study	Primary Reason for Exclusion
Gukas et al. 2000 [326]	Less than 50% of enrolled patients completed the study
Hatada et al. 2000 [327]	Fine-needle aspiration results were used in decisions about verification of results
Lamm et al. 2000 [328]	Did not address Key Question 1
Lee et al. 2000 [329]	Retrospective case study
Liberman et al. 2000 [330]	Retrospective case study
Melotti et al. 2000 [331]	Did not address Key Question 1
Mok and Keepin 2000 [332]	Enrolled a high-risk population
Moritz et al. 2000 [333]	Did not address any of the Key Questions
Nisbet et al. 2000 [334]	Did not verify diagnoses
O'hea and Tornos 2000 [335]	Retrospective case study
Philpotts et al. 2000 [336]	Retrospective case study
Philpotts et al. 2000 [337]	Retrospective case study
Portincasa et al. 2000 [338]	Used a core-needle instrument that is no longer commercially available
Schwatzberg et al. 2000 [339]	Used a core-needle instrument that is no longer commercially available
Simon et al. 2000 [340]	Less than 50% of enrolled patients completed the study
Sneige and Tulbah 2000 [341]	Did not address Key Question 1
Stolier et al. 2000 [342]	Did not address Key Question 1
Teh et al. 2000 [343]	Did not verify benign diagnoses
Whitlock et al. 2000 [344]	Less than 50% of enrolled patients completed the study
Yang et al. 2000 [345]	Used a core-needle instrument that is no longer commercially available
Al-Sobhi et al. 1999 [346]	Did not address Key Question 1
Baker et al. 1999 [347]	Fewer than 10 patients enrolled
Bloomston et al. 1999 [348]	Used a core-needle instrument that is no longer commercially available
Bokran et al. 1 999 [349]	Retrospective case study
Brem et al. 1 999 [350]	Retrospective case study
Britton and McCann 1999 [351]	Did not address Key Question 1
Damascelli et al. 1999 [352]	Used a core-needle instrument that is no longer commercially available
Deschryver et al. 1 999 [353]	Retrospective case study
Diaz et al. 1999 [354]	Did not address Key Question 1
DiPiro et al. 1 999 [355]	Retrospective case study
El-Tamer et al. 1999 [356]	Enrolled only patients with malignant masses
Evans et al. 1999 [357]	Did not verify benign diagnoses
Ferzli et al. 1999 [358]	Used a core-needle instrument that is no longer commercially available
Fraser et al. 1999 [359]	Fine-needle aspiration results were used in decisions about verification of results

Appendix C. (Continued).

Study	Primary Reason for Exclusion
Gajdos et al. 1999 [360]	Did not address Key Question 1
Gentry and Henry 1999 [361]	Did not address Key Question 1
Gray et al. 1999 [362]	Did not address Key Question 1
Harlow et al. 1999 [363]	Did not address Key Question 1
Harvey et al. 1 999 [364]	Retrospective case study
Johnson et al. 1 999 [365]	Retrospective case study
Klem et al. 1999 [366]	Did not verify benign diagnoses
LaRaja et al. 1999 [367]	Used a core-needle instrument that is no longer commercially available
Lee et al. 1999 [365]	Enrolled only patients with benign masses
Liberman et al. 1999 [368]	Retrospective case study
Liberman et al. 1999 [369]	Retrospective case study
Liberman et al. 1999 [370]	Did not address Key Question 1
Matthews and Williams 1999 [371]	Used a core-needle instrument that is no longer commercially available
Mitnick et al. 1 999 [372]	Retrospective case study
Philpotts et al. 1999 [373]	Did not address Key Question 1
Rebner et al. 1999 [374]	Used a core-needle instrument that is no longer commercially available
Rich et al. 1999 [375]	Did not verify benign diagnoses
Rosen et al. 1 999 [376]	Retrospective case study
Roth et al. 1999 [377]	Enrolled only patients with malignant masses
Sharifi et al. 1999 [378]	Did not address Key Question 1
Sheth et al. 1999 [379]	Used a core-needle instrument that is no longer commercially available
Shin et al. 1999 [380]	Results of fine-needle aspiration were used to decide who underwent core-needle biopsy
Staren et al. 1999 [381]	Fine-needle aspiration results were used in decisions about verification of results
Tran et al. 1999 [382]	Does not address any of the Key Questions
Velanovich et al. 1999 [383]	Did not verify benign diagnoses
Williams et al. 1999 [384]	Did not verify benign diagnoses
Won et al. 1 999 [385]	Retrospective case study
Yong et al. 1999 [386]	Fine-needle aspiration results were used in decisions about verification of results
Andreu et al. 1998 [387]	Fine-needle aspiration results were used in decisions about verification of results
Antley et al. 1998 [388]	Did not report sufficient data to address Key Question 1
Bleznak et al. 1998 [389]	Did not address Key Question 1
Damascelli et al. 1998 [390]	Used a core-needle instrument that is no longer commercially available
Doyle et al. 1998 [391]	Fine-needle aspiration results were used in decisions about verification of results

Study	Primary Reason for Exclusion
Goodman et al. 1998 [392]	Did not address Key Question 1
Helbich et al. 1998 [393]	Did not address Key Question 1
Jackman et al. 1998 [394]	Enrolled only patients with benign masses
Johnson et al. 1998 [395]	Did not verify benign diagnoses
Kaufman et al. 1998 [396]	Did not address Key Question 1
Kelley et al. 1998 [397]	Used a core-needle instrument that is no longer commercially available
King et al. 1 998 [398]	Retrospective case study
Liberman et al. 1998 [399]	Enrolled only patients with malignant masses
Liberman et al. 1998 [400]	Did not address Key Question 1
Lin et al. 1 998 [401]	Retrospective case study
Lind et al. 1998 [402]	Enrolled only patients with benign masses
Meyer et al. 1998 [403]	Enrolled only patients with benign masses
Mitnick et al. 1 998 [404]	Retrospective case study
Seoudi et al. 1998 [405]	Did not verify benign diagnoses
Slanetz et al. 1998 [406]	Did not address Key Question 1
Soo et al. 1998 [407]	Fewer than 10 patients enrolled
Woodcock et al. 1998 [408]	Did not verify benign diagnoses
Zardawi 1998 [409]	Did not verify benign diagnoses
Zonderland et al. 1998 [410]	Fine-needle aspiration results were used in decisions about verification of results
Acheson et a. 1997 [411]	Less than 50% of enrolled patients completed the study
Anania et al. 1997 [412]	Did not address Key Question 1
Burbank 1997 [413]	Retrospective case study
Burbank 1997 [414]	Did not address Key Question 1
Burbank 1997 [415]	Enrolled only patients with benign masses
Cerwenka et al. 1997 [416]	Did not verify benign diagnoses
D'Angelo et al. 1997 [417]	Used a core-needle instrument that is no longer commercially available
Devia et al. 1997 [418]	Did not address Key Question 1
Fenoglio et al. 1997 [419]	Did not address Key Question 1
Ferzli et al. 1997 [420]	Used a core-needle instrument that is no longer commercially available
Florentine et al. 1997 [421]	Fine-needle aspiration results were used in decisions about verification of results
Gadzala et al. 1997 [422]	Retrospective case study
Hirst and Davis 1997 [423]	Did not verify benign diagnoses
Howisey et al. 1997 [424]	Did not address Key Question 1
Jackman and Marzoni 1997 [425]	Did not address Key Question 1
Jackman et al. 1 997 [426]	Retrospective case study
Liberman et al. 1997 [427]	Did not address Key Question 1

Appendix C. (Continued).

Study	Primary Reason for Exclusion
Liberman et al. 1997 [428]	Did not address Key Question 1
Lifrange et al. 1997 [429]	Fine-needle aspiration results were used in decisions about verification of results
Meyer et al. 1997 [430]	Did not address Key Question 1
Pijnappel et al. 1997 [431]	Fine-needle aspiration results were used in decisions about verification of results
Roe et al. 1997 [432]	Did not report sufficient data to address Key Question 1
Smith et al. 1997 [433]	Did not address Key Question 1
Stolier et al. 1997 [434]	Did not address Key Question 1
Whitten et al. 1997 [435]	Did not address Key Question 1
Written et al. 1997 [436]	Did not address Key Question 1
Ballo and Sneige 1996 [437]	Fine-needle aspiration results were used in decisions about verification of results
Burbank et al. 1996 [438]	Did not address Key Question 1
Caines et al. 1996 [439]	Did not verify benign diagnoses
Chare et al. 1996 [440]	Fine-needle aspiration results were used in decisions about verification of results
Crotch-Harvey and Loughran 1996 [441]	Fine-needle aspiration results were used in decisions about verification of results
Dershaw et al. 1996 [442]	Did not address Key Question 1
Di et al. 1996 [443]	Enrolled only patients with malignant masses
Frayne et al. 1996 [444]	Fine-needle aspiration results were used in decisions about verification of results
Handy et al. 1996 [445]	Did not address Key Question 1
Hillhouse et al. 1996 [446]	Did not address Key Question 1
Hunter et al. 1996 [447]	Did not address Key Question 1
Liberman et al. 1996 [448]	Did not address Key Question 1
Pillsbury et al. 1996 [449]	Did not verify benign diagnoses
Poole et al. 1996 [450]	Fine-needle aspiration results were used in decisions about verification of results
Taft et al. 1996 [451]	Did not verify benign diagnoses
Tocino et al. 1 996 [452]	Retrospective case study
Wallace et al. 1996 [453]	Did not verify benign diagnoses
Yim et al. 1996 [454]	Did not address Key Question 1
Hann et al. 1995 [455]	Did not address Key Question 1
Israel and Fine1995 [456]	Did not verify benign diagnoses
Liberman et al. 1995 [457]	Retrospective case study
Liberman et al. 1995 [458]	Retrospective case study
Liberman et al. 1995 [459]	Enrolled patients with recurrent breast cancer
McCombs et al. 1995 [460]	Did not verify benign diagnoses
Nath et al. 1995 [461]	Fewer than 10 patients enrolled
Rubin et al. 1995 [462]	Did not address Key Question 1

Study	Primary Reason for Exclusion
Strong et al. 1995 [463]	Did not verify benign diagnoses
Vega et al. 1995 [464]	Enrolled high-risk patients
Vega et al. 1995 [465]	Did not verify benign diagnoses
Youngson et al. 1995 [466]	Did not address Key Question 1
Caines et al. 1994 [467]	Did not verify benign diagnoses
Jackman et al. 1994 [468]	Did not verify benign diagnoses
Janes and Bouton 1994 [469]	Did not verify benign diagnoses
Kaye et al. 1994 [470]	Did not address Key Question 1
Liberman et al. 1994 [471]	Did not address Key Question 1
Liberman et al. 1994 [472]	Did not address Key Question 1
Mikhail et al. 1994 [473]	Enrolled a high-risk population
Morrow et al. 1994 [474]	Did not verify benign diagnoses
Sadler et al. 1994 [475]	Fine-needle aspiration results were used in decisions about verification of results
Youngson et al. 1994 [476]	Did not address Key Question 1
Rotten et al. 1993 [477]	Fine-needle aspiration results were used in decisions about verification of results
Dronkers 1992 [478]	Did not verify benign diagnoses
Elliot et al. 1992 [479]	Did not verify benign diagnoses
Harter et al. 1992 [480]	Fewer than 10 patients enrolled
Pezner et al. 1992 [481]	Did not address any of the Key Questions
Khanna et al. 1991 [482]	Fine-needle aspiration results were used in decisions about verification of results

Appendix D. Data Abstraction Forms

Quality Assessment

- Was patient recruitment either consecutive or random?
- Were at least 85% of the patients recruited for enrollment actually enrolled?
- Were the patient inclusion/ exclusion criteria consistently applied to all patients?
- Was the study free from obvious spectrum bias? Obvious spectrum bias was defined as more than 40% or less than 10% of the breast lesions were diagnosed as malignant; and/or the mean or median age of the enrolled population was less than 50 or greater than 70.
- Was the study prospective in design?
- Was a complete set of data reported for at least 85% of enrolled lesions?
- Were the patients assessed by the gold standard (open surgical procedure) regardless of the initial biopsy results?
- Were patients assessed by a reference standard regardless of the biopsy results?
- Was funding for this study provided by a source that doesn't have an obvious financial interest in the findings of the study?
- Did the study account for inter-reader/score differences?

- Were the reader(s) of the biopsies blinded to the results of the reference standard?
- Were readers of the reference standard blinded to the results of the biopsy?
- Were the readers of the biopsy blinded to all other clinical information?
- Were readers of the reference standard blinded to all other clinical information?

Study Design

- Design of study
- Study was prospective or retrospective?
- Number of centers
- Care setting
- Country study conducted in
- Study funded by
- How many different people performed core-needle biopsies during the course of the study?
- What is the training of the persons performing the core-needle biopsies?
- What is the experience of the persons performing the core-needle biopsies?
- Describe in detail the methods used to perform the biopsies
- Who is interpreting the biopsy specimens, and what kind of training do they have?
- Biopsy results confirmed by comparing them to what?
- Describe in detail the reference standard

Patient Details

- Describe the inclusion criteria
- Describe the exclusion criteria
- Number of patients recruited/approached about enrollment
- Number of patients and lesions enrolled
- Number of lesions completing the study
- Age, median or mean, range
- Other reported age discriptors such as % post-menopausal
- Ethnicity
- Types of lesions enrolled and number of each

Accuracy Data

- Enter the type of biopsy being used for the following set of data
- How many lesions were biopsied?
- How many technical failures/ inadequate biopsies occurred?
- How many were lost to followup?
- How many lesions were diagnosed as benign and what was the final diagnosis for each

- How many lesions were diagnosed as invasive and what was the final diagnosis for each
- How many lesions were diagnosed as DCIS and what was the final diagnosis for each
- How many lesions were diagnosed as Atypical, Suspicious, or High Risk, and what was the final diagnosis for each
- Where there any other diagnoses on core-needle biopsy and if so what were they and what was the final diagnosis for each
- Enter information about accuracy by lesion characteristics
- Enter information about accuracy by patient characteristics
- Enter information about accuracy by biopsy methodology characteristics
- Enter any other reported information affected biopsy accuracy

Harms Data

- Requirement for a repeated biopsy procedure, rate
- Complications of the biopsy procedure, types and rates of
- Time to recovery or time to return to work
- Use of pain medications
- Patient satisfaction, quality of life data
- Impact of biopsy procedure on accuracy of subsequent mammography procedures . Any other harms info reported by the study

Appendix E. Evidence Tables

Table E3. Previously published systematic reviews: design.

Study	Search Dates	Types of Biopsy Evaluated	Types of Breast Abnormalities Evaluated	Reference Standard Required	Other Inclusion Criteria	Method of Rating the Quality	Statistical Methods
Fahrbach et al. 2006 [483]	1996 to June 2004	Stereotactic vacuum-assisted core-needle biopsy and stereotactic core- needle biopsy	All-comer populations referred after screening mammography	Surgical biopsy or patient followup	English language; ten or more patients; conducted in North America, Europe, Australia, or New Zealand; reported absolute numbers of each lesion type on biopsy; studies of devices no longer on the market- SiteSelect, MIBB device, ABBI device were excluded	Narrative discussion, no overall rating given	Random-effects models in SAS and SPSS, multivariate regression models
Verkooijen et al. 2000 [484]	1975 to May 1999	Large-core needle biopsy under stereotactic or ultrasound guidance	Non-palpable lesions detected on mammography	Surgical biopsy or a minimum of 2 years of followup in at least 90% of patients	The absolute number of benign and malignant lesions had to be derivable; a minimum of five large-core biopsy specimens per lesion had to be obtained; studies of fine-needle aspiration were excluded.	Not rated	Pooled by meta-analysis using SPSS. No further details provided.

Table E4. Previously Published Systematic Reviews: Quality Rating.

Study	Was an 'a priori' design provided?	Was there duplicate study selection and data extraction?	Was a comprehensive literature search performed?	Was the status of publication (i.e., grey literature) used as an inclusion criterion?	Was a list of studies (included/excluded) provided?	Were the characteristics of the included studies provided?	quality of the included studies used appropriately in formulating	Was the quality of the studies assessed and documented?	Were the methods used to combine the finding of studies appropriate?	Was the likelihood of publicationbias assessed?	Was the conflict of interest stated?	Quality Rating
Fahrbach et al. 2006 [483]	Can't tell	Yes	Yes	Yes	No	Yes	No	Yes	Yes	No	No	Moderate
Verkooijen et al. 2000 [484]	Can't tell	Yes	Yes	Yes	Yes	No	No	No	Can't tell	No	No	Moderate

Table E5. Previously Published Systematic Reviews: Results.

Study	N Studies	N Patients	Accuracy	Accuracy Affected by Patient Type/ Breast Abnormality Types	Accuracy Affected by Procedure-related Factors	Accuracy Affected by Personnel/ Facility Factors	Harms	Conclusion
Fahrbach et al. 2006 [483]	12 of vacuum-assisted biopsy and 25 of core-needle biopsy	11,355 patients, 5,119 with vacuum-assisted biopsy and 6,236 patients with automated gun core- needle biopsy	Overall agreement between vacuum-assisted and reference standard was 97.3%; overall agreement between core-needle and reference standard was 93.5%. Rate of benign lesions turning out to be malignant: vacuum-assisted: 2.02% (95% CI: 0.00 to 4.35), core-needle: 2.36% (95% CI: 1.15 to 3.58). Rate of atypia lesions turning out to be malignant: vacuum-assisted: 20.38% (15.25 to 25.52), core-needle: 36.69% (26.53 to 46.84)	For atypia to malignant upgrades the type of procedure was a significant predictor, with more underestimations occurring with core-needle as compared to vacuum-assisted	Reference standard and patient position did not influence accuracy	For benign to malignant upgrades, more benign to malignant upgrades occurred in non-North American locations than in North American locations	Frequency of technical failures: 5.7% for core-needle, 1.5% for vacuum-assisted	Vacuum-assisted biopsy may provide lower miss and underestimation rates than automated gun core-needle biopsy.

Table E5. (Continued).

Study	N Studies	N Patients	Accuracy	Accuracy Affected by Patient Type/ Breast Abnormality Types	Accuracy Affected by Procedure-related Factors	Accuracy Affected by Personnel/ Facility Factors	Harms	Conclusion
Verkooijen et al. 2000 [484]	5	865 biopsies performed	DCIS on needle biopsy upgraded to invasive cancer: 15% (95% CI: 8.0 to 26); ADH on needle biopsy upgraded to invasive cancer: 40% (95% CI: 26 to 56); sensitivity of core-needle for detecting malignancies: 97% (95% CI: 95 to 99)	Not performed	Not performed	Not performed	2 complications reported: 1 hematoma 1 infection	In a setting such as the U.S. where about 20% of cases referred for biopsy are malignant, the risk of breast cancer despite a benign diagnosis on core- needle biopsy is less than 1%. However, in a setting such as Europe where about 60% of cases referred for biopsy are malignant, the risk of breast cancer despite a benign diagnosis on core- needle biopsy is 4%.

Table E6. Studies Included to Address Key Questions 1 And 2: Design Details.

Study	Design of Study	Type of Study	Number of Centers	Care Setting	Country Conducted in	Funded by	Type(s) Core Biopsy	Core Biopsy Results Confirmed by	Number of Lesions Enrolled	Followup	% Attrition
Jackman et al. 2009 [485]	Single group (cohort or case series study)	Retrosp-ective	1	General hospital	USA	Biopsys Medical, Inc. and Ethicon Endo-Surgery	Stereotactic guidance vacuum-assisted 11 G and 14G	Combination of surgery and patient followup	1,280	2 years	10.6%
Peters et al. 2008 [486]	Single group (cohort or case series study)	Retrosp-ective	4	General hospital	Netherland s	NR	Stereotactic guidance automated gun 1 4G	Combination of surgery and patient followup	948	2 years	5%

Study	Design of Study	Type of Study	Number of Centers	Care Setting	Country Conducted in	Funded by	Type(s) Core Biopsy	Core Biopsy Results Confirmed by	Number of Lesions Enrolled	Followup	% Attrition
Schueller et al. 2008 [487]	Single group (cohort or case series study)	Retrosp-ective	1	General hospital	Austria	Authors stated no financial relationship to disclose	Ultrasound guidance automated gun 14G	Combination of surgery and patient followup	1438	2 years	5.7%
Sim and Kei 2008 [488]	Single group (cohort or case series study)	Retrosp-ective	1	General hospital	Singapore	NR	Stereotactic guidance vacuum-assisted 11 G	Combination of surgery and patient folowup	105	2 years	12.4%
Tonegutti and Girardi 2008 [489]	Single group (cohort or case series study)	Retrosp-ective	1	General hospital	Italy	NR	Stereotactic guidance vacuum-assisted 11 G	Combination of surgery and patient followup	268	2 years	0%
Youk et al. 200 [824]	Single group (cohort or case series study)	Retrosp-ective	1	General hospital	South Korea	NR	US guidance automated gun 14G	Combination of surgery and patient followup	4,359	2 years	44%
Ciatto et al. 2007 [490]	Single group (cohort or case series study)	Retrosp-ective	1	Dedicated breast cancer center	Italy	Funded in part by a National Helath and Medical Research Council (NHMRC) grant	Multiple methods	Combination of surgery and patient followup	4,035	1 year	26%
de Lucena et al. 2007 [491]	Single group (cohort or case series study)	Prospective	1	General hospital	Brazil	NR	US guidance automated gun 14G	Open surgery or surgical biopsy only	150	Immediate surgery	0%

Table E6. (Continued).

Study	Design of Study	Type of Study	Number of Centers	Care Setting	Country Conducted in	Funded by	Type(s) Core Biopsy	Core Biopsy Results Confirmed by	Number of Lesions Enrolled	Followup	% Attrition
Uematsu et al. 2007 [492]	Single group (cohort or case series study)	Prospective	1	General cancer center	Japan	NR	Stereotactic guidance vacuum-assisted 11 G	Combination of surgery and patient followup	100	Mean: 26 months Range: 5 to 44 months	0%
Vag et al. 2007 [493]	Single group (cohort or case series study)	Prospective	1	General hospital	Germany	NR	US guidance vacuum-assisted 10G	Combination of surgery and patient followup	70	2 years	0%
Chapellier et al. 2006 [494]	Single group (cohort or case series study)	Prospective	1	General cancer center	France	NR	Stereotactic guidance vacuum-assisted 11 G	Combination of surgery and patient followup	318	Range: 4 to 16 months	0%
Cipolla et al. 2006 [495]	Single group (cohort or case series study)	NR	1	General hospital	Italy	NR	Multiple methods	Combination of surgery and patient followup	426	1 year	0%
Dhillon et al. 2006 [496]	Single group (cohort or case series study)	Prospective	1	General hospital	UK	NR	Stereotactic guidance vacuum-assisted 11 G	Combination of surgery and patient followup	150	Median: 48 months	0%
Bolivar et al. 2005 [497]	Single group (cohort or case series study)	Prospective	1	General hospital	Spain	NR	US guidance automated gun 14G	Combination of surgery and patient followup	214	2 years	5%

Study	Design of Study	Type of Study	Number of Centers	Care Setting	Country Conducted in	Funded by	Type(s) Core Biopsy	Core Biopsy Results Confirmed by	Number of Lesions Enrolled	Followup	% Attrition
Crystal et al. 2005 [498]	Single group (cohort or case series study)	NR	1	General hospital	Israel	NR	US guidance automated gun 14G	Combination of surgery and patient followup	715	Median: 39 months Range: 27 to 60 months	0%
Dillon et al. 2005 [499]	Single group (cohort or case series study)	Retros-pective	1	General hospital	Ireland	NR	Multiple methods	Combination of surgery and patient followup	2,427	Median: 24 months Range: 3 to 67 months	19%
Koskela et al. 2005 [500]	Single group (cohort or case series study)	Prospective	1	General hospital	Finland	Kuopio University Hospital (the center it was conducted in)	Stereotactic guidance automated gun 14G	Combination of surgery and patient followup	213	Mean: 24 months Range: 6 to 39 months	4%
Sauer et al. 2005 [501]	Single group (cohort or case series study)	Retros-pective	1	General hospital	Germany	NR	US guidance automated gun 14G	Combination of surgery and patient followup	962	Mean: 22.2 months Median: 21 months Range : 8 to 36 months	13%
Weber et al. 2005 [502]	Non-randomized multiple groups study	Prospective	1	General hospital	Switzerlan d	NR	Stereotactic guidance vacuum-assisted 11 G	Combination of surgery and patient followup	225	Median: 2.1 years Range: 0.5 to 4.4 years	15%
Wu et al. 2005 [503]	Single gro-up (cohort or case ser-ies study)	NR	1	General hospital	Taiwan	NR	US guidan-ce vacuum-assisted 1 1G	Combination of surgery and patient followup	113	1 year	0%

Table E6. (Continued).

Study	Design of Study	Type of Study	Number of Centers	Care Setting	Country Conducted in	Funded by	Type(s) Core Biopsy	Core Biopsy Results Confirmed by	Number of Lesions Enrolled	Followup	% Attrition
Alonso-Bartolome et al. 2004 [504]	Single group (cohort or case series study)	Prospective	2	General hospital	Spain	NR	US guidance vacuum-assisted 1 1G	Combination of surgery and patient followup	102	6 to 12 months	0%
Delle and Terinde 2004 [505]	Single group (cohort or case series study)	NR	1	General hospital	Germany	NR	US guidance automated gun 14G	Combination of surgery and patient followup	169	2 years	0%
Fajardo et al. 2004 [506]	Some pati-ents were randomized to stereo-tactic or US guidance but data were reported as if the study was a single-group cohort study	Prospective	22	Academic and community practice clinical sites	USA	National Cancer Institute	Multiple methods	Combination of surgery and patient followup	2,403	2 years	30%
Kettritz et al. 2004 [507]	Single group (cohort or case series study)	Prospective	5	General hospital	Germany	NR	Stereotactic guidance vacuum-assisted 11 G	Combination of surgery and patient followup	2,893	Mean: 25 months Range: 6 to 67 months	22%
Lomoschitz et al. 2004 [508]	Non-randomized multiple	Prospective	1	General hospital	Austria	One author partially supported by both	Stereotactic guidance vacuum-	Combination of surgery and patient	100	2 years	0%

Study	Design of Study	Type of Study	Number of Centers	Care Setting	Country Conducted in	Funded by	Type(s) Core Biopsy	Core Biopsy Results Confirmed by	Number of Lesions Enrolled	Followup	% Attrition
	groups study					Ethicon Edonsurgery and Biopsys Medical	assisted 11G	followup			
Abdsaleh et al. 2003 [509]	Single group (cohort or case series study)	Prospective	1	General hospital	Sweden	NR	Multiple methods	Combination of surgery and patient followup	180	1 year	21%
Ambrogetti et al. 2003 [510]	Single group (cohort or case series study)	Retrosp-ective	1	General hospital	France	NR	Stereotactic guidance vacuum-assisted 11 G	Combination of surgery and patient followup	364	Mean: 15.8 months Range: 6 to 36 months	35%
Fishman et al. 2003 [511]	Single group (cohort or case series study)	Prospective	1	General hospital	USA	NR	US guidance automated gun 14G	Combination of surgery and patient followup	73	Mammogr aphic and US followup Median: 21 months Range: 4 to 30 months	33%
Han et al. 2003 [512]	Single group (cohort or case series study)	Retrosp-ective	1	General hospital	Korea	NR	Stereotactic guidance automated gun 14G	Combination of surgery and patient followup	271	At least 6 months	27%

Table E6. (Continued).

Study	Design of Study	Type of Study	Number of Centers	Care Setting	Country Conducted in	Funded by	Type(s) Core Biopsy	Core Biopsy Results Confirmed by	Number of Lesions Enrolled	Followup	% Attrition
Kirshenbaum et al. 2003 [513]	Single group (cohort or case series study)	Retrosp-ective	1	General hospital	USA	NR	Multiple methods	Combination of surgery and patient followup	506	Mean: 2.1 years Range: 3 months to 5 years	23%
March et al. 2003 [514]	Single group (cohort or case series study)	Prospective	2	Dedicated breast cancer center	USA	RSNA Seed Grant and the Rays of Hope charitable fund	US guidance vacuum-assisted 1 1G	Combination of surgery and patient followup	34	6 months	9%
Pfleiderer et al. 2003 [515]	Single group (cohort or case series study)	Prospective	1	General hospital	Germany	NR	MRI guidance automated gun 14G	Combination of surgery and patient followup	14	2 years	0%
Philpotts et al. 2003 [516]	Non-randomized multiple groups study	Retrosp-ective	1	General hospital	USA	NR	Multiple methods	Combination of surgery and patient followup	281	Mean: 19 months Range: 3 to 53 months for 14G Mean: 13 months Range: 1 to 24 for 11G	24%
Wong and Hisham 2003 [517]	Single gro-up (cohort or case ser-ies study)	Prospective	1	General hospital	Malaysia	NR	Freehand automated gun 14 or 16G	Combination of surgery and patient followup	150	Range: 6 to 13 months	0%

Study	Design of Study	Type of Study	Number of Centers	Care Setting	Country Conducted in	Funded by	Type(s) Core Biopsy	Core Biopsy Results Confirmed by	Number of Lesions Enrolled	Followup	% Attrition
Apesteguia et al. 2002 [518]	Single group (cohort or case series study)	Prospective	1	General hospital	Spain	NR	Stereotactic guidance vacuum-assisted 11 G	Combination of surgery and patient followup	132	1 year	0%
Georgian-Smith et al. 2002 [519]	Single group (cohort or case series study)	Retrosp-ective	4	General hospital	USA	NR	Stereotactic guidance vacuum-assisted 11 G	Combination of surgery and patient followup	185	Range: 6 to 12 months	21%
Jackman and Lamm 2002 [520]	Single group (cohort or case series study)	Retrosp-ective	1	General hospital	USA	Funded in part by Biopsys Medical	Multiple methods	Combination of surgery and patient followup	31	At least 6 months	0%
Johnson et al. 2002 [521]	Single group (cohort or case series study)	NR	1	General hospital	USA	Fashion Footwear of NY	US guidance vacuum-assisted 11 or 8G	Combination of surgery and patient followup	101	Mean: 9.5 months	24%
Liberman et al. 2002 [522]	Single group (cohort or case series study)	Retrosp-ective	1	General cancer center	USA	NR	Stereotactic guidance vacuum-assisted 11 G	Combination of surgery and patient followup	800	At least 1 year	29%
Meloni et al. 2002 [523]	Single group (cohort or case series study)	Retrosp-ective	1	General hospital	Italy	NR	Stereotactic guidance vacuum-assisted	Combination of surgery and patient followup	129	Mean: 18.7 mon-ths Range: 14 to 26 months	0%

Table E6. (Continued).

Study	Design of Study	Type of Study	Number of Centers	Care Setting	Country Conducted in	Funded by	Type(s) Core Biopsy	Core Biopsy Results Confirmed by	Number of Lesions Enrolled	Followup	% Attrition
Morris et al. 2002 [524]	Single group (cohort or case series study)	Prospective	1	Dedicated breast cancer center	USA	NR	Stereotactic guidance vacuum-assisted 14G	Combination of surgery and patient followup	21	Median: 46 months Range: 40-54 months	10%
Pfarl et al. 2002 [525]	Single group (cohort or case series study)	Retrosp-ective	1	General hospital	Austria	NR	Stereotactic guidance vacuum-assisted 11 G	Open surgery or surgical biopsy only	332	Immediate surgery	4%
Verkooijen et al. COBRA 2002 [526]	Single group (cohort or case series study)	Prospective	5	General hospital	Netherland s	Dutch National Health Insurance Fund Council	Stereotactic guidance automated gun 1 4G	Open surgery or surgical biopsy only	984	Immediate surgery	11%
Becker et al. 2001 [527]	Single gro-up (cohort or case ser-ies study)	Retrosp-ective	1	General hospital	Canada	NR	Stereotactic guidance automated gun 1 4G	Combination of surgery and patient followup	232	Range: 6 to 12 months	27%
Brenner et al. 2001 [528]	Single group (cohort or case series study)	Prospective	7	Cancer centers and hospitals	USA	NR	Stereotactic guidance automated gun 1 4G	Combination of surgery and patient followup	1,003	Mean: 19.3 months Range: 0 to 36 months	1%
Cangiarella et al. 2001 [529]	Single gro-up (cohort or case ser-ies study)	NR	1	General hospital	USA	NR	Stereotactic guidance vacuum-assisted 11 G	Combination of surgery and patient followup	160	Mean: 20.5 mon-ths Range: 6 to 35 months	38%

Study	Design of Study	Type of Study	Number of Centers	Care Setting	Country Conducted in	Funded by	Type(s) Core Biopsy	Core Biopsy Results Confirmed by	Number of Lesions Enrolled	Followup	% Attrition
Dahlstrom and Jain 2001 [530]	Single group (cohort or case series study)	NR	1	General hospital	Australia	NR	Stereotactic guidance automated gun 1 4G	Combination of surgery and patient followup	301	Range: 2.4 to 7.5 years	0%
Lai et al. 2001 [531]	Single group (cohort or case series study)	NR	1	General hospital	Canada	NR	Stereotactic guidance vacuum-assisted 11 G	Combination of surgery and patient followup	673	Mean: 6.7 months Range: 6 to 24 months	29%
Levin et al. 2001 [532]	Single group (cohort or case series study)	Prospective	1	General hospital	Canada	Physician's Services Incorporated Foundation	Stereotactic guidance automated gun 14G	Open surgery or surgical biopsy only	70	Immediate surgery	0%
Margolin et al. 2001 [533]	Single group (cohort or case series study)	Retrospective	1	General hospital	USA	NR	Multiple methods	Combination of surgery and patient followup	1,333	Mean: 14 months Range: 6 to 24 months; missing data were collected from SEER database; at the time of accession of SEER data followup ranged from 15 to 75 months	3%

Table E6. (Continued).

Study	Design of Study	Type of Study	Number of Centers	Care Setting	Country Conducted in	Funded by	Type(s) Core Biopsy	Core Biopsy Results Confirmed by	Number of Lesions Enrolled	Followup	% Attrition
Perez-Fuentes et al. 2001 [534]	Single group (cohort or case series study)	NR	1	Dedicated breast cancer center	Venezuela	NR	US guidance vacuum-assisted 1 1G	Combination of surgery and patient followup	88	Median: 11.1 mon-ths Range: 4 to 24 months	33%
Smith et al. 2001 [535]	Single gro-up (cohort or case ser-ies study)	NR	1	General hospital	USA	NR	US guidance automated gun 14G	Combination of surgery and patient followup	500	Mean: 22 months Median: 14 months Range: 12 to 60 months	21%
White et al. 2001 [536]	Single gro-up (cohort or case ser-ies study)	Retros-pective	1	General hospital	USA	NR	Multiple methods	Combination of surgery and patient followup	1,042	Median: 29 months, minimum of one year	29%
Wunderbaldinger et al. 2001 [537]	Single group (cohort or case series study)	Prospective	1	General hospital	Austria	author supported by Erwin Schroedinger Auslandsstipenium of the Austrian Science Fund	US guidance automated gun 14G	Open surgery or surgical biopsy only	45	Immediate surgery	0%
Yeow et al. 2001 [538]	Single gro-up (cohort or case ser-ies study)	Prospective	1	General hospital	China	NR	US guida-nce autom-ated gun 14 or 16G	Combination of surgery and patient followup	98	Mean: 4 years Range: 3 to 5 years	0%

Study	Design of Study	Type of Study	Number of Centers	Care Setting	Country Conducted in	Funded by	Type(s) Core Biopsy	Core Biopsy Results Confirmed by	Number of Lesions Enrolled	Followup	% Attrition
Kirwan et al. 2000 [540]	Single group (cohort or case series study)	Retrospective	1	General hospital	UK	NR	Stereotactic guidance automated gun 1 4G	Open surgery or surgical biopsy only	72	Immediate surgery	13%
Latosinsky et al. 2000 [541]	Single group (cohort or case series study)	Retrospective	1	General hospital	USA	NIH grant	Multiple methods	Combination of surgery and patient followup	692	Median: 17.2 months Range: 2.8 to 43 months	42%
Liberman et al. 2000 [542]	Single group (cohort or case series study)	Retrospective	1	General cancer center	USA	NR	Multiple methods	Combination of surgery and patient followup	155	Median: 53 months Range: 24 to 69 months	32%
Makoske et al. 2000 [543]	Single group (cohort or case series study)	Retrospective	1	General hospital	USA	NR	Multiple methods	Combination of surgery and patient followup	817	Mean: 1.7 years	30%
Ward et al. 2000 [544]	Single group (cohort or case series study)	NR	1	General hospital	Canada	NR	Stereotactic guidance automated gun 14G	Combination of surgery and patient followup	121	Mean: 16 months Range: 4 to 36 months	7%
Welle et al. 2000 [545]	Single group (cohort or case series study)	Retrospective	3	General hospital	USA	NR	Multiple methods	Combination of surgery and patient followup	225	Range: 6 to 24 months	20%

Table E6. (Continued).

Study	Design of Study	Type of Study	Number of Centers	Care Setting	Country Conducted in	Funded by	Type(s) Core Biopsy	Core Biopsy Results Confirmed by	Number of Lesions Enrolled	Followup	% Attrition
Helbich et al. 1 999 [546]	Randomized controlled trial	Prospective	1	General hospital	Austria	Ludwig-Boltzmann Institute for Radiologic Tumor Research; one author was supported by a grant from the Max Kade Foundation	Multiple methods	Open surgery or surgical biopsy only	44	Immediate surgery	0%
Jackman et al. 1999 [547]	Single group (cohort or case series study)	Retrospective	1	General hospital	USA	NR	Stereotactic guidance automated gun 1 4G	Combination of surgery and patient followup	483	Median: 55 months	1%
Meyer et al. 1 999 [548]	Single group (cohort or case series study)	Retrospective	1	General hospital	USA	NR	Multiple methods	Combination of surgery and patient followup	1,836	At least 1 year	25%
Puglisi et al. 1999 [549]	Single group (cohort or case series study)	Retrospective	1	General hospital	Italy	NR	Perforated compression grid automated gun 1 4G	Combination of surgery and patient followup	106	At least 6 months	1%
Soo et al. 1999 [550]	Non-randomized multiple groups study	Retrospective	1	General hospital	USA	NR	Multiple methods	Combination of surgery and patient followup	116	Mean: 16 months Range: 5 to 31 months	19%
Caruso et al. 1998 [551]	Single group (cohort or case series study)	Prospective	1	General hospital	Italy	NR	Multiple methods	Open surgery or surgical biopsy only	92	Immediate surgery	13%

Study	Design of Study	Type of Study	Number of Centers	Care Setting	Country Conducted in	Funded by	Type(s) Core Biopsy	Core Biopsy Results Confirmed by	Number of Lesions Enrolled	Followup	% Attrition
Doyle et al. 1998 [552]	Single group (cohort or case series study)	Retrospective	1	Dedicated breast cancer center	New Zealand	NR	Stereotactic guidance automated gun 14G	Combination of surgery and patient followup	151	Range: 6 to 36 months	11%
Fuhrman et al. 1 998 [553]	Single group (cohort or case series study)	Retrospective	1	General hospital	USA	NR	Multiple methods	Combination of surgery and patient followup	1,440	At least 6 months	18%
Heywang-Kobrunner et al. 1 998 [554]	Single group (cohort or case series study)	NR	1	General hospital	Germany	NR	Stereotactic guidance vacuum-assisted 11 or 14G	Combination of surgery and patient followup	261	6 months	31%
Ioffe et al. 1998 [555]	Single group (cohort or case series study)	NR	1	General hospital	USA	NR	Multiple methods	Combination of surgery and patient followup	224	Range: 6 to 12 months	14%
Liberman et al. 1 998 [556]	Single group (cohort or case series study)	NR	1	General cancer center	USA	NR	US guidance automated gun 14G	Combination of surgery and patient followup	151	Median: 20 months Range: 6 to 48 months	23%
Schulz-Wendtland et al. 1998 [557]	Single group (cohort or case series study)	NR	1	General hospital	Germany	NR	US guidance automated gun 14G	Combination of surgery and patient followup	307	2 years	0%
Vega-Bolivar et al. 1998 [558]	Single group (cohort or case series study)	Retrospective	1	General hospital	Spain	NR	Stereotactic guidance Surecut 1 5G	Combination of surgery and patient followup	182	Mean: 27 months Range: 6 to 47 months	6%

Table E6. (Continued).

Study	Design of Study	Type of Study	Number of Centers	Care Setting	Country Conducted in	Funded by	Type(s) Core Biopsy	Core Biopsy Results Confirmed by	Number of Lesions Enrolled	Followup	% Attrition
Whitman et al. 1 998 [559]	Single gro-up (cohort or case seri-es study)	Retros-pective	2	General hospital	USA	NR	Stereotactic guidance automated gun 1 6G	Open surgery or surgical biopsy only	12	Immediate surgery	0%
Zannis and AliaNo 1 998 [560]	Non-randomized multiple gr-oups study	Retros-pective	1	Ambulator y surgical center	USA	NR	Multiple methods	Combination of surgery and patient followup	424	At least 6 months	31%
Bauer et al. 1997 [561]	Single gro-up (cohort or case ser-ies study)	Retros-pective	NR	NR	USA	NR	Stereotactic guidance automated gun 14G	Combination of surgery and patient followup	799	Mean: 9 months	0%
Britton et al. 1 997 [562]	Single gro-up (cohort or case seri-es study)	NR	1	General hospital	UK	NR	Multiple methods	Combination of surgery and patient followup	202	Mean: 20.1 months Range: 5.3 to 30.8 months	2%
Helbich et al. 1 997 [563]	Single gro-up (cohort or case ser-ies study)	Prospective	1	General hospital	Austria	NR	Multiple methods	Open surgery or surgical biopsy only	210	Immediate surgery	0%
Khattar et al. 1 997 [564]	Single gro-up (cohort or case seri-es study)	Prospective	1	General hospital	Denmark	NR	US guid-ance auto-mated gun	Open surgery or surgical biopsy only	106	Immediate surgery	43%
Liberman et al. 1997 [565]	Single gro-up (cohort or case ser-ies study)	Retros-pective	1	General cancer center	USA	NR	Stereotactic guidance automated gun 14G	Combination of surgery and patient followup	442	Median: 18 months Range: 6 to 46 months	34%

Study	Design of Study	Type of Study	Number of Centers	Care Setting	Country Conducted in	Funded by	Type(s) Core Biopsy	Core Biopsy Results Confirmed by	Number of Lesions Enrolled	Followup	% Attrition
Pitre et al. 1997 [566]	Single group (cohort or case series study)	Retrospective	1	General hospital	USA	NR	Stereotactic guidance automated gun	Combination of surgery and patient followup	128	1 year	8%
Stolier et al. 1997 [567]	Single group (cohort or case series study)	Retrospective	1	General hospital	USA	NR	Multiple methods	Combination of surgery and patient followup	244	Mean: 12.8 months Range: 6 to 39 months	NR
Sutton, et al. 1 997 [568]	Single group (cohort or case series study)	Retrospective	1	Screening clinic	Australia	NR	Stereotactic guidance automated gun 1 4G	Combination of surgery and patient followup	206	1 year	32%
Walker et al. 1 997 [569]	Single group (cohort or case series study)	NR	1	General hospital	UK	NR	Stereotactic guidance automated gun 1 4G	Combination of surgery and patient followup	200	Range: 6 to 36 months	10%
Frazee et al. 1 996 [570]	Non-randomized multiple groups study	Prospective	1	General hospital	USA	NR	Stereotactic guidance automated gun	Combination of surgery and patient followup	103	At least 6 months	0%
Fuhrman et al. 1996 [571]	Single group (cohort or case series study)	NR	1	General hospital	USA	NR	Stereotactic guidance automated gun 1 4G	Combination of surgery and patient followup	451	1 year	22%
Head and Haynes 1996 [572]	Single group (cohort or case series study)	Prospective	1	Dedicated breast cancer center	USA	NR	Stereotactic guidance automated gun 1 8G	Combination of surgery and patient followup	115	2 years	8%

Table E6. (Continued).

Study	Design of Study	Type of Study	Number of Centers	Care Setting	Country Conducted in	Funded by	Type(s) Core Biopsy	Core Biopsy Results Confirmed by	Number of Lesions Enrolled	Followup	% Attrition
Mainiero et al. 1 996 [573]	Single group (cohort or case series study)	Retrospective	1	General hospital	USA	NR	Stereotactic guidance automated gun 1 4G	Combination of surgery and patient followup	138	At least 6 months	14%
Meyer et al. 1 996 [574]	Single group (cohort or case series study)	NR	1	General hospital	USA	NR	Stereotactic guidance automated gun 1 4G	Combination of surgery and patient followup	388	1 year	30%
Nguyen et al. 1 996 [575]	Single group (cohort or case series study)	NR	1	General hospital	USA	American Cancer Society, UCLA Jonsson Comprehensive Cancer Center, and the Stein-Oppenheim Foundation	Multiple methods	Combination of surgery and patient followup	431	At least 6 months	10%
Pettine et al. 1996 [576]	Single group (cohort or case series study)	Retrospective	1	General hospital	USA	NR	Stereotactic guidance automated gun 1 4G	Open surgery or surgical biopsy only	25	6 month repeat mammography for benign	0%
Rosenblatt et al. 1 996 [577]	Single group (cohort or case series study)	Retrospective	1	General hospital	USA	NR	Stereotactic guidance automated gun 1 4G	Combination of surgery and patient followup	25	1 year	16%
Scopa et al. 1996 [578]	Non-randomized multiple groups study	NR	1	General hospital	Greece	NR	Freehand TruCut	Open surgery or surgical biopsy only	120	Immediate surgery	0%

Study	Design of Study	Type of Study	Number of Centers	Care Setting	Country Conducted in	Funded by	Type(s) Core Biopsy	Core Biopsy Results Confirmed by	Number of Lesions Enrolled	Followup	% Attrition
Doyle et al. 1995 [580]	Non-randomized multiple gr-oups study	Prospective	1	General Hospital	USA	NR	Multiple methods	Combination of surgery and patient followup	150	Range: 6 to 24 months	3%
Hamed et al. 1995 [581]	Randomi-zed contro-lled trial	Prospective	1	General hospital	UK	NR	Freehand Biopty- cut	Open surgery or surgical biopsy only	122	Immediate surgery	0%
Burbank et al. 1 994 [582]	Non-randomized multiple gr-oups study	NR	1	General hospital	USA	NR	Multiple methods	Combination of surgery and patient followup	105	At least 6 months	0%
Gisvold et al. 1 994 [583]	Single gro-up (cohort or case seri-es study)	Prospective	1	General hospital	USA	NR	Stereotactic guidance automated gun 1 4G	Open surgery or surgical biopsy only	160	Immediate surgery	0%
Parker et al. 1 994 [584]	Non-randomized multiple gr-oups study	Retros-pective	20	Various hospitals, breast care centers, clinics	USA	NR	Multiple methods	Combination of surgery and patient followup	6,152	At least 6 months	39%
Smyth and Cederbom 1 994 [585]	Single gro-up (cohort or case seri-es study)	NR	1	General hospital	USA	NR	Stereotactic guidance automated gun 1 4G	Open surgery or surgical biopsy only	58	Immediate surgery	0%
Elvecrog et al. 1993 [586]	Non-randomized multiple gr-oups study	Prospective	1	General hospital	USA	NR	Stereotactic guidance automated gun 1 4G	Open surgery or surgical biopsy only	100	Immediate surgery	0%

Table E6. (Continued).

Study	Design of Study	Type of Study	Number of Centers	Care Setting	Country Conducted in	Funded by	Type(s) Core Biopsy	Core Biopsy Results Confirmed by	Number of Lesions Enrolled	Followup	% Attrition
Parker et al. 1993 [587]	Single group (cohort or case series study)	NR	1	Specialized imaging center	USA	NR	US guidance automated gun 14G	Combination of surgery and patient followup	181	Range: 12 to 36 months	0%
McMahon et al. 1 992 [588]	Randomized controlled trial	Prospective	1	General hospital	UK	NR	Multiple methods	Combination of surgery and patient followup	151	Median: 11 months Range: 1 to 24 months	0%
Barreto et al. 1991 [589]	Single group (cohort or case series study)	NR	1	General hospital	UK	NR	Freehand automated gun 1 8G	Open surgery or surgical biopsy only	107	Immediate surgery	0%
Cusick et al. 1 990 [590]	Single group (cohort or case series study)	NR	1	General hospital	USA	NR	Freehand	Open surgery or surgical biopsy only	96	Immediate surgery	0%
Parker et al. 1990 [591]	Single group (cohort or case series study)	NR	1	General hospital	USA	NR	Stereotactic guidance automated gun	Open surgery or surgical biopsy only	103	Immediate surgery	0%

NR = Not Reported
US = Ultrasound
UK = United Kingdom
USA = United States of America

Table E7. Quality Assessment Instrument.

1. Was patient recruitment either consecutive or random?
2. Were more than 85% of the patients approached for recruitment enrolled in the study?
3. Were the patient inclusion/ exclusion criteria consistently applied to all patients?
4. Was the study free from obvious spectrum bias? Obvious spectrum bias was defined as more than 40% or less than 10% of the breast lesions were diagnosed as malignant; and/or the mean or median age of the enrolled population was less than 50 or greater than 70.
5. Was the study prospective in design?
6. Was a complete set of data reported for at least 85% of enrolled lesions?
7. Were the patients assessed by the gold standard (open surgical procedure) regardless of the initial biopsy results?
8. Were patients assessed by a reference standard regardless of the biopsy results?
9. Was funding for this study provided by a source that doesn't have an obvious financial interest in the findings of the study?
10. Did the study account for inter-reader/scorer differences?
11. Were the reader(s) of the biopsies blinded to the results of the reference standard?
12. Were readers of the reference standard blinded to the results of the biopsy?
13. Were the readers of the biopsy blinded to all other clinical information?
14. Were readers of the reference standard blinded to all other clinical information?

Table E8. Quality of Studies Addressing Key Questions 1 and 2 (See Table E7 for the Wording of the Questions).

Study	1	2	3	4	5	6	7	8	9	10	11	12	13	14	Raw Score	Standardize
Jackman et al. 2009 [485]	Yes	Yes	Yes	NR	No	Yes	No	Yes	No	No	Yes	NR	No	NR	1	5.4
Peters et al. 2008 [486]	Yes	NR	Yes	No: over 40% malignant	No	Yes	No	Yes	NR	No	Yes	No	No	No	-1	4.6
Schueller et al. 2008 [487]	Yes	Yes	Yes	No: over 40% malignant	No	Yes	No	Yes	Yes	NR	Yes	No	No	No	1	5.4
Sim and Kei 2008 [488]	Yes	Yes	Yes	Yes	No	Yes	No	Yes	NR	NR	Yes	No	NR	No	3	6.1
Tonegutti and Girardi 2008 [489]	Yes	Yes	Yes	No: 41.6% malignant	No	Yes	No	Yes	NR	NR	NR	NR	NR	NR	3	6.1

Table E8. (Continued).

Study	1	2	3	4	5	6	7	8	9	10	11	12	13	14	Raw Score	Standardize
Youk et al. 200824	Yes	Yes	Yes	No: mean 45.3 years of age	No	No	No	Yes	NR	NR	Yes	No	No	No	-1	4.6
Ciatto et al. 2007 [490]	Yes	Yes	Yes	NR	No	No	No	Yes	Yes	No	Yes	No	No	No	-1	4.6
de Lucena et al. 2007 [491]	NR	NR	NR	No: 67% malignant	Yes	Yes	Yes	Yes	NR	NR	Yes	NR	NR	NR	5	6.8
Uematsu et al. 2007 [492]	Yes	Yes	Yes	Yes	Yes	Yes	No	Yes	NR	No	Yes	NR	NR	NR	6	7.1
Vag et al. 2007 [493]	NR	NR	NR	No: 41.4% malignant	Yes	Yes	No	Yes	NR	NR	Yes	NR	NR	NR	3	6.1
Chapellier et al. 2006 [494]	NR	NR	NR	Yes	Yes	Yes	No	Yes	NR	NR	Yes	NR	NR	NR	4	6.4
Cipolla et al. 2006 [495]	Yes	Yes	Yes	No: 43% malignant	NR	Yes	No	Yes	NR	NR	Yes	NR	NR	NR	5	6.8
Dhillon et al. 2006 [496]	Yes	Yes	Yes	Yes	Yes	Yes	No	Yes	NR	NR	Yes	NR	NR	NR	7	7.5
Bolivar et al. 2005 [497]	Yes	Yes	Yes	No: 58% malignant	Yes	Yes	No	Yes	NR	No	Yes	NR	NR	NR	5	6.8
Crystal et al. 2005 [498]	Yes	Yes	Yes	No: 45% malignant	NR	Yes	No	Yes	NR	NR	Yes	NR	NR	NR	5	6.8
Dillon et al. 2005 [499]	Yes	Yes	Yes	No: 57% malignant	No	No	No	Yes	NR	NR	Yes	No	No	No	-1	4.6
Koskela et al. 2005 [500]	Yes	Yes	Yes	No: 42% malignant	Yes	Yes	No	Yes	Yes	No	Yes	No	No	No	3	6.1
Sauer et al. 2005 [501]	Yes	Yes	Yes	No: 64.2% malignant	No	Yes	No	Yes	NR	No	Yes	No	No	No	0	5.0
Weber et al. 2005 [502]	Yes	Yes	Yes	Yes	Yes	Yes	No	Yes	NR	Yes	Yes	NR	NR	NR	8	7.9
Wu et al. 2005 [503]	Yes	Yes	Yes	No: 0% malignant	NR	Yes	No	Yes	NR	NR	Yes	NR	NR	NR	5	6.8

Study	1	2	3	4	5	6	7	8	9	10	11	12	13	14	Raw Score	Standardize
Alonso-Bartolome et al. 2004 [504]	NR	Yes	Yes	No: 0.9% malignant, mean age 42	Yes	Yes	No	Yes	NR	NR	Yes	NR	NR	NR	5	6.8
Delle and Terinde 2004 [505]	Yes	Yes	Yes	No: 77% malignant	NR	Yes	No	Yes	NR	NR	Yes	NR	NR	NR	5	6.8
Fajardo et al. 2004 [506]	Yes	Yes	Yes	Yes	Yes	Yes	No	Yes	Yes	Yes	Yes	NR	NR	NR	9	8.2
Kettritz et al. 2004 [507]	NR	NR	No	NR	Yes	No	No	Yes	NR	NR	Yes	NR	No	NR	-1	4.6
Lomoschitz et al. 2004 [508]	Yes	Yes	Yes	No: 47% malignant	Yes	Yes	No	Yes	No	No	NR	NR	NR	NR	3	6.1
Abdsaleh et al. 2003 [509]	Yes	Yes	Yes	No: 74% malignant	Yes	Yes	No	Yes	NR	NR	Yes	NR	NR	NR	6	7.1
Ambrogetti et al. 2003 [510]	Yes	Yes	Yes	No: 43.4% malignant	No	No	No	Yes	NR	NR	Yes	No	No	No	-1	4.6
Fishman et al. 2003 [511]	Yes	Yes	No	NR	Yes	No	No	Yes	NR	No	Yes	NR	Yes	NR	2	5.7
Han et al. 2003 [512]	Yes	Yes	Yes	No: mean age 47 years	No	No	No	Yes	NR	NR	NR	NR	NR	NR	1	5.4
Kirshenbaum et al. 2003 [513]	Yes	Yes	Yes	Yes	No	No	No	Yes	NR	NR	Yes	No	No	No	0	5.0
March et al. 2003 [514]	Yes	No: 67%	Yes	NR	Yes	Yes	No	Yes	Yes	No	Yes	No	No	No	2	5.7
Pfleiderer et al. 2003[515]	No	NR	Yes	No: 42% malignant	Yes	Yes	No	Yes	NR	NR	Yes	NR	NR	NR	4	6.4
Philpotts et al. 2003 [516]	Yes	Yes	Yes	NR	No	No	No	Yes	NR	NR	Yes	No	No	No	-1	4.6
Wong and Hisham 2003 [517]	Yes	Yes	Yes	No: 46% malignant	Yes	Yes	No	Yes	NR	NR	Yes	NR	NR	NR	6	7.1
Apesteguia et al. 2002 [518]	Yes	Yes	Yes	Yes	Yes	Yes	No	Yes	NR	NR	NR	NR	NR	NR	6	7.1

Table E8. (Continued).

Study	1	2	3	4	5	6	7	8	9	10	11	12	13	14	Raw Score	Standardize
Georgian-Smith et al. 2002 [519]	Yes	Yes	Yes	Yes	No	Yes	No	Yes	NR	NR	Yes	No	No	No	2	5.7
Jackman and Lamm 2002 [520]	Yes	Yes	Yes	Yes	No	Yes	No	Yes	No	NR	Yes	No	No	No	1	5.4
Johnson et al. 2002 [521]	Yes	Yes	Yes	No: 5% malignant	NR	No	No	Yes	Yes	NR	Yes	NR	NR	NR	4	6.4
Liberman et al. 2002 [522]	Yes	Yes	Yes	No	No	No	No	Yes	NR	NR	Yes	No	No	No	-2	4.3
Meloni et al. 2002 [523]	Yes	Yes	Yes	NR	Yes	Yes	No	Yes	NR	NR	Yes	No	No	No	3	6.1
Morris et al. 2002 [524]	NR	NR	Yes	Yes	Yes	Yes	No	Yes	NR	No	Yes	NR	NR	NR	4	6.4
Pfarl et al. 2002 [525]	Yes	Yes	Yes	No: 65% malignant	No	Yes	Yes	Yes	NR	NR	Yes	No	No	No	3	6.1
Verkooijen et al. COBRA 2002 [526]	Yes	NR	Yes	Yes	Yes	Yes	Yes	Yes	Yes	No	Yes	NR	NR	NR	8	7.9
Becker et al. 2001 [527]	Yes	Yes	Yes	Yes	No	No	No	Yes	NR	NR	Yes	No	No	No	0	5.0
Brenner et al. 2001 [528]	NR	NR	NR	NR	Yes	Yes	No	Yes	NR	NR	Yes	NR	NR	NR	3	6.1
Cangiarella et al. 2001 [529]	Yes	Yes	Yes	No: 9% malignant	NR	No	No	Yes	NR	NR	Yes	NR	NR	NR	3	6.1
Dahlstrom and Jain 200 1530	Yes	Yes	Yes	NR	NR	Yes	No	Yes	NR	NR	Yes	NR	NR	NR	5	6.8
Lai et al. 2001 [531]	Yes	Yes	Yes	Yes	NR	No	No	Yes	NR	NR	Yes	NR	NR	NR	4	6.4
Levin et al. 2001 [532]	NR	NR	Yes	NR	Yes	Yes	Yes	Yes	Yes	No	Yes	NR	NR	NR	6	7.1
Margolin et al. 2001 [533]	Yes	Yes	Yes	No: mean age less than 50	No	Yes	No	Yes	NR	NR	Yes	No	No	No	1	5.4
Perez-Fuentes et al. 2001 [534]	No	NR	No	No: mean age 48	NR	No	No	Yes	NR	NR	Yes	NR	NR	NR	-1	4.6

Study	1	2	3	4	5	6	7	8	9	10	11	12	13	14	Raw Score	Standardize
Smith et al. 2001 [535]	Yes	Yes	Yes	No: mean age 47	NR	No	No	Yes	NR	NR	Yes	NR	NR	NR	3	6.1
White et al. 2001 [536]	Yes	Yes	Yes	Yes	No	No	No	Yes	NR	No	Yes	No	No	No	-1	4.6
Wunderbaldinger et al. 2001 [537]	No	NR	Yes	No: 49% malignant	Yes	Yes	Yes	Yes	Yes	No	No	No	NR	NR	3	6.1
Yeow et al. 2001 [538]	Yes	Yes	Yes	No: mean age 46	Yes	Yes	No	Yes	NR	NR	Yes	NR	NR	NR	6	7.1
Beck et al. 2000 [539]	Yes	Yes	Yes	NR	NR	Yes	No	Yes	NR	NR	Yes	NR	NR	NR	5	6.8
Kirwan et al. 2000 [540]	NR	NR	NR	NR	No	Yes	Yes	Yes	NR	NR	Yes	No	No	No	0	5.0
Latosinsky et al. 2000 [541]	Yes	Yes	Yes	NR	No	No	No	Yes	Yes	NR	NR	Yes	No	No	1	5.4
Liberman et al. 2000 [542]	Yes	Yes	Yes	No: median age 47 years	No	No	No	Yes	NR	NR	Yes	No	No	No	-1	4.6
Makoske et al. 2000 [543]	Yes	Yes	Yes	NR	Yes	No	No	Yes	NR	NR	Yes	No	No	No	1	5.4
Ward et al. 2000 [544]	Yes	Yes	Yes	Yes	NR	Yes	No	Yes	NR	NR	Yes	No	No	No	3	6.1
Welle et al. 2000 [545]	NR	NR	NR	NR	No	No	No	Yes	NR	NR	Yes	No	No	No	-4	3.6
Helbich et al. 1999 [546]	Yes	NR	Yes	No: 86% malignant	Yes	Yes	Yes	No	NR	No	Yes	NR	No	NR	3	6.1
Jackman et al. 1999 [547]	Yes	Yes	Yes	Yes	No	Yes	No	Yes	NR	Yes	No	No	No	No	0	5.0
Meyer et al. 1999548	Yes	Yes	Yes	Yes	No	No	No	Yes	NR	No	Yes	No	No	No	-1	4.6
Puglisi et al. 1999 [549]	Yes	Yes	Yes	Yes	No	Yes	No	Yes	NR	No	Yes	No	No	No	1	5.4
Soo et al. 1999 [550]	Yes	Yes	Yes	NR	No	No	No	Yes	NR	Yes	Yes	No	No	No	0	5.0
Caruso et al. 1998 [551]	Yes	NR	Yes	No: 85% malignant	Yes	Yes	Yes	Yes	NR	No	Yes	NR	No	NR	5	6.8
Doyle et al. 1998 [552]	Yes	Yes	Yes	NR	No	Yes	No	Yes	NR	No	Yes	No	No	No	0	5.0

Table E8. (Continued).

Study	1	2	3	4	5	6	7	8	9	10	11	12	13	14	Raw Score	Standardize
Fuhrman et al. 1 998 [553]	Yes	Yes	Yes	Yes	No	No	No	Yes	NR	No	Yes	No	No	No	-1	4.6
Heywang-Kobrunner et al. 1 998 [554]	Yes	Yes	Yes	NR	NR	No	No	Yes	NR	NR	Yes	NR	NR	NR	3	6.1
Ioffe et al. 1998 [555]	Yes	NR	Yes	Yes	NR	NR	No	Yes	NR	NR	NR	NR	NR	NR	3	6.1
Liberman et al. 1998 [556]	Yes	Yes	Yes	Yes	NR	No	No	Yes	NR	NR	Yes	NR	NR	NR	4	6.4
Schulz-Wendtland et al. 1998 [557]	Yes	Yes	Yes	No: 52% malignant	NR	Yes	No	Yes	NR	NR	Yes	NR	NR	NR	5	6.8
Vega-Bolivar et al. 1998 [558]	Yes	NR	Yes	No: over 40% were malignant	No	Yes	No	Yes	NR	No	Yes	No	No	No	-1	4.6
Whitman et al. 1 998 [559]	NR	Yes	NR	No: 50% malignant	No	Yes	No	Yes	NR	NR	NR	NR	NR	NR	1	5.4
Zannis and AliaNo 1998 [560]	Yes	Yes	Yes	Yes	No	Yes	No	Yes	NR	NR	Yes	No	No	No	2	5.7
Bauer et al. 1997 [561]	Yes	Yes	Yes	Yes	No	Yes	No	Yes	NR	Yes	Yes	No	No	No	2	5.7
Britton et al. 1997 [562]	Yes	Yes	Yes	No: 50% malignant	NR	Yes	No	Yes	NR	NR	Yes	NR	NR	NR	5	6.8
Helbich et al. 1997 [563]	Yes	Yes	Yes	No: 47% malignant	Yes	Yes	Yes	Yes	NR	No	Yes	No	NR	NR	6	7.1
Khattar et al. 1997[564]	NR	NR	Yes	No: 44% malignant	Yes	No	Yes	Yes	NR	NR	Yes	NR	NR	NR	4	6.4
Liberman et al. 1997 [565]	Yes	NR	Yes	NR	No	No	No	Yes	NR	NR	Yes	No	No	No	-2	4.3
Pitre et al. 1997 [566]	Yes	Yes	Yes	No: 8.6% malignant	No	Yes	No	Yes	NR	NR	Yes	No	No	No	1	5.4
Stolier et al. 1997 [567]	Yes	Yes	Yes	NR	No	Yes	No	Yes	NR	NR	Yes	No	No	No	1	5.4

Study	1	2	3	4	5	6	7	8	9	10	11	12	13	14	Raw Score	Standardize
Sutton, et al. 1997 [568]	NR	NR	No	Yes	No	No	No	Yes	NR	NR	Yes	No	No	No	-4	3.6
Walker et al. 1997 [569]	Yes	Yes	Yes	No: 54% malignant	NR	Yes	No	Yes	NR	NR	Yes	NR	NR	NR	5	6.8
Frazee et al. 1996 [570]	Yes	Yes	Yes	Yes	Yes	Yes	No	Yes	NR	NR	NR	NR	NR	NR	6	7.1
Fuhrman et al. 1996 [571]	NR	Yes	Yes	NR	NR	No	No	Yes	NR	NR	NR	NR	NR	NR	1	5.4
Head and Haynes 1996 [572]	NR	NR	NR	Yes	Yes	Yes	No	Yes	NR	NR	Yes	NR	NR	NR	4	6.4
Mainiero et al. 1996 [573]	NR	Yes	Yes	Yes	No	Yes	No	Yes	NR	NR	NR	NR	NR	NR	3	6.1
Meyer et al. 1996 [574]	Yes	No: 67.7%	Yes	No: median age 49	NR	No	No	Yes	NR	NR	NR	NR	NR	NR	1	5.4
Nguyen et al. 1996 [575]	NR	NR	Yes	No: 43% malignant	NR	Yes	No	Yes	Yes	NR	Yes	NR	NR	NR	4	6.4
Pettine et al. 1996 [576]	NR	Yes	Yes	NR	No	Yes	Yes	NR	NR	NR	NR	NR	NR	NR	3	6.1
Rosenblatt et al. 1996 [577]	Yes	Yes	Yes	No: 52% malignant	No	No	No	Yes	NR	NR	Yes	No	No	No	-1	4.6
Scopa et al. 1996 [578]	NR	Yes	Yes	No: 65% malignant	NR	Yes	Yes	Yes	NR	NR	NR	NR	NR	NR	5	6.8
Cross et al. 1995 [579]	NR	NR	NR	Yes	NR	Yes	No	Yes	NR	NR	Yes	No	No	No	0	5.0
Doyle et al. 1995 [580]	Yes	Yes	Yes	Yes	Yes	No	No	Yes	NR	NR	NR	NR	NR	NR	4	6.4
Hamed et al. 1995 [581]	Yes	Yes	Yes	No: 88% malignant	Yes	Yes	No	No	NR	NR	NR	NR	NR	NR	3	6.1
Burbank et al. 1994 [582]	NR	Yes	NR	NR	NR	Yes	No	Yes	NR	NR	NR	NR	NR	NR	2	5.7
Gisvold et al. 1994 [583]	Yes	No: 33.6%	No	No: 42% malignant	Yes	Yes	Yes	Yes	NR	No	Yes	NR	NR	NR	4	6.4

Table E8. (Continued).

Study	1	2	3	4	5	6	7	8	9	10	11	12	13	14	Raw Score	Standardize
Parker et al. 1994 [584]	NR	NR	Yes	NR	No	No	No	Yes	NR	NR	No	No	NR	NR	-3	3.9
Smyth and Cederbom 1994 [585]	NR	NR	NR	Yes	NR	Yes	Yes	No	NR	No	No	No	NR	NR	-1	4.6
Elvecrog et al. 1993 [586]	Yes	Yes	Yes	NR	Yes	Yes	Yes	Yes	Yes	NR	NR	NR	NR	NR	8	7.9
Parker et al. 1993 [587]	Yes	Yes	Yes	NR	NR	Yes	No	Yes	NR	NR	Yes	NR	NR	NR	5	6.8
McMahon et al. 1992 [588]	Yes	Yes	Yes	NR	Yes	Yes	No	Yes	NR	No	Yes	NR	NR	NR	5	6.8
Barreto et al. 1991 [589]	NR	NR	Yes	No: 90% malignant	NR	Yes	Yes	Yes	NR	NR	Yes	NR	NR	NR	5	6.8
Cusick et al. 1 990 [590]	NR	Yes	Yes	No: 81.3% malignant	NR	Yes	Yes	No	NR	NR	NR	NR	NR	NR	3	6.1
Parker et al. 1990[591]	Yes	No	Yes	NR	NR	Yes	Yes	No	NR	NR	NR	NR	NR	NR	2	5.7

NR = Not Reported

Table E9. Details of the Core-Needle Biopsies Performed in the Studies Addressing Key Questions 1 and 2.

Study	Number of Different People Performing Biopsies	Training of Persons Performing Biopsies	Experience of Persons Performing Biopsies	Method of Imaging Guidance	Patient Position	Biopsy Device	Number of Cores
Jackman et al. 2009[485]	4	Radiologists	0.25 to 3.75 years of experience performing stereotactic biopsies but no experience with vacuum-assisted biopsies before the study began	Stereotactic	Prone	Mammotome 11 G or 1 4G	12 or more

Study	Number of Different People Performing Biopsies	Training of Persons Performing Biopsies	Experience of Persons Performing Biopsies	Method of Imaging Guidance	Patient Position	Biopsy Device	Number of Cores
Peters et al. 2008 [486]	NR	NR	NR	Stereotactic	Prone	Biopty automated gun 14G	Range: 5 to 8
Schueller et al. 2008 [487]	2	Radiologists	Performed 100 or more biopsies before the study period began	US	Supine or decubitus	Bard automated gun 14G	Mean: 5.9 Range: 5 to 10
Sim and Kei 2008 [488]	1	Radiologist	NR	Stereotactic	Seated	Mammotome 1 1G	Mean: 13.5 Range: 2 to 36
Tonegutti and Girardi 2008 [489]	1	Radiologists	Short training period with 30 patients	Stereotactic	Prone	Mammotome 11 G	20
Youk et al. 2008[24]	9	Radiologists	7 had fellowship training, 2 had extensive clinical experience in breast imaging and biopsy	US	Supine	Pro-Mag automated gun, 14G	Mean: 5.4 cores Range: 3 to 8
Ciatto et al. 2007 [490]	13	Radiologists	NR	US or stereotactic guidance	NR	Automated gun 14G or Mammotome 11G	2 to 4
de Lucena et al. 2007 [491]	1	NR	NR	US	NR	Pro-Mag automated gun 14G	6
Uematsu et al. 2007 [492]	1	Radiologists	1 year of prior experience with the procedure	Stereotactic	Prone	Mammotome 1 1G	NR
Vag et al. 2007 [493]	NR	Radiologists	reports the device is new and they are trying it out, but the radiologist was highly experienced in breast interventions	US	NR	VACORA 10G	NR
Chapellier et al. 2006 [494]	NR	Radiologists	Device was newly acquired at start of the study	Stereotactic	NR	Mammotome	NR
Cipolla et al. 2006 [495]	NR	NR	NR	Stereotactic or US	NR	14G needle	Mean: 3 Range: 2 to 5

Table E9. (Continued).

Study	Number of Different People Performing Biopsies	Training of Persons Performing Biopsies	Experience of Persons Performing Biopsies	Method of Imaging Guidance	Patient Position	Biopsy Device	Number of Cores
Dhillon et al. 2006 [496]	NR	NR	NR	Stereotactic	Prone	Mammotome 11G	Mean: 12 Range: 6 to 18
Bolivar et al. 2005 [497]	NR	NR	NR	US	Supine	Automated gun 14G	Mean: 3.5 cores Range: 1 to 7
Crystal et al. 2005 [498]	NR	NR	NR	US	NR	Biopty automated gun 14G	Median: 4 cores Range: 1 to 8
Dillon et al. 2005 [499]	NR	NR	NR	US or stereotactic guidance or freehand	Supine or seated	Automated 14G or 16G needles	NR
Koskela et al. 2005 [500]	5	Radiologists	4 to 6 years of experience	Stereotactic	Seated	Biopty automated gun 14G	Mean: 7 cores Range: 4 to 15
Sauer et al. 2005 [501]	3	NR	Undergone dedicated training in the biopsy method	US	NR	Biopty automated gun 14G	Mean: 2
Weber et al. 2005 [502]	NR	Surgeons	5 month training period with the device before the study commenced	Stereotactic	Prone	Mammotome 11 G	NR
Wu et al. 2005 [503]	1	Surgeons	Reported to be “skilled”	US	NR	Mammotome 1 1G	NR
Alonso-Bartolome et al. 2004 [504]	NR	NR	NR	US	Supine	NR	NR
Delle and Terinde 2004 [505]	NR	NR	NR	US	NR	Automated gun	Median: 2 Range: 1 to 4
Fajardo et al. 2004 [506]	NR	Radiologists	Radiologists at each participating site performed at least 50	Stereotactic	NR	14G needle	Minimum: 5

Study	Number of Different People Performing Biopsies	Training of Persons Performing Biopsies	Experience of Persons Performing Biopsies	Method of Imaging Guidance	Patient Position	Biopsy Device	Number of Cores
			procedures before enrolling patients into the trial				
Kettritz et al. 2004 [507]	NR	Radiologists	NR	Stereotactic	Prone	Mammotome 11 G	At least 20 or remove entire lesion
Lomoschitz et al. 2004 [508]	4	Radiologists	Two were highly experienced with the procedure, two were not	Stereotactic	Prone	Mammotome 11 G	20
Abdsaleh et al. 2003 [509]	1	Radiologists	NR	Stereotactic or US	NR	Semi-automated 14G	NR
Ambrogetti et al. 2003 [510]	1	NR	NR	Stereotactic	Prone	NR	Mean: 10.2 Range: 4 to 25
Fishman et al. 2003 [511]	1	Radiologists	Person performing procedure was a resident supervised by an attending radiologist	US	NR	Bard automated gun 14G	5
Han et al. 2003 [512]	2	Radiologists	NR	Stereotactic	Prone	Biopty automated gun 14G	Mean: 7 Range: 5 to 20
Kirshenbaum et al. 2003 [513]	3	Radiologists	NR	Stereotactic	72% seated	Bard automated gun 14G or Mammotome 11G	Bard gun Mean: 5.9 Range: 1 to 11 Mammotome Mean: 5.1 Range: 4 to 8
March et al. 2003 [514]	3	Radiologists	Reports the procedure is not their usual practice	US	NR	Mammotome 11 G	Mean: 29 Range: 10 to 70
Pfleiderer et al. 2003 [515]	NR	NR	NR	MRI	Prone	Magnum automated gun 14G	Range: 3 to 6

Table E9. (Continued).

Study	Number of Different Peopl Performing Biopsies	Training of Persons Performing Biopsies	Experience of Persons Performing Biopsies	Method of Imaging Guidance	Patient Position	Biopsy Device	Number of Cores
Philpotts et al. 2003 [516]	More than 5	Radiologists	Majority of the procedures appear to have been performed by fellows and residents under the supervision of 5 experienced breast radiologists	US	Supine	US Biopty automated gun 14G or Mammotome 1 1G	Biopty Mean: 4.7 Range: 1 to 17 Mammotome Mean: 5.8 Range: 1 to 12
Wong and Hisham 2003 [517]	NR	NR	NR	Freehand	NR	Bard automated gun 14 or 16G	NR
Apesteguia et al. 2002 [518]	NR	Radiologists	NR	Stereotactic	Prone	Mammotome 1 1G	Mean: 10.7 Range: 1 to 26
Georgian-Smith et al. 2002 [519]	NR	Radiologists	NR	Stereotactic	Most seated	Mammotome 11 G	Mean: 9.5 Range: 5 to 26
Jackman and Lamm 2002 [520]	NR	Radiologists	NR	Stereotactic	Prone	Biopty automated gun 14G or Mammotome 11G or 14G	Median 14 Range: 5 to 30
Johnson et al. 2002 [521]	NR	NR	No experience at the beginning of the study	US	Supine	Mammotome 11 G or 8G	Attempt to completely remove lesion
Liberman et al. 2002522	NR	NR	NR	Stereotactic	Prone	Mammotome 11G	Median: 15 Range: 4 to 47
Meloni et al. 2002523	NR	NR	NR	Stereotactic	Seated	Vacuum-assisted	Mean: 12 Range: 3 to 14
Morris et al. 2002 [524]	NR	NR	NR	Stereotactic	Prone	Mammotome 14G	NR
Pfarl et al. 2002 [525]	More than 7	Radiologists	7 had an average of 2.6 (Range: 0 to 18) procedures before the study commenced; non specified number of residents in training	Stereotactic	Prone	Mammotome 1 1G	15 to 20

Study	Number of Different People Performing Biopsies	Training of Persons Performing Biopsies	Experience of Persons Performing Biopsies	Method of Imaging Guidance	Patient Position	Biopsy Device	Number of Cores
			had no experience before the study commenced				
Verkooijen et al. COBRA 2002 [526]	More than 5	Radiologists	radiologists first attended 10 biopsy procedures and subsequently they performed another 10 under the supervision of a radiologist with considerable experience	Stereotactic	Prone	Bard automated gun 14G	NR
Becker et al. 2001 [527]	4	Radiologists	NR	Stereotactic	Seated	14G needle	NR
Brenner et al. 2001 [528]	NR	NR	All took a two-day course	Stereotactic	Prone	Automated gun 14G	5 or more
Cangiarella et al. 2001529	NR	Radiologists	NR	Stereotactic	Prone	Mammotome 11 G	Mean: 11 Range: 7 to 15
Dahlstrom and Jain 2001 [530]	NR	NR	NR	Stereotactic	NR	Biopty automated gun 14G	5
Lai et al. 2001 [531]	NR	NR	NR	Stereotactic	Prone	Mammotome 11G	Mean: 17.2
Levin et al. 2001 [532]	3	Radiologists	2 of 3 radiologists had prior training in stereotactic core biopsy and attended a two-day course on use of the add-on unit; these two taught the third radiologist	Stereotactic	Seated	BIP automated gun 14G	5
Margolin et al. 2001 [533]	3	Radiologists	NR	Stereotactic or US	Prone	Automated 14G, 16G, or 18G gun or Mammotome 11G or 14G	NR

Table E9. (Continued).

Study	Number of Different People Performing Biopsies	Training of Persons Performing Biopsies	Experience of Persons Performing Biopsies	Method of Imaging Guidance	Patient Position	Biopsy Device	Number of Cores
Perez-Fuentes et al . 2001 534	NR	NR	NR	US	Supine	Mammotome 11G	Median: 17 Range: 8 to 40
Smith et al. 2001 [535]	NR	NR	NR	US	NR	Automated 14G gun	NR
White et al. 2001 [536]	NR	Radiologists	NR	Stereotactic or US	Prone or supine	Automated 14G gun or Mammotome 11G or 14G	NR
Wunderbaldinger et al. 2001 [537]	1	Radiologists	Performed 30 procedures on phantoms prior to the study	US	Seated	Magnum automated gun 14G	Mean: 6 Range: 3 to 10
Yeow et al. 2001538	1	Radiologists	NR	US	NR	Automated gun 14G or 16G	Mean: 3.4 Range: 1 to 7
Beck et al. 2000 [539]	NR	NR	NR	Stereotactic	Prone	Mammotome 11G	NR
Kirwan et al. 2000540	NR	NR	NR	Stereotactic	Prone	Automated gun 14G	NR
Latosinsky et al. 2000 [541]	NR	NR	NR	Stereotactic or US	Prone for stereotactic	Automated gun or vacuum-assisted 1 4G	NR
Liberman et al. 2000542	NR	NR	NR	US or stereotactic	NR	Automated 14G gun	Median: 4 Range: 1 to 7
Makoske et al. 2000 [543]	More than 1	Radiologists and surgeons	No experience in the procedure at the beginning of study; they were, however, trained and credentialed.	Stereotactic	NR	Automated gun or Mammotome	Minimum: 5
Ward et al. 2000 [544]	2	Radiologists	Radiologists described as "specialize in breast imaging and diagnosis"	Stereotactic	NR	Bard automated gun 14G or 16G	Mean: 11 Range: 4 to 18
Welle et al. 2000 [545]	NR	NR	NR	Stereotactic	Most decubitus	Bard automated gun 14G or Mammotome 11 G	3 to 16

Study	Number of Different People Performing Biopsies	Training of Persons Performing Biopsies	Experience of Persons Performing Biopsies	Method of Imaging Guidance	Patient Position	Biopsy Device	Number of Cores
Helbich et al. 1999 [546]	1	Radiologists	NR	Stereotactic	Seated	Patients randomized to various automated biopsy guns with different needle G	NR
Jackman et al. 1999 [547]	NR	NR	NR	Stereotactic	Prone	Biopty automated gun 14G	Mean: 8.1 Range: 2 to 20
Meyer et al. 1999 [548]	NR	NR	NR	Stereotactic	Prone	Automated gun 14G or Mammotome 11G or 14G	Mean: 5 to 8
Puglisi et al. 1999 [549]	NR	NR	NR	Perforated compression grid	NR	Automated gun 14G	Median: 5
Soo et al. 1999 [550]	4	Radiologists	NR	Stereotactic	Prone	Magnum automated gun 14G or Mammotome 14G	Automated gun Mean: 5.8 Mammotome Mean: 15.8
Caruso et al. 1998 [551]	1	Surgeons	Reports "experienced surgeon"	Freehand	NR	Trucut 18G	NR
Doyle et al. 1998 [552]	NR	NR	No experience with the procedure at the beginning of the study	Stereotactic	Decubitus	Pro-Mag automated gun 14G	NR
Fuhrman et al. 1998 [553]	3	Radiologists	Reports "radiologists with expertise in breast imaging"	Stereotactic or US	Stereotactic prone, US supine	Automated gun 14G	At least 5
Heywang-Kobrunner et al. 1998554	NR	NR	NR	Stereotactic	Prone	Mammotome 11G or 14G	NR
Ioffe et al. 1998 [555]	NR	NR	NR	Stereotactic or US	NR	Bard automated gun 14G	At least 5

Table E9. (Continued).

Study	Number of Different People Performing Biopsies	Training of Persons Performing Biopsies	Experience of Persons Performing Biopsies	Method of Imaging Guidance	Patient Position	Biopsy Device	Number of Cores
Liberman et al. 1998 [556]	NR	NR	NR	US	Supine	Pro-Mag automated gun 14G	Median: 4 Range: 2 to 7
Schulz-Wendtland et al. 1998 [557]	NR	NR	NR	US	NR	14G needle	1 to 3
Vega-Bolivar et al. 1998 [558]	1	Radiologists	NR	Stereotactic	NR	Surecut 15G	At least 2
Whitman et al. 1998 [559]	NR	NR	NR	Stereotactic	NR	Monopty 16G	NR
Zannis and AliaNo 1998 [560]	1	Surgeons	NR	Stereotactic	Prone	Trucut 14G or Mammotome 14G or 11G	Trucut Mean: 4.8 cores Range: 1 to 7 Mammotome at least 16
Bauer et al. 1997 [561]	NR	NR	NR	Stereotactic	Prone or seated	BIP automated gun 14G	Mean: 9 Range: 1 to 13
Britton et al. 1997 [562]	4	Radiologists	NR	Stereotactic or US	Supine for US	Automated gun 14, 16, or 18G	Mean: 5
Helbich et al. 1997 [563]	1	Radiologists	Described as an "expert"	Stereotactic or US	Prone or supine or seated	Automated gun 14G	NR
Khattar et al. 1997 [564]	NR	Surgeons	NR	US	Supine	Pro-Mag automated gun	2 or 3
Liberman et al. 1997 [565]	NR	NR	NR	Stereotactic	Prone	Biopty-cut 14G	Mean: 6 Range: 1 to 22
Pitre et al. 1997 [566]	NR	NR	NR	Stereotactic	Prone	Pro-Mag automated gun	Mean: 5
Stolier et al. 1997 [567]	1	Surgeons	No experience in the procedure at the beginning of study	Stereotactic	Prone	Automated gun 14G or Mammotome	Minimum: 5

Study	Number of Different People Performing Biopsies	Training of Persons Performing Biopsies	Experience of Persons Performing Biopsies	Method of Imaging Guidance	Patient Position	Biopsy Device	Number of Cores
Sutton, et al. 1997 [568]	5	Radiologists	All involved radiologists have experience in mammography and interventional techniques in breast disease diagnosis	Stereotactic	Prone	Biopty automated gun 14G	NR
Walker et al. 1997 [569]	NR	NR	NR	Stereotactic	NR	Automated gun 14G	Minimum: 5
Frazee et al. 1996 [570]	NR	Radiologists	NR	Stereotactic	Prone	NR	Minimum: 5
Fuhrman et al. 1996 [571]	NR	NR	NR	Stereotactic	Prone	Automated gun 14G	Minimum: 5
Head and Haynes 1996 [572]	NR	NR	NR	Stereotactic	Prone	Biopty automated gun 18G	NR
Mainiero et al. 1996 [573]	NR	NR	NR	Stereotactic	Prone	Biopty automated gun 14G	NR
Meyer et al. 1996 [574]	NR	Radiologists	NR	Stereotactic	Prone	Biopty automated gun 14G	NR
Nguyen et al. 1996 [575]	NR	NR	NR	Stereotactic or US	Prone	Automated gun 14G	5 to 10
Pettine et al. 1996 [576]	NR	NR	NR	Stereotactic	Prone	Biopty automated 14G gun	5 to 9
Rosenblatt et al. 1996 [577]	NR	NR	NR	Stereotactic	Prone	Biopty automated gun 14G	NR
Scopa et al. 1996 [578]	NR	NR	NR	Freehand	NR	TruCut	NR
Cross et al. 1995 [579]	NR	NR	NR	Stereotactic	Prone	Bard automated gun 14G	Mean: 3.4 Range: 1 to 8

Table E9. (Continued).

Study	Number of Different People Performing Biopsies	Training of Persons Performing Biopsies	Experience of Persons Performing Biopsies	Method of Imaging Guidance	Patient Position	Biopsy Device	Number of Cores
Doyle et al. 1995 [580]	NR	NR	NR	Stereotactic or US	Prone	Automated gun 14G or 15G	NR
Hamed et al. 1995 [581]	NR	NR	NR	Freehand	NR	Biopty automated gun 14G or 18G	Mean: 3
Burbank et al. 1994 [582]	NR	NR	NR	Stereotactic or US	NR	NR	NR
Gisvold et al. 1994 [583]	7	Radiologists	All attended a training session before performing any procedures	Stereotactic	Prone	Biopty automated gun 14G	Minimum: 5
Parker et al. 1994 [584]	NR	Radiologists	The radiologists participated in a two-day training session before the study commenced	Freehand	NR	Biopty automated gun 14G	NR
Smyth and Cederbom 1994 [585]	NR	NR	NR	Stereotactic	Prone	Automated gun	NR
Elvecrog et al. 1993 [586]	2	Radiologists	NR	Stereotactic	Prone	Biopty automated gun 14G	Minimum: 5
Parker et al. 1993 [587]	NR	Radiologists	NR	US	Supine	Biopty automated gun 14G	4 to 5
McMahon et al. 1992 [588]	More than 8	Surgeons	NR	Freehand	NR	Various 14 to 18G devices	1
Barreto et al. 1991 [589]	NR	NR	No experience at the beginning of the study	Freehand	NR	Biopty automated gun 18G	1
Cusick et al. 1990 [590]	NR	NR	NR	Freehand	NR	NR	NR
Parker et al. 1990 [591]	4	Radiologists	NR	Stereotactic	NR	Biopty automated gun 14, 16, or 18G	NR

NR = Not Reported

Table E 10. Patient Inclusion/Exclusion Criteria for Studies Addressing Key Questions 1 and 2.

Study	Patient Inclusion Criteria	Patient Exclusion Criteria
Jackman et al. 2009485	Consecutive patients referred for core-needle biopsy between March 1995 through December 2001	Weighed more than 300 lbs; had bleeding diathesis; use of anti-coagulants that could not be discontinued (but no patients had these conditions during the study period).
Peters et al. 2008486	All patients with nonpalpable lesions referred for core-needle biopsy between February 2000 and June 2002	Coagulopathies or the use of anti-coagulants that could not be discontinued and an inability to stay in the prone positionfor one hour
Schueller et al. 2008487	All patients referred to the center for core-needle biopsy between January 1995 and February 2004	Patients unable to cooperate with the procedure or had a bleeding diathesis
Sim and Kei et al. 2008488	All patients with microcalcifications referred for core-needle biopsy between November 2002 and August 2005	NR
Tonegutti and Girardi 2008489	Women with suspicious nonpalpable mammographic lesions (microcalcifications, mass with or without microcalcifications, architectural distortion) not recognisable by ultrasound	NR
Youk et al. 200824	All patients undergoing US-guided core-needle biopsy between February 2000 and June 2005	NR
Ciatto et al. 2007490	All consecutive core-needle biopsies performed at the study center between January 1996 and March 2005	NR
de Lucena et al. 2007491	NR	NR
Uematsu et al. 2007492	Consecutivepatients with mammographically-detected microcalcifications BIRADS 3, 4, or 5 whose lesions were not visible on US	Unable to provide consent or undergo MRI imaging due to pacemaker, claustrophobia, or metallic clip; blood coagulation disorder; currently being treated with anti-coagulants; unable to cooperate with the biopsy procedure
Vag et al. 2007493	NR	NR
Chapellier et al. 2006494	Core-needle biopsies performed between January 2001 to November 2002	NR
Cipolla et al. 2006495	Consecutive patients undergoing core-needle biopsy at the center between September 1999 to February 2004	NR
Dhillon et al. 2006496	The first 150 consecutive patients who met these criteria: all indeterminate calcifications; distortions or masses not seen on US; a non-diagnostic biopsy on US; problem cases referred from other units	NR

Table E 10. (Continued).

Study	Patient Inclusion Criteria	Patient Exclusion Criteria
Bolivar et al. 2005497	All patients with suspicious non-palpable breast lumps who underwent US-guided biopsy between August 1997 to April 2001	NR
Crystal et al. 2005498	Patients with US visible solid breast lesions referred for biopsy between October 1, 1998 and September 1, 2001	Lesions that appeared to be radial scars were excluded
Dillon et al. 2005499	All women who underwent biopsy at the center between January1999 to September 2003	NR
Koskela et al. 2005500	Between June 1998 and January 2001, all patients with lesions not visible on US who were scheduled for core-needle stereotactic biopsy	Lesions located too high or too close to the chest wall such that it could not be reached by the stereotactic equipment
Sauer et al. 2005501	All patients undergoing US biopsy of lesions detected on routine screening over a 28 month period	NR
Weber et al. 2005 [502]	All patients between October 1999 to August 2003 with mammographically suspicious but nonpalpable lesions	Breast too small, lesion too close to the chest wall, lesion not evident on image
Wu et al. 2005 [503]	Patients suspected of having benign lesions who underwent vacuum-assisted biopsy between July 2000 and July 2003	NR
Alonso-Bartolome et al. 2004 [504]	Patients with "probably benign" lesions	NR
Delle and Terinde 2004 [505]	Patients referred to the clinic because of palpable or non-palpable lesions or because of suspicion of cancer on mammography between September 2000 and September 2001	NR
Fajardo et al. 2004 [506]	NR	Lesions located in prior lumpectomy or radiation therapy site, known bleeding disorder or anticoagulant therapy, pregnancy, allergy to local anesthesia, breast implants, psychiatric or neurologic conditions limiting patient's ability to cooperate during biopsy and/or provide informed consent
Kettritz et al. 2004 [507]	NR	NR
Lomoschitz et al. 2004 [508]	Consecutive women with solitary non-palpable lesions referred for 1 1G mammotome between February 1999 and July 2000, consecutive until 50 women with mammographic masses and 50 women with microcalcifications were enrolled	NR
Abdsaleh et al. 2003 [509]	Consecutive patients between August 2000 and December 2001	NR
Ambrogetti et al. 2003 [510]	Consecutive nonpalpable isolated microcalcifications detected in routine screening considered suspicious enough to warrant investigation between	NR

Study	Patient Inclusion Criteria	Patient Exclusion Criteria
	February 1999 and June 2002	
Fishman et al. 2003 [511]	Consecutive patients referred for an US-guided biopsy over a 7-month period	Lesion turned out to be a cyst, pathological material was lost in one case, and in two cases ad hoc exclusion because the pathologist involved in the study had come to a different diagnosis than the "routine" pathology reading
Han et al. 2003 [512]	Nonpalpable calcifications referred between April 1997- March 2002	NR
Kirshenbaum et al. 2003 [513]	All patients undergoing stereotactic core-needle biopsy between October 1994 and February 2001 with nonpalpable lesions.	NR
March et al. 2003 [514]	Patients referred to two outpatient centers between August 2000 and October 2001 for US-guided biopsy of a single breast lesion well-visualized on US and located at least 0.5 cm from the skin and pectoralis margin and at least 2 cm from the nipple with the lesion measuring 1.2 cm or less in diameter	Lesion turned out to be a cyst
Pfleiderer et al. 2003 [515]	Women were invited after an MRI exam that found lesions with suspicious contrast enhancement, reasons why they had the MRI exam not reported	Pregnancy or lactation, coagulation abnormalities, allergies to local anesthetics or MRI contrast agents, compressed breast thickness less than 25 mm
Philpotts et al. 2003 [516]	All patients who underwent US-guided biopsy between January 1997 and August 2001	NR
Wong and Hisham 2003 [517]	Consecutive biopsies of palpable breast lesions from May 2000 to May 2001	Nonpalpable lesion, less than 6 months followup
Apesteguia et al. 2002 [518]	All cases detected between April and December 1999 with suspicious non-palpable lesion which could not be reliably detected by US	NR
Georgian-Smith et al. 2002 [519]	Consecutive patients between June 1999 and August 2000	NR
Jackman and Lamm 2002 [520]	All patients who underwent core-needle biopsy between July 1991 and December 1999 who had breast implants	NR
Johnson et al. 2002 [521]	All patients with probably benign lesions scheduled for US-guided mammotome excisional attempt between April 2000 to January 2002	NR
Liberman et al. 2002 [522]	Consecutive lesions undergoing stereotactic biopsy between October 31, 1996 to March 8, 2001. Indications for biopsy were nonpalpable lesions suspicious of malignancy, calcifications or masses 0.5 cm or less or masses that could not be viewed on US	Bleeding diathesis, patient unable to cooperate, lesion could not be targeted
Meloni et al. 2002 [523]	All cases of non-palpable mammographically detected lesions undergoing	NR

Table E 10. (Continued).

Study	Patient Inclusion Criteria	Patient Exclusion Criteria
	vacuum-assisted core-needle biopsy at the center between December 1999 and November 2000	
Morris et al. 2002 [524]	Twenty-one nonpalpable masses seen on mammography in 19 women who gave informed consent.The masses on mammography had no associated calcifications and were classified as either BI-RADS 4 (n = 17) or 5 (n = 4) lesions.	NR
Pfarl et al. 2002 [525]	All patients undergoing 1 1G Mammotome biopsy from September 1997 to December 2001	Unable to cooperate with the procedure, had a bleeding diathesis
Verkooijen et al. COBRA 2002 [526]	Nonpalpable breast lesions requiring histologic exam enrolled in 19 Dutch hospitals	Coagulotherapies or use of anticoagulants that could not be discontinued, inability to maintain prone position for one hour, inability to comprehend study protocol
Becker et al. 2001 [527]	Biopsies performed for microcalcifications at the center between November 1993 and January 1997	NR
Brenner et al. 2001 [528]	NR	NR
Cangiarella et al. 2001 [529]	Patients with indeterminate microcalcifications that had been detected by routine screening and had no evidence of a mammographic density or mass biopsied between January 1997 and December 1997	NR
Dahlstrom and Jain 2001 [530]	Women with suspicious calcifications detected on routine screening between July 1993 and August 1998	NR
Lai et al. 2001 [531]	Consecutive patients who underwent biopsy between September 1997 and March 2000	NR
Levin et al. 2001 [532]	Women with a single non-palpable lesion detected during a routine mammography and scheduled for a lumpectomy. Spiculated lesions, indeterminate nodules, indeterminate calcifications, and localized asymmetric density were eligible.	Palpable lesion, radial scar, bleeding diathesis, lesion not well visualized, in a difficult location
Margolin et al. 2001 [533]	All patients who underwent core biopsy between January 1994 and December 1998	NR

Study	Patient Inclusion Criteria	Patient Exclusion Criteria
	benign. Selectively used for solid lesions that were suspicious and measured 2 cm or less. Solid lesions that were suggestive of malignancy and measured 1 cm or less. Complex lesions, intraductal lesions, subtle lesions, cysts with mural thickening, intramural nodules, or thick septations regardless of size; lesions suspected of being radial scars or papillomas; other lesions; occasional probably benign lesions 2 cm or less.	
Smith et al. 2001 [535]	Betweeen August 1991 and February 1998, women referred for US-guided biopsy because of non-calcificied US visible masses	NR
White et al. 2001 [536]	All patients who had image-guided core-needle biopsy at the center between August 1992 and February 1999	NR
Wunderbaldinger et al. 2001 [537]	Patients scheduled to undergo open biopsy for non-palpable breast lesions	NR
Yeow et al. 2001 [538]	Consecutive patients referred for needle biopsy January 1995 to October 1997 with palpable breast masses	Lesion was identified as a cyst
Beck et al. 2000 [539]	Until April 1999 patients with indeterminate lesions who were sent for biopsy	NR
Kirwan et al. 2000 [540]	Women with mammographically-detected stellate lesions with or without microcalcifications	NR
Latosinsky et al. 2000 [541]	Between November 1994 to May 1998, all patients who underwent core biopsy	NR
Liberman et al. 2000 [542]	Patients with palpable lesions who underwent core-needle biopsy betweeen August 1992 and May 1998	NR
Makoske et al. 2000 [543]	All eligible patients from 1993 through 1998, those with nonpalpable lesions found on mammography who were sent for biopsy	NR
Ward et al. 2000 [544]	Patients with indeterminate microcalcifications sent for core biopsy between November 1993 and January 1997	Cases with associated mass, distortion, or palpable lesion were excluded
Welle et al. 2000 [545]	Patients with stereotactic core-needle biopies performed between September 1995 trhough March 1999	NR
Helbich et al. 1999 [546]	NR	NR
Jackman et al. 1999 [547]	Consecutive patients with nonpalpable lesions who had stereotactic core-needle biopsy between July 1991 and December 1993	NR
Meyer et al. 1999 [548]	Patients seen between August 1991 and December 31, 1997 for suspicious nonpalpable breast abnormalities	NR

Table E 10. (Continued).

Study	Patient Inclusion Criteria	Patient Exclusion Criteria
Puglisi et al. 1999 [549]	Consecutive patients seen from July 1992-December 1997	US-guided procedures
Soo et al. 1999 [550]	Patients with noncalcified, nonpalpable, mammographically-detected lesions referred for biopsy between October 1995 and August 1997	NR
Caruso et al. 1998[551]	From 1990 to 1995, a consecutive series of 91 patients	NR
Doyle et al. 1998 [552]	Patients who underwent stereotactic core-needle biopsy between September 1994 and March 1998	NR
Fuhrman et al. 1998 [553]	All nonpalpable breast lesions from July 1993-February 1997 that underwent image-guided core needle breast biopsy.	Palpable masses, lesions not clearly visualized in the stereotactic unit (usually lesions deep in the breast along the chest wall), lesions found in small breasts which compress to <2 cm in the stereotactic unit, asymmetric dense breast tissue, unable to tolerate the prone position for 30 minutes.
Heywang-Kobrunner et al. 1998 [554]	Patients referred for biopsy up to March 1997	NR
Ioffe et al. 1998 [555]	Consecutive core-needle biopsies between July 1995 and January 1997	NR
Liberman et al. 1998 [556]	Patients with a solitary, nonpalpable mass who underwent US-guided biopsy between May 1993 and June 1997	The parenchyma was too thin to support the excursion of the needle, a hemorrhagic diathesis, unable to cooperate, or the lesion was less than 5 mm
Schulz-Wendtland et al. 1998 [557]	Patients who underwent US-guided biopsies between May 1992 and April 1993	NR
Vega-Bolivar et al. 1998 [558]	Patients seen between October 1993-October 1996 for nonpalpable breast lesions	NR
Whitman et al. 1998 [559]	Mammographically-guided coaxial core-needle biopsy procedures performed with a fenestrated alphanumeric compression device between 1995-1997	NR
Zannis and AliaNo 1998 [560]	Consecutive records of patients undergoing a stereotactic procedure and biopsy by the same surgeon for a non-palpable, mammographically-detected lesion between January 1993 and August 1997	NR
Bauer et al. 1997 [561]	Mammographically-detected breast lesions considered worrisome enough to require biopsy, such as clustered microcalcifications, a spiculated mass, or an area of architectural distortion during the 30 months from July 1, 1993 to January 1, 1996.	NR
Britton et al. 1997 [562]	All patients after April 1994 who were recalled for core-needle biopsy after routine mammographic screening	NR

Study	Patient Inclusion Criteria	Patient Exclusion Criteria
Helbich et al. 1997 [563]	Consecutive patients with solid breast lesions over 20 months	NR
Khattar et al. 1997 [564]	Between February 1993 and March 1995, patients over 18 years of age with a palpable mass scheduled for surgical excision	Lesion was revealed to be a simple cyst on US
Liberman et al. 1997565	Patients who underwent stereotactic core biopsy between August 7, 1992 and December 14, 1995	Thickness of compressed breast was inadequate to accommodate the needle; the lesion measured less than 5 mm in diameter; the lesion could not be targeted accurately; the patient had a bleeding diathesis; the patient was on anticoagulants; the patient was unable to cooperatewith the procedure.
Pitre et al. 1997566	Patients who had stereotactic core-needle biopsy for a nonpalpable unicentric mammographically-detected breast lesion between January 1994 and February 1995	NR
Stolier et al. 1997567	All patients who underwent core-needle biopsy at the center by the study author from August 1993 through May 1996	NR
Sutton, et al. 1997568	Women who elected to have stereotactic-guided large-gauge core biopsy between July 1993 and June 1995 after detection of suspicious non-palpable abnormalities at a mammographic screening clinic	Initially, women with abnormalities considered to be obviously malignant were excluded from the series (from July to December 1993) but after the first 70 patients, thesehighly suspicious lesions were offered core biopsy
Walker et al. 1997569	All patients who had stereotactic core-needle for a nonpalpable lesion since 1993	NR
Frazee et al. 1996570	Patients with nonpalpable mammographic abnormality between July1994 to June 1995	NR
Fuhrman etal. 1996571	All non-palpable suspicious masses and calcifications noted on mammography from July 1993 - January 1995	Lesions not clearly visualized in the stereotactic unit, usually lesions deep within the breast along the chest wall, lesions found in small breasts which compress to less than 2cm in the stereotactic unit, asymmetric dense breast tissue, and patients unable to tolerate the prone position for30 minutes
Head and Haynes 1996572	Patients with nonpalpable breast lesions discovered during routine mammography	NR
Mainiero et al. 1996573	Patients with microcalcifications were considered indeterminate or suspicious for malignancy	Lesions in which calcifications were within a mass or an area of architectural distortion
Meyer et al. 1996574	Clinically occult suspicious mammographic abnormalities. The mass must be at least 6mm in diameter and be clearly visible on mammography	NR
Nguyen et al.1996575	All core-needle biopsies performed between December 1992 andJune 1995	NR

Table E 10. (Continued).

Study	Patient Inclusion Criteria	Patient Exclusion Criteria
Pettine et al. 1996576	Patients with nonpalable lesions discovered on mammogram followed immediately by wire localized biopsy	NR
Rosenblatt et al. 1996577	All patients who underwent biopsy of multiple unilateral lesions between January 1994 and September 1995	NR
Scopa et al. 1996578	Patients undergoing Tru-Cut biopsies who had not been previously investigated with fine-needle aspiration	NR
Cross et al. 1995579	Patients who were referred to the center for stereotactic biopsy of a nonpalpable mammographic abnormality	NR.
Doyle et al. 1995 [580]	Mammographically-detected impalpable breast lesions, completely well-circumscribed masses less than 8mm in diameter with smooth borders. Opacities containing fat or with concave margins, clusters or uniform tiny rounded calcifications, scattered calcifications, and scattered nodules. Lesions considered strongly suggestive of cancer included new spiculated masses, new clustered pleomorphic calcifications, or both.	Inability to provide informed consent and irreversible bleeding diathesis
Hamed et al. 1995 [581]	Female patients with clinically suspected breast carcinoma	Patients with locally advanced breast carcinoma
Burbank et al. 1994 [582]	NR	Patients who underwent bone biopsies
Gisvold et al. 1994 [583]	All patients referred for wire-localized open surgery between October 19, 1991 and January 15, 1993 were considered for the study. The inclusion criteria are: If it appeared the lesion and patient were suitable (patient could lie prone for an hour, no bleeding problems, and no allergy to local anesthesia; lesions thought to be visualizable and were not too superficial or close to the nipple).	Equipment or radiologist not available, lesion visualizable only on US
Parker et al. 1994 [584]	Core-needle biopsies performed at sites at which the radiologists and assisting technologists had undergone dedicated training in larger core breast biopsy and had followed a standard protocol	NR
Smyth and Cederbom 1994 [585]	Patients with mammographically suspicious non palpable lesions	NR
Elvecrog et al. 1993 [586]	Patients with single non-palpable mammographic lesion; study restricted to patients who would have undergone open biopsy if core biopsy wasn't available	Lesions less than 5 mm in diameter
Parker et al. 1993 [587]	Consecutive patients with solid or indeterminate breast lesions visualized by US between August 1989 and July 1991	NR

Study	Patient Inclusion Criteria	Patient Exclusion Criteria
McMahon et al. 1992 [588]	Consecutive patients with palpable breast lumps between September 1989 and August 1991	NR
Barreto et al. 1991 [589]	Symptomatic patients with palpable breast lumps suspected of having early breast cancer who were scheduled for open surgical excision	NR
Cusick et al. 1990 [590]	Patients with suggestive mammary lumps seen at the surgery clinic of San Bernardino County Medical Center	NR
Parker et al. 1990 [591]	During a 13-month period, consecutive patients who underwent stereotactic-needle core breast biopsies	NR

NR = Not Reported

Table E 11. Characteristics of Patients Enrolled in Studies Addressing Key Questions 1 and 2.

Study	Number of Patients Recruited for Enrollment	Number of Patients Enrolled	Number of Lesions Enrolled	Age	Age Dispersion	Ethnicity
Jackman et al. 2009 [485]	1,152	1,152	1,280	NR	NR	NR
Peters et al. 2008 [486]	955	948	948	NR	NR	NR
Schueller et al. 2008 [487]	1390	1390	1438	Median: 51	Range: 15 to 93	NR
Sim and Kei et al. 2008 [488]	106	97	105	Mean: 53.2	Range: 36 to 81	Asian: 100%
Tonegutti and Girardi 2008 [489]	268	268	268	Mean: 52	Range: 22-79	NR
Youk et al. 200824	4,359	4,359	4,359	Median: 45 Mean: 45.3	Range: 12 to 88	NR
Ciatto et al. 2007 [490]	4,035	4,035	4,035	NR	NR	NR
de Lucena et al. 2007 [491]	NR	144	150	Mean: 50	Range: 15 to 89 Standard deviation:16	NR

Table E 11. (Continued).

Study	Number of Patients Recruited for Enrollment	Number of Patients Enrolled	Number of Lesions Enrolled	Age	Age Dispersion	Ethnicity
de Lucena et al. 2007 [491]	NR	144	150	Mean: 50	Range: 15 to 89 Standard deviation:16	NR
Uematsu et al. 2007 [492]	NR	96	100	Mean: 49.4	Range: 28 to 85	NR
Vag et al. 2007 [493]	NR	65	70	Median: 57	Range: 31 to 82	NR
Chapellier et al. 2006 [494]	NR	301	318	Mean: 56	Range: 35 to 78, 64% postmenopausal	NR
Cipolla et al. 2006 [495]	426	426	426	64% post-menopausal	NR	NR
Dhillon et al. 2006 [496]	150	150	150	Median: 56	Range: 37 to 77	NR
Bolivar et al. 2005 [497]	208	208	214	Mean: 55	Range: 32 to 87	NR
Crystal et al. 2005 [498]	652	652	715	NR	NR	NR
Dillon et al. 2005 [499]	2,427 (lesions)	NR	2,427	NR	NR	NR
Koskela et al. 2005 [500]	212	205	213	Mean: 56	Range: 32 to 88	NR
Sauer et al. 2005 [501]	906	906	962	NR	NR	NR
Weber et al. 2005 [502]	239	225	225	Median: 56.1	Range: 30 to 84	NR
Wu et al. 2005 [503]	113	113	113	Median: 31	Range: 18 to 35	NR
Alonso-Bartolome et al. 2004 [504]	97	97	102	Mean: 42	Range: 18 to 77	NR
Delle and Terinde 2004 [505]	146	146	169	NR	NR	NR
Fajardo et al. 2004 [506]	2,403	2,403	2,403	Mean: 54.6	Range: 25 to 89	% White European descent: 1,313

Study	Number of Patients Recruited for Enrollment	Number of Patients Enrolled	Number of Lesions Enrolled	Age	Age Dispersion	Ethnicity
						(78.1%) % Black African descent: 265 (15.8%) % Asian descent: 27 (1.6%) % Hispanic descent: 62 (3.7%) % other, please specify: 6 Native American (0.4%), 8 another race (0.5%)
Kettritz et al. 2004 [507]	2,939	NR	2,893	NR	NR	NR
Lomoschitz et al. 2004 [508]	100	100	100	Median: 55	Range: 31 to 81	NR
Abdsaleh et al. 2003 [509]	180	180	180	NR	Range: 35 to 93	NR
Ambrogetti et al. 2003 [510]	364	364	364	Mean: 54.9	Range: 33 to 81	NR
Fishman et al. 2003 [511]	75	70	73	NR	NR	NR
Han et al. 2003 [512]	284 (lesions)	267	271	Mean: 47 yrs	Range: 23 to 72	NR
Kirshenbaum et al. 2003 [513]	492	492	506	Mean: 59.1	Range: 27 to 78	NR
March et al. 2003 [514]	57	34	34	NR	NR	NR
Pfleiderer et al. 2003 [515]	NR	14	14	Mean: 47.9	Standard deviation: 13.1	NR
Philpotts et al. 2003 [516]	271	271	281	NR	NR	NR

Table E 11. (Continued).

Study	Number of Patients Recruited for Enrollment	Number of Patients Enrolled	Number of Lesions Enrolled	Age	Age Dispersion	Ethnicity
Wong and Hisham 2003 [517]	NR	145	150	NR	Range: 20 to 80	% Asian descent: 80% % other, please specify: 18% Indian 2% "other"
Apesteguia et al. 2002 [518]	126	126	132	Mean: 50.5	Range: 29 to 81 Standard deviation: 10.2	NR
Georgian-Smith et al. 2002 [519]	179	179	185	Mean: 54.6	Range: 35 to 85	NR
Jackman and Lamm 2002 [520]	25	25	31	Median: 58	Range: 35 to 75	NR
Johnson et al. 2002 [521]	81	81	101	Mean: 46.8	Range: 21 to 72	NR
Liberman et al. 2002 [522]	797	797	800	Median: 57	Range: 28 to 88	NR
Meloni et al. 2002 [523]	138	129	129	NR	NR	NR
Morris et al. 2002 [524]	NR	19	21	Mean: 57	Range: 36 to 75	NR
Pfarl et al. 2002 [525]	332 (lesions)	325	332	Median: 56	Range: 28 to 83	NR
Verkooijen et al. COBRA 2002 [526]	973	928	984	Mean: 58	Range: 29 to 85	NR
Becker et al. 2001 [527]	218	218	232	Mean: 57.3	Range: 33 to 84	NR
Brenner et al. 2001 [528]	NR	1003	1003	NR	NR	NR
Cangiarella et al. 2001 [529]	142	142	160	Mean: 53.5	Range: 34 to 79	NR

Study	Number of Patients Recruited for Enrollment	Number of Patients Enrolled	Number of Lesions Enrolled	Age	Age Dispersion	Ethnicity
Dahlstrom and Jain 2001 [530]	266	discrepancy: study reports data for 301 core biopsies but states in methods that 266 women with 274 lesions were enrolled	310	NR	NR	NR
Lai et al. 2001 [531]	650	650	673	Mean: 54.7	Range: 22 to 89 Standard deviation: 11.6	NR
Levin et al. 2001 [532]	NR	70	70	NR	Range: 39 to 80	NR
Margolin et al. 2001 [533]	1,183	1,183	1,333	Mean: split into three groups 55, 52, 40	Range: 17 to 93	NR
Perez-Fuentes et al. 2001 [534]	88 (lesions)	83	88	Median: 48	Range: 25 to 78	NR
Smith et al. 2001 [535]	446	446	500	Median: 46 Mean: 47	Range: 18 to 89	NR
White et al. 2001 [536]	939	939	1042	Median: 60	Range: 32 to 85	NR
Wunderbaldinger et al. 2001 [537]	NR	45	45	Mean: 50	Range: 20 to 77	NR
Yeow et al. 2001 [538]	104	98	98	Mean: 46.5	Range: 23 to 85 Standard deviation: 12.3	NR
Beck et al. 2000 [539]	560	560	594	NR	NR	NR
Kirwan et al. 2000 [540]	NR	72	72	NR	NR	NR
Latosinsky et al. 2000 [541]	607	607	692	NR	NR	NR
Liberman et al. 2000 [542]	155 (lesions)	NR	155	Median: 47	Range: 19 to 88	NR

Table E 11. (Continued).

Study	Number of Patients Recruited for Enrollment	Number of Patients Enrolled	Number of Lesions Enrolled	Age	Age Dispersion	Ethnicity
Makoske et al. 2000 [543]	817	817	887	NR	NR	NR
Ward et al. 2000 [544]	161	NR	121	Mean: 58	Range: 33 to 83	NR
Welle et al. 2000 [545]	NR	225	225	NR	NR	NR
Helbich et al. 1999 [546]	NR	44	44	NR	Range: 20 to 77	NR
Jackman et al. 1999 [547]	410	410	483	Median: 55	Range: 29 to 89	NR
Meyer et al. 1999 [548]	NR	1,643	1,836	Mean: 50	Range: 20 to 85	NR
Puglisi et al. 1999 [549]	NR	99	106	Median: 57	Range: 33 to 84	NR
Soo et al. 1999 [550]	110	110	116	NR	NR	NR
Caruso et al. 1998 [551]	NR	91	92	Median: 65	Range: 29 to 81	NR
Doyle et al. 1998 [552]	151 (lesions)	NR	151	NR	NR	NR
Fuhrman et al. 1998 [553]	1,440	1,440	1,440	NR	NR	NR
Heywang-Kobrunner et al. 1998 [554]	238	238	261	NR	NR	NR
Ioffe et al. 1998 [555]	NR	198	224	Mean: 51	Range: 14 to 87	NR
Liberman et al. 1998 [556]	179	151	151	Median: 50	Range: 23 to 80	NR
Schulz-Wendtland et al. 1998 [557]	307	307	2,307	NR	NR	NR
Vega-Bolivar et al. 1998 [558]	180	180	182	Mean: 55	Range: 30 to 79	NR
Whitman et al. 1 998 [559]	11	11	12	Mean: 55	Range: 31 to 75, 8.3% older than age 65	NR

Study	Number of Patients Recruited for Enrollment	Number of Patients Enrolled	Number of Lesions Enrolled	Age	Age Dispersion	Ethnicity
Zannis and AliaNo 1998 [560]	372	372	424	Mean: 57.7	Range: 25 to 90	NR
Bauer et al. 1997 [561]	799 (lesions)	NR	799	Mean: 61	Range: 38 to 87	NR
Britton et al. 1997 [562]	202	202	202	NR	NR	NR
Helbich et al. 1997 [563]	205	205	210	Mean: 52.2	Range: 23 to 88	NR
Khattar et al. 1997 [564]	117	106	106	Median: 52	Range: 19 to 85	NR
Liberman et al. 1997 [565]	NR	NR	442	NR	NR	NR
Pitre et al. 1997 [566]	128	128	128	Mean: 56.4	NR	NR
Stolier et al. 1997 [567]	242	242	244	NR	NR	NR
Sutton, et al. 1997 [568]	200	200	206	Mean: 59	Range: 41 to 85	NR
Walker et al. 1997 [569]	200	200	200	NR	Range: 35 to 86	NR
Frazee et al. 1996 [570]	103	103	103	Mean: 60	NR	NR
Fuhrman et al. 1996 [571]	451 (lesions)	NR	451	NR	NR	NR
Head and Haynes 1996 [572]	115	115	115	NR	NR	NR
Mainiero et al. 1996 [573]	128	124	138	Mean: 56.2	Range: 30 to 87	NR
Meyer et al. 1996 [574]	545 (lesions)	369	388	Median: 49 yrs Mean: 51 yrs	Range: 24 to 81	NR

Table E 11. (Continued).

Study	Number of Patients Recruited for Enrollment	Number of Patients Enrolled	Number of Lesions Enrolled	Age	Age Dispersion	Ethnicity
Nguyen et al. 1996 [575]	NR	408	431	NR	NR	NR
Pettine et al. 1996 [576]	25	25	25	NR	NR	NR
Rosenblatt et al. 1996 [577]	156	25	58	NR	NR	NR
Scopa et al. 1996 [578]	109	109	120	Mean: 51.2	Range: 21 to 85	NR
Cross et al. 1995 [579]	NR	225	250	Mean: 54	Range: 26 to 89	NR
Doyle et al. 1995 [580]	366	365	365	Mean: 57 years	NR	NR
Hamed et al. 1995 [581]	122	122	122	NR	NR	NR
Burbank et al. 1994 [582]	105 (lesions)	NR	105	NR	NR	NR
Gisvold et al. 1994 [583]	471	158	160	NR	NR	NR
Parker et al. 1994 [584]	6,152 (lesions)	NR	6,152	NR	NR	NR
Smyth and Cederbom 1994 [585]	52	52	58	Mean: 57	NR	NR
Elvecrog et al. 1993 [586]	107	100	100	NR	NR	NR
Parker et al. 1993 [587]	164	164	181	NR	NR	NR
McMahon et al. 1992 [588]	151	152	151	Median: 57 Trucut 50 Bipopty 14G 56 Biopty 18G	Range: 24 to 87	NR
Barreto et al. 1991 [589]	NR	107	107	Mean: 60.5 one group, 57.9 other group	SE 1.3 one group, 2.4 other group	NR

Study	Number of Patients Recruited for Enrollment	Number of Patients Enrolled	Number of Lesions Enrolled	Age	Age Dispersion	Ethnicity
Cusick et al. 1990 [590]	95	95	96	Mean: 52 years	Range: 24 to 78	NR
Parker et al. 1990 [591]	103	103	103	NR	NR	NR
	Sum		**55,936**			

NR = Not Reported

Table E12. Characteristics of the Breast Lesions in the Studies Addressing Key Questions 1 and 2.

Study	Number of Lesions Enrolled	% Non-palpable Lesions	Number of Non-palpable Lesions	Number of Microcalcifi-cations	Number with Mammo-graphic Masses	Number with Mammo-graphic Distortions	Lesion Size	BIRADS 5	BIRADS 4	BIRADS 3
Jackman et al. 2009 [485]	1,280	NR	NR	NR	NR	NR	NR	NR	NR	NR
Peters et al. 2008 [486]	948	100%	948	NR	NR	NR	NR	NR	NR	NR
Schueller et al. 2008 [487]	1438	100%	0	NR	NR	NR	Median:17 mmRange: 5 to 55 mm	36.0%	50.6%	13.4%
Sim and Kei et al. 2008 [488]	105	NR	NR	105	NR	NR	NR	0%	89%	1.9%
Tonegutti and Girardi 2008 [489]	268	100%	268	186	36	18	67% were 10 mm or less	7%	40%	19%
Youk et al. 200824	4,359	NR	NR	NR	NR	NR	NR	NR	NR	NR
Perez- Fuentes et al. 2001 [534]	88	73%	64	NR	NR	NR	NR	9.10%	81 .80%	8.00%

Table E 12. (Continued).

Study	Number of Lesions Enrolled	% Non-palpable Lesions	Number of Non-palpable Lesions	Number of Microcalcifi-cations	Number with Mammo-graphic Masses	Number with Mammo-graphic Distortions	Lesion Size	BIRADS 5	BIRADS 4	BIRADS 3
Ciatto et al. 2007 [490]	4,035	67%	2,714	1,887	NR	NR	NR	NR	NR	NR
de Lucena et al. 2007 [491]	150	NR	NR	NR	NR	NR	44% were 2 cm or less 52% were 2 to 5 cm	NR	NR	NR
Uematsu et al. 2007 [492]	100	NR	NR	100	NR	NR	NR	18%	27%	55%
Vag et al. 2007 [493]	70	63%	44	NR	NR	NR	Median:12 mmRange:5 to 35 mm	15.70%	33%	51 .40%
Chapellier et al. 2006 [494]	318	NR	NR	288	30	NR	NR	11%	53.50%	34.90%
Cipolla et al. 2006 [495]	426	71%	302	NR	NR	NR	NR	10.10%	10.60%	50.20%
Dhillon et al. 2006 [496]	150	NR	NR	130	12	8	NR	NR	NR	NR
Bolivar et al. 2005 [497]	214	95%	204	9	152	34	53 lesions 1 to 10 mm 119 lesions 11 to 20 mm 32 lesions larger than 20 mm	NR	NR	NR
Crystal et al. 2005 [498]	715	NR	NR	NR	NR	NR	NR	NR	NR	NR
Dillon et al. 2005 [499]	2,427	NR	NR	NR	NR	NR	NR	NR	NR	NR
Koskela et al. 2005 [500]	213	NR	NR	108	NR	NR	NR	22.10%	56.80%	16.40%
Sauer et al. 2005 [501]	962	75%	726	NR	NR	NR	Mean: 2.5 cm Range: 0.2 to 11 cm	NR	NR	NR

Study	Number of Lesions Enrolled	% Non-palpable Lesions	Number of Non-palpable Lesions	Number of Microcalcifi-cations	Number with Mammo-graphic Masses	Number with Mammo-graphic Distortions	Lesion Size	BIRADS 5	BIRADS 4	BIRADS 3
Weber et al. 2005 [502]	225	100%	225	NR	NR	NR	NR	NR	NR	NR
Wu et al. 2005 [503]	113	27%	30	NR	NR	NR	Median size: 1.4 cm Range: 0.5 to 2.0 cm	NR	NR	NR
Alonso-Bartolome et al. 2004 [504]	102	61%	62	NR	NR	NR	Mean: 14.7 mm Range: 6-30 mm	NR	NR	100%
Delle and Terinde 2004 [505]	169	NR	NR	NR	NR	NR	Mean 1.5 cm	NR	NR	NR
Fajardo et al. 2004 [506]	2,403	70%	1,681	NR	NR	NR	NR	NR	NR	NR
Kettritz et al. 2004 [507]	2,893	NR	NR	2,013	NR	61	1,677 were less than 10 mm, 809 were 11 to 20 mm, and 388 were larger	5.90%	84.30%	9.80%
Lomoschitz et al. 2004 [508]	100	100%	100	50	50	NR	NR	NR	NR	NR
Abdsaleh et al. 2003 [509]	180	NR	NR	15	130	NR	6 to 80 mm	NR	NR	NR
Ambrogetti et al. 2003 [510]	364	100%	364	326	NR	NR	NR	NR	NR	NR

Table E 12. (Continued).

Study	Number of Lesions Enrolled	% Non-palpable Lesions	Number of Non-palpable Lesions	Number of Microcalcifi-cations	Number with Mammo-graphic Masses	Number with Mammo-graphic Distortions	Lesion Size	BIRADS 5	BIRADS 4	BIRADS 3
Fishman et al. 2003 [511]	73	78%	57	NR	NR	NR	Mean: 1.7 cm Range: 0.6 to 6 cm	Fishman et al. 2003 [511]	73	78%
Han et al. 2003 [512]	271	100%	271	228	NR	NR	NR	NR	NR	NR
Kirshenbaum et al. 2003 [513]	506	100%	506	228	212	75	Mean: 0.8 cm Range: 0.3 to 2.3 cm	NR	NR	NR
March et al. 2003 [514]	34	71%	24	3	NR	NR	Mean: 0.7 cm Range: 0.4 to 1.2 cm	NR	NR	NR
Pfleiderer et al. 2003 [515]	14	NR	NR	NR	NR	NR	NR	28.60%	64.30%	NR
Philpotts et al. 2003 [516]	281	NR	NR	NR	NR	NR	NR	NR	NR	NR
Wong and Hisham 2003 [517]	150	0%	0	NR	NR	NR	NR	NR	NR	NR
Apesteguia et al. 2002 [518]	132	100%	132	82	NR	24	NR	NR	NR	NR
Georgian- Smith et al. 2002 [519]	185	NR	NR	159	16	5	NR	NR	NR	NR
Verkooijen et al. COBRA 2002 [526]	984	100%	984	533	310	26	NR	NR	NR	NR
Pfarl et al. 2002 [525]	332	NR	NR	166	152	NR	NR	NR	NR	NR

Study	Number of Lesions Enrolled	% Non-palpable Lesions	Number of Non-palpable Lesions	Number of Microcalcifi-cations	Number with Mammo- graphic Masses	Number with Mammo-graphic Distortions	Lesion Size	BIRADS 5	BIRADS 4	BIRADS 3
Pfarl et al. 2002 [525]	332	NR	NR	166	152	NR	NR	NR	NR	NR
Verkooijen et al. COBRA 2002 [526]	984	100%	984	533	310	26	NR	NR	NR	NR
Johnson et al. 2002 [521]	101	27%	27	NR	NR	NR	Mean: 1.15 cm	NR	NR	NR
Liberman et al. 2002 [522]	800	100%	800	606	194	NR	Median: 0.8 cm Range: 0.2 to 10 cm	NR	NR	NR
Meloni et al. 2002 [523]	129	100%	129	NR	NR	NR	NR	NR	NR	NR
Morris et al. 2002 [524]	21	100%	21	NR	21	NR	Mean: 1.8 cm Range: 0.8 to 5.5 cm	NR	NR	NR
Becker et al. 2001 [527]	232	NR	NR	232	NR	NR	NR	NR	NR	NR
Brenner et al. 2001 [528]	1,003	100%	1003	355	630	92	NR	11.10%	39.10%	35.70%
Cangiarella et al. 2001 [529]	160	NR	NR	160	NR	NR	NR	NR	NR	NR
Dahlstrom and Jain 2001 [530]	310	NR	NR	301	NR	NR	NR	NR	NR	NR
Lai et al. 2001 [531]	673	NR	NR	NR	NR	NR	NR	NR	NR	NR
Levin et al. 2001 [532]	70	100%	70	27	NR	NR	NR	NR	NR	NR
Margolin et al. 2001 [533]	1,333	NR	NR	NR	NR	NR	NR	NR	94%	NR
Perez-Fuentes et al. 2001 [534]	88	73%	64	NR	NR	NR	NR	9.10%	81 .80%	8.00%

Table E 12. (Continued).

Study	Number of Lesions Enrolled	% Non-palpable Lesions	Number of Non-palpable Lesions	Number of Microcalcifi-cations	Number with Mammo- graphic Masses	Number with Mammo-graphic Distortions	Lesion Size	BIRADS 5	BIRADS 4	BIRADS 3
Smith et al. 2001 [535]	500	95%	475	0	NR	NR	Mean: 15 mm Range: 4 to 60 mm	NR	NR	NR
White et al. 2001536	1,042	NR	NR	NR	NR	NR	NR	NR	NR	NR
Wunderbaldinger et al. 2001 [537]	45	100%	45	4	41	NR	Mean: 18 mm Range: 8 to 41 mm	NR	NR	NR
Yeow et al. 2001 [538]	98	0%	0	NR	NR	NR	Mean: 2.6 cm Range: 0.9 to 10 cm	NR	NR	NR
Beck et al. 2000 [539]	594	NR	NR	NR	NR	NR	NR	16.50%	83.50%	NR
Kirwan et al. 2000 [540]	72	NR	NR	NR	NR	NR	NR	NR	NR	NR
Latosinsky et al. 2000 [541]	692	NR	NR	313	426	4	NR	NR	NR	NR
Liberman et al. 2000 [542]	155	0%	0	NR	NR	NR	Median: 1.7 cm Range: 0.5 to 15 cm	NR	NR	NR
Makoske et al. 2000 [543]	887	100%	887	NR	NR	NR	NR	NR	NR	NR
Ward et al. 2000 [544]	121	100%	121	121	NR	NR	NR	NR	NR	NR
Welle et al. 2000 [545]	225	NR	NR	90	135	NR	NR	NR	NR	NR
Helbich et al. 1999 [546]	44	NR	NR	24	5	5	Mean 12.9 mm Range: 8 to 27 mm	NR	NR	NR

Study	Number of Lesions Enrolled	% Non-palpable Lesions	Number of Non-palpable Lesions	Number of Microcalcifi-cations	Number with Mammo-graphic Masses	Number with Mammo-graphic Distortions	Lesion Size	BIRADS 5	BIRADS 4	BIRADS 3
Jackman et al. 1999 [547]	483	100%	483	234	249	NR	NR	NR	NR	NR
Meyer et al. 1999 [548]	1,836	100%	1,836	643	1,194	NR	NR	NR	NR	NR
Puglisi et al. 1999 [549]	106	75%	79	66	59	NR	NR	NR	NR	NR
Soo et al. 1999 [550]	116	100%	116	0	NR	NR	NR	NR	NR	NR
Caruso et al. 1998551	92	0%	0	11	92	NR	NR	NR	NR	NR
Doyle et al. 1998 [552]	151	100%	151	88	71	5	NR	NR	NR	NR
Fuhrman et al. 1998 [553]	1,440	100%	1,440	749	691	NR	NR	NR	NR	NR
Heywang- Kobrunner et al. 1998 [554]	261	NR	NR	134	127	NR	NR	1.90%	10.00%	88.10%
Ioffe et al. 1998 [555]	224	NR	NR	51	173	NR	NR	NR	NR	NR
Liberman et al. 1998 [556]	151	100%	151	NR	NR	NR	NR	NR	NR	NR
Schulz- Wendtland et al. 1998 [557]	2,307	NR	NR	NR	NR	NR	NR	NR	NR	NR
Vega-Bolivar et al. 1998 [558]	182	100%	182	75	33	24	NR	NR	NR	NR
Whitman et al. 1998 [559]	12	NR	NR	NR	NR	NR	NR	NR	NR	NR
Zannis and AliaNo 1998 [560]	424	100%	424	NR	424	NR	NR	NR	NR	NR
Britton et al. 1997 [562]	202	NR	NR	NR	NR	NR	NR	NR	NR	NR

Table E 12. (Continued).

Study	Number of Lesions Enrolled	% Non-palpable Lesions	Number of Non-palpable Lesions	Number of Microcalcifi-cations	Number with Mammo-graphic Masses	Number with Mammo-graphic Distortions	Lesion Size	BIRADS 5	BIRADS 4	BIRADS 3
Helbich et al. 1997 [563]	210	NR	NR	NR	NR	NR	Mean: 14 mm Range: 7 to 30 mm	NR	NR	NR
Khattar et al. 1997 [564]	106	0%	0	NR	NR	NR	NR	NR	NR	NR
Liberman et al. 1997 [565]	442	NR	NR	196	246	NR	NR	NR	NR	NR
Pitre et al. 1997 [566]	128	100%	128	NR	NR	NR	NR	3.90%	NR	NR
Stolier et al. 1997567	244	NR	NR	65	173	4	NR	NR	NR	44.70%
Sutton, et al. 1997 [568]	206	100%	206	81	125	NR	Mean: 14 mm Range: 2 mm to 30 mm	NR	NR	NR
Walker et al. 1997 [569]	200	100%	200	136	28	36	NR	NR	NR	NR
Frazee et al. 1996 [570]	103	100%	103	NR	NR	NR	NR	NR	NR	NR
Fuhrman et al. 1996 [571]	451	NR	NR	NR	NR	NR	NR	NR	NR	NR
Head and Haynes 1996 [572]	115	100%	115	22	85	NR	NR	NR	NR	NR
Mainiero et al. 1996 [573]	138	NR	NR	138	NR	NR	NR	NR	NR	NR
Meyer et al. 1996 [574]	388	100%	388	NR	NR	NR	NR	NR	NR	NR

Study	Number of Lesions Enrolled	% Non-palpable Lesions	Number of Non-palpable Lesions	Number of Microcalcifi-cations	Number with Mammo-graphic Masses	Number with Mammo-graphic Distortions	Lesion Size	BIRADS 5	BIRADS 4	BIRADS 3
Pettine et al. 1996 [576]	25	100%	25	NR	NR	NR	NR	NR	NR	NR
Rosenblatt et al. 1996 [577]	58	NR	NR	22	14	NR	Median: 1.5 cm Range: 0.8 to 3.0 cm	NR	NR	NR
Scopa et al. 1996 [578]	120	NR	NR	NR	NR	NR	Range: 0.7 to 5 cm	NR	NR	NR
Cross et al. 1995 [579]	250	100%	250	NR	NR	NR	NR	NR	NR	NR
Doyle et al. 1995 [580]	365	62%	225	59	225		Larger than 5 mm	NR	NR	NR
Hamed et al. 1995 [581]	122	NR	NR	NR	NR	NR	NR	NR	NR	NR
Burbank et al. 1994 [582]	105	NR	NR	NR	NR	NR	NR	NR	NR	NR
Gisvold et al. 1994 [583]	160	NR	NR	NR	NR	NR	Range: 3 to 70 mm	NR	NR	NR
Parker et al. 1994 [584]	6,152	93%	5,702	1,637	4,515		NR	NR	NR	NR
Smyth and Cederbom 1994 [585]	58	100%	58	NR	NR	NR	NR	NR	NR	NR
Elvecrog et al. 1993 [586]	100	100%	100	26	100		NR	NR	NR	NR
Parker et al. 1993 [587]	181	46%	84	NR	NR	NR	NR	NR	NR	NR
McMahon et al. 1992 [588]	151	0%	0	NR	NR	NR	NR	NR	NR	NR

Table E 12. (Continued).

Study	Number of Lesions Enrolled	% Non-palpable Lesions	Number of Non-palpable Lesions	Number of Microcalcifi-cations	Number with Mammo-graphic Masses	Number with Mammo-graphic Distortions	Lesion Size	BIRADS 5	BIRADS 4	BIRADS 3
Barreto et al. 1991 [589]	107	0%	0	NR	NR	NR	NR	NR	NR	NR
Cusick et al. 1990 [590]	96	NR	NR	NR	NR	NR	NR	NR	NR	NR
Parker et al. 1990 [591]	103	NR	NR	NR	NR	NR	NR	NR	NR	NR
Sum	55,936		25,760	13,303	11,186	421				

NR = Not Reported

Table E13. Studies of the Dissemination Of Cancerous Cells During Biopsy Procedures.

Reference	Design of Study	Number of Patients	Biopsy Methods	Conclusion
Michalopoulos et al. 2008[33]	Prospective study. Patients under-went core-needle biopsy followed by open surgery 6-8 days later. The needle track was excised and examined by a pathologist.	21 with DCIS and 10 with invasive ductal carcinoma	Vacuum-assisted 1 1G Mammotome device	No cases of dissemination of cancerous cells were observed. In two cases benign epithelial displacement was observed. The duration of the core-needle procedure was significantly longer in these two cases than for cases with no displacement observed.
Uematsu and Kasami 2007[96]	The exterior of the core needles was washed immediately following withdrawl and the washings were examined for cells.	207	US-guided 18G automated Bard Magnum gun	65% of the washings were positive for cells. Lesions diagnosed as invasive lobular carcinoma were significantly less likely to have had cells in the washings than lesions diagnosed as DCIS or invasive ductal carcinoma. Biopsies that had been performed using multiple passes were slightly but not significantly more likely to yield cells in the washings than biopsies performed with a single pass.

Reference	Design of Study	Number of Patients	Biopsy Methods	Conclusion
Fitzal et al. 2006 [110]	Retrospective case-control study of patients treated with breast-conserving surgery and radiotherapy, with or without chemotherapy/hormonal therapy.	189 with preoperative core- needle biopsy, 530 without preoperative core-needle biopsy	14G or 1 1G; stereotactic or US guidance; vacuum-assisted or not.	In patients with preoperative core-needle biopsy, the local recurrence rate was 1.1% with a median followup of 78 months (range 46 to 108 months); the mortality rate was 0%. In patients without preoperative core-needle biopsy, the local recurrence rate was 2.1% with a median followup of 71 months (range 8 to 128 months); the mortality rate was 4.7%.
Newman et al. 2006 [130]	Retrospective chart review of women who underwent sentinel lymph node biopsy	279 with core-needle biopsy, 41 with fine-needle biopsy, and 217 with open excisional biopsy	Not described	The method of biopsy did not correlate with metastasis to the sentinel lymph node; however, patients who underwent excisional biopsy were more likely to have micrometastases to the sentinel lymph node than patients who underwent needle biopsies.
Uriburu et al. 2006 [139]	Case report	3	14G under stereotactic guidance	Three women treated with skin-sparing mastectomy are reported on. All three developed recurrences of their breast tumors at the core-needle biopsy scar. Two of the three had invasive ductal carcinomas and one had a mucinous carcinoma.
Hansen et al. 2004 [188]	Retrospective chart review of women who underwent sentinel lymph node biopsy	126 with fine-needle biopsy, 227 with core-needle biopsy and 323 with open excisional biopsy	11 or 14G, under stereotactic or US guidance	The incidence of metastases to the sentinel lymph node was significantly higher in women who underwent needle biopsies compared to women who had excisional biopsy.
Hoorntje et al. 2004 [190]	Prospective study. Patients under-went core-needle biopsy followed by open surgery a mean of 21 days later. The needle track was excised and examined by a pathologist.	13	14G automated device Bard under stereotactic guidance	Needle tracks were visible in 11 cases, and of these, 7 had displaced cells in the needle track.

Table E 13. (Continued).

Reference	Design of Study	Number of Patients	Biopsy Methods	Conclusion
Peters-Engl et al. 2004 [195]	Retrospective review of women who underwent sentinel lymph node biopsy	1,048 with fine-needle or core-needle biopsy, 842 with open excisional biopsy	Not described	Patients who had undergone a needle biopsy had a 1.37 times increased risk of metastases to the lymph nodes, but after adjusting for known risk factors of axillary node metastases this result was overturned, 1.09 times increased risk (95% CI: 0.85% to 1.40%).
Chen et al. 2002 [244]	Retrospective review of women treated with breast-conserving surgery and radiation therapy	86 with core-needle biopsy, 465 with open excisional biopsy	14G Bard device or 11 G vacuum-assisted device Mammotome, all under stereotactic guidance	At a mean followup of 4.9 years (range 2.0 to 8.9 years), tumor recurrence rate was 2.3% in the core-needle group and 7.7% in the open biopsy group.
Knight et al. 2002 [256]	Retrospective review of women treated with breast-conserving surgery; 78.6% had radiation therapy as well	297 with core-needle biopsy, 101 with open excisional biopsy	14G Bard device under stereotactic or ultrasound guidance	At a mean followup of 29.7 months (range: 2 to 90 months), 3.7% of the patients with core-needle biopsy had a tumor recurrence compared to 3.96% of patients with open biopsy who had a tumor recurrence.
Chao et al. 2001 [282]	Case report	3	14G under stereotactic guidance	Two of the patients developed tumor recurrences at the site of the core-needle biopsy; the third patient had the needle track excised 1 month after biopsy and cancer cells were detected in the needle track. None of the patients received radiation therapy for the primary tumor.
King et al. 2001 [295]	Retrospective review of women diagnosed with breast cancer by either core-needle biopsy or wire-localized open excisional biopsy and then treated with breast-conserving surgery; 91% had radiation therapy as well	132 with core-needle biopsy, 79 with open excisional biopsy	14G under US or stereotactic guidance	At a median followup of 44.4 months, 3.0% of patients with core-needle biopsy had tumor recurrences; at a median followup of 50.1 months, 2.5% of patients with open biopsy had tumor recurrences.

Table E14. Surgical Procedures Avoided.

Reference	Design of Study	Number of Patients	Biopsy Methods	Conclusion
Friese et al. 2009 [592]	Analysis of data from the SEER data of women diagnosed with DCIS or stage I/II breast cancer between 1991 and 1999	45,542	Needle or surgical	Needle biopsy use was associated with a reduced likelihood of multiple breast surgeries (odds ratio 0.35, 95% CI: 0.34 to 0.37)
Altomare et al. 2005 [145]	Retrospective chart review of patients with nonpalpable breast lesions who underwent core-needle biopsy between January 2001-January 2004.	591	US- or stereotactic-guided vacuum-assisted biopsy (Mammotome) 11-gauge needle or ABBI	Core-needle biopsy spared a surgical procedure for 128 cancer patients and 134 non-cancer patients, but did not spare a procedure in 17 women
Bolivar et al. 2005 [497]	Prospective case series of patients with non-palpable suspicious breast lesions who underwent core-needle biopsy from August 1997-August 2001.	198	US-guided (7.5 MHz linear array transducer) using a freehand technique with patient in supine or supine oblique position.	Core-needle biopsy spared 155/1 98 (or 78%) women a surgical procedure.
Chapellier et al. 2005 [494]	Prospective case series of the first 318 aspiration-guided macrobiopsy procedures performed at one institution. The majority of patients had microcalcifications; approximately 50% were BIRADS 4 while 35% were BIRADS 3 but had risk factors.	301	Fischer stereotactic imaging table, vacuum-assisted biopsy (AND).	128 BIRADS 4 patients and six BIRADS 5 patients were spared an additional operation by use of core- needle biopsy.
Carmon et al. 2004 [176]	Retrospective chart review of patients with nonpalpable breast lesions who were ultimately operated on for primary breast carcinoma between 1997- mid-	167	Percutaneous image-guided core biopsy	From 1997 to 2001, the percent of patients requiring a second operation decreased from 56.2% to 11.1%, with increased availability of a preoperative diagnosis. 79.2% of subjects with a preoperative

Table E 14. (Continued).

Reference	Design of Study	Number of Patients	Biopsy Methods	Conclusion
	2001.			diagnosis of invasive duct carcinoma had axillary lymph node dissection vs. 37.7% of those without a preoperative CNB diagnosis.
Apesteguia et al. 2002 [518]	Prospective consecutive case series of patients with nonpalpable breast lesions non-visible or non- accessible by US.	126	Vacuum-assisted core biopsy on a digital stereotaxic table with an 11-gauge needle.	Second surgical procedures due to involved margins were required in 17.4% of cases and 5 additional lymphadenectomy procedures were needed based on core-needle biopsy's inability to predict invasion.
Liberman et al. 2002 [522]	Retrospective study. Rate of spared surgical procedures was compared for those whose lesion was completely excised compared to those whose lesion was only sampled.	800 (565 calcifications, 194 mass, 41 both)	Vacuum-assisted core biopsy (Mammotome) with 11-gauge needle	466 lesions were totally removed by the core-needle procedure. Surgery was spared in 80.6% of lesions. There was not a significant difference between the excised versus sampled lesion groups in spared surgery rates (81.5% vs. 82%, $p = 0.95$).
Becker et al. 2001 [527]	Retrospective chart review of lesions with indeterminate microcalcifications	218	DMR regular mammog-raphy machine plus either a Stereotix 2 conventional add-on unit or a SenoVision digital add-on unit. Core-needle biopsy was perfor-med with a 14-gauge needle in all but 5 cases (in which a 16-gauge needle was used)	Open biopsy was avoided in 78 (69.6%) of patients in the conventional treatment group and in 78 (73.6%) of the digital treatment group.
Liberman et al. 2001 [298]	Retrospective review of women with calcifications highly suggestive of malignancy who underwent a diagnostic biopsy procedure from 1993-2000.	139	Stereotactic vacuum-assisted biopsy with 11 or 14-gauge needle	The mean number of surgical procedures was 1.2 and 1.6 for core-needle biopsy vs. surgical biopsy. 62% of surgical biopsy patients overall and 83.8% of diagnostic surgical biopsy with cancer needed two
				procedures. The likelihood of requiring a single operation was greater for women who had core-

Reference	Design of Study	Number of Patients	Biopsy Methods	Conclusion
				needle biopsy. A surgical procedure was spared in 58.4% of this group.
Perez-Fuentes et al. 2001 [534]	Prospective case series of patients seen between August 1998-December 2000 with palpable or nonpalpable breast masses	83	US-guided vacuum-assisted biopsy (Mammotome) with 11- gauge needle	Of the 83 patients studied, 79 were spared a surgical procedure (95.2%).
Verkooijen et al. 2001 [593]	Prospective comparison of patients with nonpalpable breast lesions	164	Patient prone, 14-gauge needle	In 75% of core-needle cases, only a single surgical procedure was needed, while this was true in only 16% of open biopsy cases ($p < 0.001$). Mean number of surgical procedures was 1.31 vs. 1.91 ($p < 0.001$) in the core-needle and open biopsy groups, respectively.
Liberman et al. 2000 [542]	Retrospective chart review of patients with breast masses that were palpable on physical examination from 1992 to 1998.	107	Stereotactic- or US-guided core biopsy with a 14-gauge needle.	Core-needle biopsy spared 74% of subjects in this study an additional diagnostic tissue sampling
Morrow et al. 2000 [305]	Prospective nonrandomized comparative study of patients with nonpalpable mammographically- detected abnormalities	1,550	Core-needle or open biopsy	Among those with cancer, a single procedure was performed in 33% of the excisional biopsy subjects versus 84% of the core- needle group ($p < 0.001$). The core-needle group consistently had a larger proportion of subjects treated with a single procedure, regardless of lesion type: for architectural distortions 71% vs. 46% and for highly suspicious lesions 83% vs. 45%.
Al-Sobhi et al. 1999 [346]	Retrospective review of patients found to have cancer	67	Vacuum-assisted with an 11 or 14-gauge needle	The number of surgical procedures performed in an operating room differed significantly for the two groups overall (CNB mean 1.1 ±0.3 and wire localization mean 1.8 ±0.4). For the subset who underwent breast-conserving treatment a significant difference between groups was also

Table E 14. (Continued).

Reference	Design of Study	Number of Patients	Biopsy Methods	Conclusion
				evident, mean surgical procedures were 1.2 ±0.4 and 2.1 ±0.2, respectively.
Williams et al. 1999 [384]	Prospective case series of patients with impalpable breast lesions diagnosed by stereotactic CNB on a prone table vs. a historical cohort of patients with similar lesions diagnosed prior to the use of prone stereotactic CNB.	222	Stereotactic prone core-needle with Mammotest and 14-gauge needle.	More patients in the prone group required only a single operation ($p < 0.03$). The average number of operations was 1.33 (SE 0.053) vs.1 .47 (SE 0.054) in the prone and control groups, respectively.
Johnson et al. 1998 [395]	Retrospective review of patients with malignant-appearing microcalcifications without an associated parenchymal abnormality on mammography.	167	Stereotactic biopsy was performed using Lorad Stereotactic prone biopsy table with 14-gauge needle. Digital mammography was used to localize the lesions. US biopsies were performed using a 7.5 MHz probe with real-time imaging using the same CNB device.	The mean number of procedures required until definitive treatment was 2.4 and 1.7 for the initial IGBB and initial NLOB, respectively ($p = 0.0002$)
Kaufman et al. 1998396	Retrospective review of consecutive mammographically-detected nonpalpable breast lesions ultimately diagnosed as in situ or invasive carcinoma.	113	Core-needle or open biopsy	Negative margins were achieved twice as often in thecore-needle group as in the open biopsy group after the first surgical procedure (77% vs. 38%, $p < 0.001$). A one- stage surgical procedure was possible in many more of the core-needle patients than in the open biopsy group (79% vs. 21%, $p < 0.001$). On average, 2.2 procedures (surgery and biopsy) were needed in the core-needle group vs. 1.8 among the open biopsy patients. However, the average number of surgeries was 50% higher in the open biopsy group (1.8 vs. 1.2).

Reference	Design of Study	Number of Patients	Biopsy Methods	Conclusion
Liberman et al. 1998556	Retrospective review of patients with nonpalpable breast masses.	151	US-guided biopsy was performed in the supine or supine oblique position using high resolution (7.5 MHz linear array transducer) equipment with a 14-gauge cutting needle.	85% of patients in this study were spared a surgical procedure by use of core-needle biopsy.
Lind et al. 1998402	Retrospective review ofpatients with mammographically-detected breast cancer that underwent breast-conserving surgery	117	Biopsies were performed on a dedicated prone table with 14-gauge needle	Only 6% of patients in the core-needle group had positive margins vs. 55% of the open biopsy patients ($p < 0.01$). One patient with positive margins in the core-needle group was re-excised vs. 34/38 of those with positive margins in the open group ($p < 0.01$).
Fenoglio et al. 1997 [419]	Retrospective chart review of patients with mammographically-detected breast cancer	40	14-gauge long throw Biopty gun plus Mammotest Stereotactic System	All 20 patients diagnosed with core-needle biopsy required one surgical procedure only whereas among the 20 initially diagnosed with open biopsy a total of 41 procedures were required to diagnose and treat their cancers
Liberman et al. 1997 [428]	Retrospective chart review of nonpalpable breast cancers	197	Stereotactic CNB were done with patient in prone position using StereoGuide; sonographically-guided CNB were done with patients in supine or supine oblique using a 7.5 MHz linear array transducer and high resolution sonographic equipment; all CNB used a 14-gauge needle or an ultra-core biopsy needle.	84% of patients in the CNB group underwent a single surgical procedure vs. 29% of those diagnosed by surgical biopsy ($p < 0.00001$). 16% of the CNB patients required two surgical procedures while 66% of the open-biopsy patients needed two surgeries and 5% underwent three surgical procedures.

Table E 14. (Continued).

Reference	Design of Study	Number of Patients	Biopsy Methods	Conclusion
Smith et al. 1997 [433]	Retrospective review.	677	US-guided Mammotest (67) or wire localized excisional biopsy (610)	On average, 1.25 surgical procedures were required by the core-needle group versus 2.01 in the surgical biopsy group ($p < 0.001$).
Sutton et al. 1997 [568]	Retrospective review of patients with nonpalpable mammographic abnormalities detected at routine screening in a community-based clinic.	200	Biopsies were performed on a dedicated prone stereotactic table (Mammotest) with an autoguide attachment and 14-gauge 22 mm-throw Bard Biopty-cut needles held in a Bard Biopty gun.	The authors estimated that open biopsy was avoided in 82% of cases by using core-needle biopsy for diagnosis.
Whitten et al. 1997 [435]	Retrospective review	171	Stereotactic- or US-guided biopsy with a 14-gauge needle	Among the 86 subjects diagnosed by image-guided core-needle biopsy, 98 surgical procedures were completed (1.1 surgeries per patient) compared with 1.9 operations on average for the 85 patients undergoing a diagnostic needle localized biopsy (157 surgeries total in 85 subjects).
Yim et al. 1996 [454]	Retrospective review	52	Stereotactic biopsy with a 14-gauge needle was performed on a dedicated prone table	At the time of excision, surgical margins were more frequently positive in the open biopsy group (55%) vs. the CNB group (0%); the distance of the tumor from the surgical margin was greater for the CNB vs. open biopsy patients among the negative margins; and, among those having breast conservation surgery, the rate of re-excision was higher for the open biopsy group (74%) vs. no patients in the CNB treatment group.
Liberman et al. 1995 [458]	Retrospective chart review of patients with impalpable speculated masses.	43	Biopsies were performed with patients prone on a dedicated table using either	The use of core-needle biopsy in the diagnosis of breast cancer reduced the number of procedures required in 33 (77%) patients.

Reference	Design of Study	Number of Patients	Biopsy Methods	Conclusion
			a 14-gauge Bard Biopty needle or a 14-gauge Manan needle and either a Bard Biopty gun with 23 mm throw or Manan ProMag 2.2 gun with a 22 mm throw.	
Strong et al. 1995 [463]	Prospective study of patients with mammographically-detected, asymptomatic, nonpalpable breast lesions	97	Mammotest stereotactic device using 14-gauge Manan needle.	In eight benign cases, open biopsy was performed, adding an extra procedure to the diagnostic protocol for these patients. However, 74 women (76%) were spared an open biopsy by core-needle biopsy. As the 15 women with carcinoma went directly to mastectomy without an open biopsy, core- needle biopsy did not add a diagnostic procedure in these cases.
Elliott et al. 1992 [479]	Retrospective review of 12-month period of patients with nonpalpable breast lesions.	115	Mammotest II with 18-gauge Bard biopsy needle using Bard Biopty gun	Core-needle biopsy spared 97 patients an open surgical biopsy.

Table E15. Patient Procedure Preference.

Reference	Design of study	Number of patients	Biopsy methods	Conclusion
Duschesne et al. 200761	Prospective trial of new device	113	US-guided radiofreq-uency tipped vacuum-assisted with 9-gauge needle (SenoCor 360 Biopsy System).	They rated patient comfort as equivalent with other types of biopsies.
Krainick-Strobel et al. 200773	Prospective case series of patients with benign lesions undergoing biopsy for the purpose of complete extirpation.	45	Hand-held US-guided vacuum-assisted biopsy (Mammotome) using	Ninety-five percent of respondents said they would prefer core-needle to open excisional biopsy if they needed a future procedure. A minimum of 7 days post-procedure,

Table E15. (Continued).

Reference	Design of study	Number of patients	Biopsy methods	Conclusion
			either an 8- or 11-gauge needle.	patients were given a questionnaire about their experience. The mean level of satisifaction with the procedure, on a scale of 0-10, was 9.2 (range 3-10).
Killebrew et al. 2006120	Retrospective comparison study of patients with BIRADS 4 or 5 and mammographic lesions presenting as microcalcifications.	1600	Vacuum-assisted procedure (Mammot-ome) with 11-gauge needle vs. vacuum-assisted intact specimen biopsy with 10 or 15 mm probe.	Self-reports by patients showed that those undergoingboth treatments tolerated theirrespective procedures equally. Patients were asked to rate the biopsy procedure for comfort and to rate comfort of lying on stereotactic table, as a comparison. In the vacuum-assisted arm, ratings of 5.8 and 2.0 (with 10 = extreme pain) were given for lying on table and actual biopsy procedure, respectively. In theother group, the ratings were 4.1 and 1.9,respectively.
Chapellier et al. 2005 [494]	Prospective case series of the first 318 aspiration-guided macrobiopsy procedures performed at one institution. The majority of patients had microcalcifications; approximately 50% were BIRADS 4 while 35% were BIRADS 3 but had risk factors.	301	Fischer stereotactic imaging table, vacuum-assisted	Patient tolerance of procedure was excellent, as measured by a self-administered patient questionnaire. The authors also found that the postprocedure psychological state was associated with the procedure outcome, the information given to patients and the attitudes of medical staff members.
Weber et al. 2005 [502]	Retrospective comparison study of patients with nonpalpable breast lesions	387	Stereotactically-guided vacuum-assisted (Mammotome) technique with 11-gauge needle or ABBI	Three patients in this series underwent both procedures but they did not indicate a preference for one over the other.
Wong et al. 2005 [171]	Prospective trial of Asian patients with nonpalpable mammographic abnormalities	114	Vacuum-assisted (Mammotome) on a prone biopsy table with 8- to 11-gauge needle	Bruising (one week post- procedure) occurred in 79 patients (46 minimal, 25 mild, 5 moderate and 3 severe). All patients were able to be discharged after 2-3 hours following the procedure and all reported the procedure was acceptable without undo discomfort.
Alonso-Bartolome et al. 2004 [504]	Prospective study of women with probably benign breast lesions who refused radiologic followup and, instead, insisted on removal. Complete lesion	97	US-guided vacuum-assisted biopsy (Mammotome) with 11-gauge needle	Patients estimated that the time lost to core-needle biopsy is less than 20% of the time required for a surgical biopsy.

Reference	Design of study	Number of patients	Biopsy methods	Conclusion
	removal was the intended goal for all lesions.			
Geller et al. 2004 [183]	Survey of women with nonpalpable breast lesions	315	US-guided core-needle biopsy or open excisional biopsy	Survey results 1-3 months post procedure measured convenience of the procedure (distance travelled, procedure time, and number of days of work missed post procedure). No difference was found between two groups in terms of miles travelled for procedure, but the excisional biopsy group missed more work.
March et al. 2003 [514]	Prospective study of women with breast masses who underwent biopsy in which complete removal of the lesion was attempted.	34	US-guided vacuum-assisted biopsy with an 11-gauge biopsy device	Radiologists examined the biopsy site 2-5 days post-procedure and found 24 subjects (71%) had ecchymosis, nine (26%) had no visible abnormality aside from the skin incision and one (3%) had slight skin convexity without ecchymosis at the biopsy site. Twenty-one subjects who did not undergo an open procedure were examined at 6 months post core-needle biopsy. All 21 said they would recommend the procedure to others.
Mariotti et al. 2003 [228]	Retrospective study of patients with suspicious non palpable mammographic lesions not confirmed by ultrasonography.	360	Vacuum-assisted (Mammotome) with an 11-gauge needle or ABBI	Patient acceptance of the biopsy procedure was high.
Fineet al. 2003217	Women with low risk palpable masses were assessed prospectively.	216	Vacuum-assisted (Mammotome) with US guidance with either an 8- or 11-gauge probe	A majority of patients stated that they would recommend the procedure to others in a survey conducted 10 days post-procedure (82% and 92%, respectively).By the 6-month follow-up visit, 100% stated they would recommend the procedure to others, while 97% stated they themselves would have the procedure again, if needed.
Chun et al. 2002245	Retrospective review and survey of patients who had undergone a Mammotome, ABBI or wire localized biopsy more than 2 years ago for benign disease.	59	Stereotactic vacuum-assisted 11-gauge (Mammotome) or stereotactic excisional biopsy with ABBI (15	The biopsy experience was rated as satisfactory by 90%, 75% and 80% of patients in the open, ABBI, and Mammotome groups, respectively. Complaints about the procedures included uncomfortable (2 Mammotome, 4 ABBI), pain (2 each open and Mammotome), painful breast

Table E 15. (Continued).

Reference	Design of study	Number of patients	Biopsy methods	Conclusion
			or 20 mm cannula) or wire localized open biopsy	compression (3 ABBI), delay in getting results (1 each Mammotome and ABBI), rude doctors (2 Mammotome) and length of procedure (1open).
Hui et al. 2002252	Prospective case series of patients with nonpalpable breast lesions requiring a biopsy procedure.	79	Stereotactic-guided breast biopsy (StereoGuide with Digital Spot Mammography): Trucut with a 14-gauge needle, vacuum-assisted (Mammotome) with 11-gauge probe	31.6% of patients were very satisfied with the procedure; 73.7% felt the level of pain associated with the biopsy was less severe than erect mammography; 34.2% felt thepain experienced was less severe than needle pricking; and 14.5% felt it was less severe than previous free-hand or ultrasound-guided breast biopsy.
Beck et al. 2000 [539]	Retrospective review of first experience using vacuum- assisted core-needle biopsy.	560	Digital stereotaxic biopsy table, vacuum-assisted (Mammotome) with 11-gauge needle.	A majority of patients tolerated the procedure well.
Gukas et al. 2000 [326]	Prospective study of 112 consecutive patients with palpable breast lesions	108	Tru-Cut and excisional biopsies.	A majority of patients, 90.7%, accepted the procedure. The authors note that patients experienced more apprehension about the procedure than actual discomfort.
Welle et al. 2000 [545]	Retrospective review of patients who underwent a stereotactic CNB in a decubitus or recumbent position from September 1995-March 1999.	225	Stereotactic-guided core- needle biopsy in a decubitus or recumbent position.	Two patients out of the 225 had experienced a traditional prone position CNB and both stated they preferred the dec-ubitus position, preferring to lie on their sides. Overall, 29% of patients reported mild discomfort or numbness in the dependent arm with the decubitis or recumbent position.
Doyle et al. 1999 [552]	Retrospective study of patients with mammographically-detected lesions	151	Senographe 600T was used for 136 biopsies; 15 using Mammomat 3000; all in decubitus position unless the patient couldn't tolerate that positioning and with a 14-gauge needle.	90% of subjects were able to tolerate the decubitus position although some developed discomfort in the dependent arm and required supporting the arm away from the body on a chair or small trolley.

Reference	Design of study	Number of patients	Biopsy methods	Conclusion
Helbich et al. 1998 [393]	Prospective randomized study of consecutive patients with indeterminate or suggestive lesions on mammography	64	Mammotest stereotactic system with 13-gauge coaxial needle.	Author reports that all patients tolerated the procedure well.
Handy et al. 1996[445]	Prospective survey of patients. Patients completed a pre-procedure survey, one immediately after the procedure, one 24 hours post-procedure and 5 days later.	58	StereoGuide SM Breast Biopsy System with 14-gauge needle. The majority of patients were in a prone position.	67% of patients reported that they understood the procedure they were about to undergo. Immediately after the procedure, 78% said they understood the procedure but the remainder still felt they did not understand it. Five of those who initially thought they understood decided they really had not after experiencing it. 38% said the clinic nurse/technologist was the best source of information about the procedure, 26% said it was the physician,15% said there was no good source of information available to them and 21 said other (books, friends, popular media). Pre-procedure, 79% were most concerned about the results of the biopsywhile 10% were most concerned about the procedure itself. 31% reportednone or slight anxiety about the impending procedure, 60% said they were mild to moderately anxious and 9% were extremely anxious. Five days post procedure, 97% said they would have the procedure again in the future, if needed.
Elliott et al. 1992[479]	Retrospective review of 12 month period	115	Mammotest II with 18-gauge Bard biopsy needle using Bard Biopty gun	The authors explain that patients are very accepting of the CNB procedure and found the test easy to perform in the office.

Table E16. Cosmetic Outcome.

Reference	Design of Study	Number of Patients	Biopsy Methods	Conclusion
Krainick-Strobel et al. 2007[73]	Prospective case series of patients with benign lesions undergoing vacuum-assisted biopsy for the purpose of complete lesion removal	45	Hand-held ultrasound-guided vacuum-assisted CNB biopsy (Mammotome) using either an 8- or 11-gauge needle.	Ninety-five percent of respondents said they would prefer CNB to open excisional biopsy if they needed a future procedure. A minimum of seven days post-procedure, patients were given a questionnaire about their experience. All patients said that the scar from the needle was cosmetically unimportant to them and, on a scale of 0-10, their mean level of satisfaction with CNB was 9.2 (range 3-10).
Weber et al. 2005 [502]	Retrospective comparison study of patients with impalpable breast lesions undergoing either Mammotome or ABBI	387	Stereotactically-guided vacuum-assisted CNB biopsy (Mammotome) technique with 11-gauge needle or ABBI	Incomplete satisfaction with the cosmetic result occurred at a higher rate in the ABBI group (6.7% vs. 1.3%, $p = 0.03$).
Wong et al. 2005 [171]	Prospective trial of Asian patients with nonpalpable mammographic abnormalities underwent either ABBI ($N = 7$) or Mammotome ($N = 107$).	114	CNB was performed on a prone biopsy table with vacuum-assisted CNB (Mammotome) with 8- to 11-gauge needle or ABBI.	Bruising (one week post- procedure) occurred in 79 patients (46 minimal, 25 mild, 5 moderate and 3 severe) and at one-month followup a scar was visible in 79 patients (40 minimal, 32 mild, 7 moderate, 0 severe).
Mariotti et al. 2003 [228]	Retrospective study of patients undergoing either ABBI or Mammotome from June 1999-December 2001 for suspicious non palpable mammographic lesions not confirmed by ultrasonography	360	Vacuum-assisted CNB (Mammotome) with 11-gauge needle or ABBI	Both surgeons and patients were pleased with the cosmetic outcome.
March et al. 2003514	Prospective study of women with breast masses who underwent CNB in which complete removal of the lesion was attempted.	34	Ultrasound-guided vacuum-assisted CNB with an 11-gauge biopsy device	The twenty-one subjects who did not undergo an open procedure following CNB were examined at 6 months post-CNB. Nineteen (90%) were very satisfied with appearance of biopsy area, 2 were satisfied and none were dissatisfied. Sixteen were very satisfied with how the biopsy area felt, 5 satisfied, none dissatisfied. At 6-month follow-up examination, four (19%) had no visible scar, 17 (81%) minimal scarring = 2-9 mm, none had skin retraction concavity, convexity, or other changes in breast contour.

Reference	Design of Study	Number of Patients	Biopsy Methods	Conclusion
Fine et al. 2003217	Women who underwent CNB for low risk palpable masses were assessed prospectively.	216	Ultrasound-guided vacuum-assisted handheld biopsy device (Mammotome) with either an 8- or 11-gauge needle	A majority of patients were both satisfied with the appearance of their incisions and stated that they would recommend the procedure to others in a survey conducted 10 days post-procedure (82% and 92%, respectively).By the6-month follow-up visit, 100% were happy with the incision'sappearance and would recommend the procedure to others, while 97% stated they themselves would have the procedure again, if needed.
Kettritz et al. 2003594	Retrospective analysis of patients who underwent a CNB between January 1996-June 2000 for indeterminate lesions and microcalcifications.	2874	Vacuum-assisted CNB on a digital prone table (Mammotest) with an 11-gauge needle.	Scarring at the latest postbiopsy visit was graded as not relevant (86%), slight (14%) or relevant (0.3%).
Chun et al. 2002245	Retrospective review and survey of patients who had undergone a Mammotome, ABBI or wire localized biopsy more than 2 years	59	Stereotactic vacuum-assisted CNB biopsy (Mammotome) with 11-gauge needle or stereotactic excisional biopsy	Patients were asked to rate the appearance of their scar, if they were satisfied with the biopsy procedure, and which mattered most to them, complete lesion removal or scar appearance. Ninety-five percent of the core-needle biopsy group and only
	ago for benign disease, 20 patients per group.		with ABBI (15 or 20 mm cannula) or wire localized open biopsy	25% of the open biopsy group were very satisfied with the appearance of their breast. None of the core-needle biopsy group said the cosmetic results were unacceptable compared to 20% of the open biopsy groupwho found the results unacceptable. Overall, eighty percent of subjects were more concerned with complete lesion removal than scar appearance.
Perez-Fuentes et al. 2001534	Prospective case series of patients seen between August 1998-December 2000 with palpable or nonpalpable breast masses diagnosed with CNB.	83	Ultrasound-guided vacuum-assisted CNB (Mammotome) with 11-gauge needle	No scarring was evident at followup.
Beck et al. 2000539	Retrospective review of first experience using vacuum-assisted CNB	560	Digital stereotaxic biopsy table and vacuum-assisted CNB (Mammotome) 11-gauge needle.	In 90% no scar was visible at final followup.

CNB = Core-needle Biopsy

Table E17. Physician Experience.

Reference	Design of Study	Number of Patients	Biopsy Methods	Conclusion
Duschesne et al. 2007[61]	Prospective trial of new device used on patients already scheduled for CNB between December 2002- April 2003.	113	US-guided radiofrequency tipped vacuum-assisted CNB with 9-gauge needle (SenoCor 360 Biopsy System).	Operators of the new device rated it in terms of ease of penetration, positioning and holding the device, acquiring a satisfactory specimen, positioning accuracy, safety, and patient comfort and compared it to existing spring and vacuum devices based on their past experiences with these. All operators of the study device were experienced in US breast biopsy techniques. Operators found the new device to be equivalent to 14-gauge biopsy devices but superior to other vacuum-assisted devices in terms of penetration of the lesion and positioning of the device at the desired location. They rated patient comfort as equivalent with other types of biopsies.
hHolloway et al. 2007[67]	Retrospective review of patients with breast abnormality seen between April 2002-December 31, 2002 who were diagnosed by CNB or fine-needle aspiration and/or surgery as the initial procedure in Ontario Canada.	17,068	Fine-needle aspiration or CNB or mastectomy	Differences in the availability of the CNB (specialized expertise) may account for some of the geographic variation in how often women received a needle-biopsy procedure rather than proceeding immediately to open surgery.
Liberman et al. 2007[80]	Retrospective chart review of patients who had lesions detected with MRI and then had an MRI-guided CNB	237 lesions	MRI-guided vacuum-assisted CNB with a 9-gauge needle	The median number of previous MRI-guided CNB performed by the radiologists was 21 (Range: 1-55).
Hoffman 2005 [115]	To compare the quality of service at a clinic only partially staffed with breast specialists in 1998 to the same clinic in 2003 after it had become fully specialized. Technologically, the only change in diagnostic equipment in that time period was more sophisticated US scanners, which were used in a majority of 2003 procedures but only a small percent of 1998 procedures.	5,451	CNB vs. excisional biopsy	Over time, excisional biopsy was used less, more women had breast-conserving surgery and complication rates decreased. It is the author's conclusion that a dedicated, specialized breast care center improved the quality of care.

Reference	Design of Study	Number of Patients	Biopsy Methods	Conclusion
Lehman et al. 2004 [160]	Retrospective review of consecutive patients with nonpalpable lesions not clearly visible on mammography or targeted sonography, many of whom had recently been diagnosed with breast cancer.	28	MRI-guided vacuum-assisted CNB with the ETEC Breast Biopsy and Excision System.	The experience level of those performing the procedures was low, with half having no prior experience and the other half having one month of experience performing the procedure only (although they had one year of experience with MRI-guided CNB).
Popiela et al. 2002 [263]	Retrospective review of asymptomatic women without pathological resistance on physical examination but with breast pathologies below 0.5 cm confirmed by complementary examination.	122	Vacuum-assisted CNB (Mammotome) biopsy with either ultrasonography or digital mammography guidance	The authors contend that a lack of experience, rather than a problem with the equipment, explains problems encountered early on in precise targeting and complete removal of the lesion.
Schneider et al. 2001 [312]	Prospective case series of patients undergoing a new unilateral MR-guided breast lesion localization and core biopsy system.	14	MR image guidance CNB using a mechanical needle guide and trajectory planning software with 14-gauge needle.	The authors report that the new device is intuitive and easy to use as well.
Wunderbaldinger et al. 2001 [537]	Prospective nonconsecutive first-experience case series of patients with nonpalpable breast lesions diagnosed by CNB followed by surgical excision.	45	New dedicated US system for computer-guided CNB (Sonopsy) with a 14-gauge needle.	The authors also comment that this new device may hold promise for non-skilled physicians.
McMahon et al. 1992 [588]	Prospective randomized trial of consecutive patients with palpable breast lumps. Patients were randomized to percutaneous biopsy using Tru-Cut 14-gauge needle, Biopty-cut 14-gauge needle or a	151	Biopty-cut needles were used with the Biopty gun. A standard technique was used for the Tru Cut.	Tru Cut's poor performance (sensitivity 68%) may be related to the fact that eight different surgeons performed the 49 Tru Cut biopsies included in this study whereas the Biopty gun, with an absolute diagnostic sensitivity of 92%, may be less dependent on operator experience.

Table E 17. (Continued).

Reference	Design of Study	Number of Patients	Biopsy Methods	Conclusion
	Biopty-cut 18-gauge needle.			
Parker et al. 1990 [591]	Prospective case series of consecutive patients referred for biopsy of nonpalpable mammographically-suggestive lesions. Subjects underwent CNB followed by wire localization and excisional surgery.	103	14-, 16-, or 18-gauge Biopty-cut needles were used in conjunction with a Biopty gun. The first 30 patients were treated with Senographe Mammographic System 600T coupled with Stereotix computerized stereotactic needle localization device. Logistical problems caused investigators to switch to the Mammotest Stereotactic System for remaining patients.	Increased operator experience brought about a reduction in procedure time.

CNB = Core-needle Biopsy

Table E18. Procedure Duration Time.

Reference	Design of Study	Number of Patients	Biopsy Methods	Conclusion
Duschesne et al. 2007[61]	Prospective trial of new device used on patients already scheduled for CNB between December 2002-April 2003.	113	US-guided radiofrequency tipped vacuum-assisted (SenoCor 360 Biopsy System) with 9-gauge needle	Procedure time is decreased for this device as the breast tissue offers no resistance to penetration, but the authors do not report a time estimate.
Liberman et al. 2007[80]	Retrospective chart review of patients who had lesions detected with MRI and then had a MRI-guided CNB	237 lesions	MRI-guided vacuum-assisted (Mammotome) with 9-gauge needle	Median procedure time was 31 minutes, with procedures ranging from 17-57 minutes in total
Michalopoulos et al. 2007[33]	Prospective review of nonpalpable mammographic lesions diagnosed by CNB as either DCIS or IDC then surgically excised.	31	Vacuum-assisted CNB (Mammotome) with 11-gauge needle	Two cases of benign epithelial cell displacement occurred. The duration of the procedure was significantly longer in the two cases with displacement (52.5 ±3.5 minutes) vs. in cases without any displacement (42.0 ±4.4 min., $p = 0.018$).
Uematsu et al. 2007[97]	Retrospective study of all patients who had had an 18-gauge CNB performed from July 2003-June 2004 followed by a surgical excision.	235 lesions	US-guided 18-gauge CNB	Average procedure time was 10 minutes.
Viehweg et al. 2006 [142]	Retrospective review of consecutive patients with a family history, but no personal history, of breast cancer.	63	Either MR-guided preoperative wire localization or vacuum-assisted CNB.	Examination time was approximately 40 minutes per wire localization and 20-30 minutes for the vacuum-assisted CNB procedure, including pre- and post-interventional imaging.

Table E 18. (Continued).

Reference	Design of Study	Number of Patients	Biopsy Methods	Conclusion
Bolivar et al. 2005 [497]	Prospective case series of patients with non-palpable suspicious breast lesions who underwent 14-gauge US-guided CNB from August 1997- August 2001.	198	US-guided (7.5 MHz linear array transducer) CNB using a freehand technique with patient in supine or supine oblique position.	Examination time did not exceed 20 minutes in any cases.
Chapellier et al. 2005 [494]	Prospective case series of the first 318 aspiration-guided macrobiopsies procedures performed at one institution.	301	Fischer stereotactic imaging table system, AND vacuum-assisted CNB	The procedure, including manual pressure application, took less than one hour in 79% of cases, 90 minutes in 16% of cases, and two hours in about 5% of cases.
Diebold et al. 2005 [152]	Prospective consecutive case series of patients with mammographic BI-RADS IV microcalcifications who underwent stereostatic vacuum-assisted CNB.	58	Vacuum-assisted CNB (Mammotome) with 8-gauge needle with the ST driver (Holster) on a Mammotest plus S biopsy table.	Mean biopsy time was 28.2 minutes (Range: 10-1 20 minutes). Removing 5 highly complicated cases from this analysis reduced the average procedure time to 16.1 minutes.
Orel et al. 2005 [131]	Retrospective review of patients with suspicious lesions identified at MR imaging who either underwent surgery or had six month follow-up imaging.	75	MR-guided vacuum-assisted CNB with a 9-gauge needle	Total MRI-guided procedure time (including pre-biopsy imaging examination, biopsy and postbiopsy care) ranged from 30-60 minutes.
Perlet et al. 2005 [132]	Prospective study of MR-guided vacuum-assisted CNB visible by CE- MRI alone or localized in 3 dimensions by MRI alone	538	Impact, Expert or Vision MR scanner guidance, vacuum-assisted CNB (Mammotome) with an 11-gauge needle	On average, MR-guided CNB lasted 70 minutes if the patient was having one lesion biopsied and 90 minutes for patients with two lesions.
Weber et al. 2005 [502]	Retrospective comparison study of patients with impalpable breast lesions undergoing either Mammotome or ABBI.	387	Stereotactically-Guided vacuum-assisted CNB (Mammotome) with 11-gauge needle or ABBI	Median duration of the Mammotome procedure was shorter than the ABBI procedure ($p < 0.0001$).

Reference	Design of Study	Number of Patients	Biopsy Methods	Conclusion
Wong et al. 2005 [171]	Prospective trial of Asian patients with nonpalpable mammographic abnormalities underwent either ABBI (N = 7) or vacuum-assisted CNB (N = 107).	114	Vacuum-assisted CNB (Mammotome) with an 8- to 11-gauge needle prone or ABBI.	Procedures lasted from 30-128 minutes (Median: 68.5).
Alonso-Bartolome et al. 2004 [504]	Prospective study of women with probably benign breast lesions who refused radiologic followup and, instead, insisted on removal. Complete lesion removal was the intended goal for all lesions.	97	US-guided vacuum-assisted CNB (Mammotome) with 11-gauge needle	Mean procedure time was one hour (Range: 40-75 minutes). Based on a cost to patient estimate in terms of hours lost, investigators report that the time lost to CNB is less than 20% of the time required for a surgical biopsy.
Geller et al. 2004 [183]	Survey of women with nonpalpable breast lesions who had an US-guided CNB or excisional biopsy between 1997-1999.	315	US-guided CNB vs. excisional biopsy.	Survey results 1-3 months post procedure measured convenience of the procedure (distance travelled, procedure time, and number of days of work missed post procedure). No difference was found between two groups in terms of miles travelled for procedure, but the excisional biopsy group missed more work.
Lehman et al. 2004 [160]	Retrospective review of consecutive patients with nonpalpable lesions not clearly visible on mammography or targeted sonography, many of whom had recently been diagnosed with breast cancer.	28	MRI-guided vacuum-assisted CNB with the ETEC Breast Biopsy and Excision System.	Time to perform procedure was defined as the start of the first MRI sequence (localizing) to the last scan sequence (clip deployment). The average time for single biopsy procedures was 38 minutes (range: 23-57 minutes). Average time for multiple biopsy procedures in a single breast was 59 minutes (51-68 minutes) and for bilateral procedures 64 (46-80 minutes).

Table E 18. (Continued).

Reference	Design of Study	Number of Patients	Biopsy Methods	Conclusion
Rotenberg et al. 2004 [200]	Prospective case series of patients with palpable tumors and patients with tumors which were visible on ultrasound imaging or radiology.	30	Spirotome System with 8- to 10-gauge needle. No stereotactic tables were used in the study.	Biopsies took a maximum of 20 minutes to complete, with 80% of the biopsies being completed in only 10 minutes.
Chen et al. 2003 [210]	Retrospective study of patients with nonpalpable breast lesions from January 1998-2001 undergoing either a CNB or open biopsy.	232	Comparison of vacuum-assisted CNB (Mammotome) with 11-gauge needle vs. ultrasound-guided excisional biopsy	Procedure times were measured from initial skin incision to wound closure or needle withdrawal. Procedure times were as follows: for benign tumor cases 44.3 and 21.5 minutes ($p < 0.001$); for malignant cases 44.0 and 27.0 ($P = .036$); for tumors <1 cm in diameter, 43.5 and 20.6 ($p < 0.001$) and for tumors 1-2 cm, 44.2 and 23.6 minutes ($p < 0.001$) for open and CNB, respectively. Procedure time for the older model Mammotome device (used in first year of study) vs. newer handheld variant , which was used in the second year, was 24 and 18 minutes on average, respectively ($p < 0.001$).
Liberman et al. 2003 [227]	Prospective case series of women with one of the following: a nonpalpable mammographically-occult lesion at high risk for breast cancer or for extent of disease assessment.	20	MRI-guided 9-gauge vacuum-assisted breast biopsy.	Imaging time was 20 minutes, on average, including three contrast enhanced acquisitions. Median MRI-guided CNB time, from localizing image to imaging after clip deployment was 35 minutes (Mean: 35, Range: 24-48 for a single lesion and 65 minutes (Mean: 69, Range: 62-86) for patients with two lesions. Median tissue acquisition time was 38 seconds (Mean: 41, Range: 29-87).

Reference	Design of Study	Number of Patients	Biopsy Methods	Conclusion
Mariotti et al. 2003 [228]	Retrospective study of patients undergoing either ABBI or CNB from June 1999-December 2001 for suspicious non palpable mammographic lesions not confirmed by ultrasonography.	360	Vacuum-assisted CNB (Mammotome) with 11-gauge needle vs. ABBI	ABBI and Mammotome procedure times were 20 and 10 minutes, on average, respectively, for the operative portion of the procedure only.
Pleiderer et al. 2003 [515]	Prospective nonconsecutive case series of patients with suspicious breast lesions who had a diagnostic CNB with a new device.	14	Remote controlled MRI compatible prototype manipulator system (ROB ITOM) using 14-gauge large core breast biopsy.	Total procedure time was between 50-70 minutes.
Apesteguia et al. 2002 [518]	Prospective consecutive case series of patients with nonpalpable breast lesions non-visible or non-accessible by US.	126	Vacuum-assisted CNB on a digital stereotaxic table with an 11-gauge needle.	Mean procedure time was 29.6 ±14 minutes (Range: 15-90 minutes).
Hui et al. 2002 [252]	Prospective case series of patients with nonpapable breast lesions requiring a biopsy procedure.	79	Stereotactic-guided breast biopsy (StereoGuide with Digital Spot Mammography): Trucut with a 14-gauge needle, Mammotome with 11-gauge probe, or FNA with a 22-gauge needle, depending on the characteristics of the lesion.	Mean duration of the biopsy procedure was 49 minutes (range: 30-90).
Mainiero et al. 2002 [259]	Prospective nonrandomized comparison study of patients with suspicious breast lesions underg-oing a CNB between 1997-1999.	193	Either freehand high resolution sonographically-guided large core biopsy with 14-gauge needle vs. stereotactic vacuum-assisted	The authors examined how much room time and physician time was expended for each type of procedure. They found stereotactic VABB took more room and physician time when all biopsies were

Table E 18. (Continued).

Reference	Design of Study	Number of Patients	Biopsy Methods	Conclusion
			CNB (Mammotest with 11-gauge needle).	examined together. When only room and physician time for patients with masses was examined, only room time significantly differed in the same direction by procedure type. The authors conclude that sonographically-guided breast biopsies reduce procedure time compared with stereotactic biopsy.
Becker et al. 2001 [527]	Retrospective chart review of 232 lesions with indeterminate microcalcifications in 218 women.	218	DMR regular mammography machine plus either a Stereotix 2 conventional add-on unit or a SenoVision digital add-on unit. CNB was performed with a 14-gauge needle in all but 5 cases (in which a 16-gauge needle was used)	Changing from a conventional to a digital add-on unit cut the procedure time by half (from 50 to 20 minutes). Most of this time savings is related to the speed of displaying digital images, 15 seconds per image, versus 3 minutes to develop radiographs.
Perez-Fuentes et al. 2001 [534]	Prospective case series of patients seen between August 1998-December 2000 with palpable or nonpalpable breast masses diagnosed with CNB.	83	Sonographically- guided vacuum-assisted CNB (Mammotome) with 11-gauge needle	Median procedure time (acquisition of prebiopsy sonogram to positioning of sterile bandage on skin) was 17 minutes (Range: 10-40)
Schneider et al. 2001 [312]	Prospective case series of patients undergoing a new unilateral MR-guided breast lesion localization and core biopsy system.	14	MR image guidance AND CNB using a mechanical needle guide and trajectory planning software with 14-gauge needle.	Mean procedure time was 15 ±5 minutes (Range: 5-24), including 3D acquisition scan, completion of the verification scan, placement of single and multiple stylettes for multiple localization wire placements, and multiple tissue sampling by CNB.

Reference	Design of Study	Number of Patients	Biopsy Methods	Conclusion
Wunderbaldinger et al. 2001 [537]	Prospective nonconsecutive first-experience case series of patients with nonpalpable breast lesions diagnosed by CNB followed by surgical excision.	45	New dedicated US system for computer-guided CNB (Sonopsy) with a 14-gauge needle.	Average procedure time (including patient positioning, biopsy, localization but not post procedural handling) was 30 ±2.7 minutes.
Beck et al. 2000 [539]	Retrospective review of first experience using vacuum-assisted CNB	560	Digital stereotaxic biopsy table and vacuum-assisted CNB (Mammotom) with 11-gauge needle.	The authors report that patient positioning took approximately 15 minutes; 30 minutes for the actual procedure; 15 minutes for compression; 10 minutes for a final mammogram; and another 30-45 for observation.
Welle et al. 2000 [545]	Retrospective review of patients who underwent a stereotactic CNB in a decubitus or recumbent position from September 1995-March 1999.	225	Stereotactic CNB in a decubitus or recumbent position.	Procedure time was recorded as minutes in compression (mean 25, range: 20-50). Procedures done with digital mammogr-aphic equipment and the Mammotome were approximately 10 minutes shorter
Bloomston et al. 1999 [348]	Prospective consecutive case series of women with nonpalpable breast abnormalities who had an ABBI.	100	Stereotactic ABBI.	Average procedure time was 20 ±8 minutes.
Doyle et al. 1999 [552]	Retrospective study of patients with mammographically-detected lesions on CNB from 1994-1998.	151	Senographe 600T was used for 136 biopsies; 15 using Mammomat 3000; all in decubitus position unless the patient couldn't tolerate that positioning and with a 14-gauge needle.	Mean procedure time was 20 minutes

Table E 18. (Continued).

Reference	Design of Study	Number of Patients	Biopsy Methods	Conclusion
Bolivar et al. 1998 [558]	Patients seen between October 1993- October 1996 having a CNB for nonpalpable breast lesions.	180	Stereotactic CNB (Stereotix localization stereotaxic device attached to Senix 500T screen film mammo-graphic unit) with the Menghini nonautomatic 15-gauge needle with multiple pass technique (Surecut).	THE CNB procedure averaged between 45-55 minutes.
Whitman et al. 1998 [559]	Retrospective chart review of 12 CNB in 11 women.	11	Mammographically- guided coaxial CNB procedure performed with a fenestrated alphanumeric compression device with a 15-gauge Tru Guide outer cannula and a 16-gauge Monopty biopsy instrument	The CNB procedure ranged in time from 30-80 minutes.
Burbank 1997 [413]	Retrospective study comparing the accuracy of directional, vacuum-assisted stereotactic CNB with stereotactic automated gun CNB	101	Prone position under stereotactic guidance on the Mammotest with 14-gauge needles	Directional, vacuum-assisted biopsy tissue harvest time was 18.6 ±15.8 minutes per lesion, on average, meaning 26.5 specimens can be obtained in that amount of time, at a tissue harvest rate of 1.4 specimens per minute. No information is given for automated procedure.
Florentine et al. 1997 [421]	Retrospective review of patients with palpable breast lesions who underwent a combined FNA/CNB procedure.	12	CNB using an 18-gauge Temno needle	The CNB procedure took approximately 20 minutes, on average.

Reference	Design of Study	Number of Patients	Biopsy Methods	Conclusion
Helbich et al. 1997 [563]	Prospective randomized trial of patients with mammographically-suspicious solid lesions. Patients were randomized to stereotactic CNB in a sitting position; stereotactic CNB in the prone position; or CNB with US guidance. CNB was followed by surgical excision.	210	CNB with either stereotactic or US guidance using a 14-gauge needle.	Acquisition of the CNB specimen took an average of 19±3 minutes with stereotactic guidance vs. 13±4 minutes with US guidance.
Howisey et al. 1997 [424]	Retrospective review of Medicare patients with mammographic abnormalities who went on to have ultrasound-guided CNB, stereotactic-guided CNB or wire localization with surgical excision between July 1994-December 1995.	139	Ultrasound or stereotactic-guided CNB	US-guided CNB had a shorter procedure time (<20 minutes per case) than stereotacticguided CNB. No time given for stereotactic procedure.
Yim et al. 1996 [454]	Retrospective chart review of subjects with invasive breast cancer diagnosed by either CNB or needle localization surgical biopsy.	52	Stereotactic CNB with a 14-gauge needle was performed on a dedicated prone table (Lorad, Danbury, CT) vs. needle localized open biopsy	Average total procedure time for the CNB was 40-50 minutes, but the biopsy time itself was shorter than for open biopsy.
Janes et al. 1994 [469]	Prospective case series of initial 300 CNBs performed by a group of five surgeons.	288	CNB using Fischer Imaging Mammotest with Auto-Guide and the Mammoscan System, 14-gauge needle Biopty-Cut Biopsy Needle.	By the 100th procedure, total procedure time, from initial image taking to completion of the acquisition, rarely exceeded 30 minutes. Acquisition times for lesions centered on the initial image were 15-20 minutes.

Table E 18. (Continued).

Reference	Design of Study	Number of Patients	Biopsy Methods	Conclusion
Elvecrog et al. 1993 [586]	Prospective study of women with a single nonpalpable breast lesion imaged by mammography who underwent CNB followed by hook-wire localization and open surgical biopsy.	100	Mammotest stereotaxic system and 14-gauge needle.	Average per case procedure time, including obtaining preliminary views, was 50-60 minutes. The CNB alone took between 30-40 minutes, on average. No data on average time for the open biopsy procedure was presented.
Parker et al. 1990[591]	Prospective case series of consecutive patients referred for biopsy of nonpalpable mammogr-aphically-suggestive lesions. Subjects underwent CNB followed by wire localization and excisional surgery.	103	14-, 16-, or 18-gauge Biopty-cut needles were used in conjunction with a Biopty gun. The first 30 patients were treated with Senographe Mammographic System 600T coupled with Stereotix computerized stereotactic needle localiz-ation device. Logistical problems caused investiga-tors to switch to the Mam-motest Stereotactic System for remaining patients.	Average procedure time by end of the study was 20-30 minutes without local-ization wire placement. No data on proce-dure time for early cases was provided.

Table E19. Wait time for test results.

Reference	Design of Study	Number of Patients	Biopsy Methods	Conclusion
Verkooijen et al. 2001 [593]	Prospective comparison of patients with nonpalpable breast lesions	164	Stereotactic guidance on a prone table with a 14-gauge needle.	Median wait time was 9 days for core-needle biopsies and 19 days for wire-localized open biopsies.
Gukas et al. 2000 [326]	Prospective study of patients with palpable lesions	108	Tru-Cut	Reduced wait time to get back a test result was, on av-erage, 7.3 days less for Tru-Cut than excisional biopsy.

Table E20. Availability of a Qualified Pathologist.

Reference	Design of study	Number of patients	Biopsy methods	Conclusion
Collins et al. 2004 [179]	Retrospective chart review of patients with nonpalpable lesions	2,004	CNB using either stereotactic mammography or ultrasound. In some cases a 14-gauge needle was used, in others a vacuum-assisted procedure was done with either a 14- or 11-gauge needle.	Local pathology diagnoses were compared to those made by a central pathologist. In 96% of CNB cases the two pathologists were in agreement. Agreement rates were as follows for the subcategories of benign lesions, invasive cancers, DCIS cases, ADH, and lobular neoplasia: 99%, 97%, 83%, 63%, and 53%, respectively. Agreement rates remained stable regardless of biopsy guidance system and biopsy device used.
Gukas et al. 2000 [326]	Prospective study of 112 consecutive patients with palp-able breast lesions.	108	Tru-Cut and excisional biopsies.	The pathologist in this study was not highly experienced with Tru-Cut, which the authors believe explains its poor diagnosis rate in this study.

Table E21. Availability of Equipment.

Reference	Design of Study	Number of Patients	Biopsy Methods	Conclusion
Deurloo et al. 2001 [285]	Retrospective review of patients with nonpalpable breast lesions.	84	StereoGuide with 14-gauge needle	Vacuum-assisted biopsy is increasingly being used in the United States. But, in Europe, acceptance of vacuum-assisted biopsy is considerably less whereas core biopsy devices are used much more.
Verkooijen et al. 2001 [593]	Prospective comparison of patients with nonpalpable breast lesions	164	Stereotactic guidance, on a prone table with a 14-gauge needle.	Median wait times for access to core-needle biopsy equipment were only 4 days while access to open surgical biopsy had a median wait time of 13 days.
Williams et al. 1999 [384]	Prospective case series of patients with impalpable breast lesions diagnosed by stereotactic core- needle biopsy on a prone table vs. a historical cohort of patients with similar lesions diagnosed prior to the availability of a prone table.	222	Stereotactic prone CNB with Mammotest and 14-gauge needle.	There was no significant difference in lag time between screening and definitive diagnosis for the two groups. However, there was a delay in having the prone procedure due to the longer waiting list.

Table E22. Resource Usage.

Reference	Design of Study	Number of Patients	Biopsy Methods	Conclusion
Mainiero et al. 2002 [259]	Prospective nonrandomized comparison study of patients with suspicious breast lesions	193	Either freehand high resolution US-guided large core biopsy with 14-gauge needle or a stereotactic-guided vacuum- assisted biopsy (Mammotest) with 11-gauge needle	The authors examined how much room time and physician time was expended for each type of procedure. They found vacuum-assisted procedures took more room and physician time when all biopsies were examined together. When only room and physician time for patients with masses was examined, only room time significantly differed in the same direction by procedure type.
Wunderbaldinger et al. 2002 [277]	Prospective randomized study	200	Stereotactic-guided biopsies in either sitting or prone position with a 14-gauge needle.	In the conclusion the authors report that prone systems require four times the amount of space as a regular unit and are often underused as their only function is breast biopsy. In addition, there is a weight limit to prone machines.

Appendix F. Data Analysis

Table F23. Accuracy Data Freehand Biopsies.

Study	Type Core Biopsy	TP	FP	FN	TN	N Atypia	N Atypia Underestimates	N DCIS	N DCIS Underestimates
Wong and Hisham 2003 [517]	Freehand automated gun 14G	42	1	3	50	NR	NR	NR	NR
Wong and Hisham 2003 [517]	Freehand automated gun 16G	23	0	1	30	NR	NR	NR	NR
Scopa et al. 1996 [578]	Freehand TruCut	83	1	10	14	6	5	NR	NR
McMahon et al. 1992 [588]	Freehand Bioptycut 14G	21	0	3	27	NR	NR	NR	NR
McMahon et al. 1992 [588]	Freehand Bioptycut 18G	23	0	1	27	NR	NR	NR	NR
McMahon et al. 1992 [588]	Freehand Trucut 14G	17	0	8	24	NR	NR	NR	NR
Barreto et al. 1991 [589]	Freehand automated gun 18G	62	0	34	11	NR	NR	NR	NR
Cusick et al. 1990 [590]	Freehand	78	0	10	6	NR	NR	NR	NR

Table F24. Accuracy Data for US-Guided Automated Gun Biopsies.

Study	Type of core biopsy	TP	FP	FN	TN	N atypia	N atypia underestimated	N DCIS	N DCIS underestimated
Schueller et al. 2008 [487]	US guidance automated gun 14G	698	59	11	584	86	27	52	19
Youk et al. 200824	US guidance automated gun 14G	1,281	68	31	1,040	93	25	126	36
de Lucena et al. 2007 [491]	US guidance automated gun 14G	95	0	6	49	0	0	0	0
Bolivar et al. 2005 [497]	US guidance automated gun 14G	118	2	4	79	2	0	NR	NR
Crystal et al. 2005 [498]	US guidance automated gun 14G	313	3	10	389	5	2	6	4
Sauer et al. 2005 [501]	US guidance automated gun 14G	604	0	11	44	2	2	18	11
Delle and Terinde 2004 [505]	US guidance automated gun 14G	124	0	4	39	NR	NR	NR	NR
Fishman et al. 2003 [511]	US guidance automated gun 14G	14	0	0	38	NR	NR	2	0
Philpotts et al. 2003 [516]	US guidance automated gun 14G	35	4	1	81	4	0	2	0
Smith et al. 2001 [535]	US guidance automated gun 14G	118	2	0	275	4	2	5	1
Wunderbaldinger et al. 2001 [537]	US guidance automated gun 14G	21	3	0	20	3	0	2	0
Yeow et al. 2001 [538]	US guidance automated gun 14 or 1 6G	66	2	0	30	2	0	2	0
Liberman et al. 1998 [556]	US guidance automated gun 14G	51	1	3	64	1	0	4	2
Schulz-Wendtland et al. 1998 [557]	US guidance automated gun 14G	155	0	3	147	1	1	8	2
Khattar et al. 1997 [564]	US guidance automated gun	41	0	3	13	NR	NR	NR	NR
Parker et al. 1993 [587]	US guidance automated gun 14G	34	4	0	143	4	0	NR	NR

Table F25. Accuracy Data Stereotactic Guidance Automated Gun Core-Needle Biopsies.

Study	Type of Core Biopsy	TP	FP	FN	TN	N Atypia	N Atypia Underestimated	N DCIS	N DCIS Underestimated
Peters et al. 2008 [486]	Stereotactic guidance automated gun 14G	483	16	0	312	22	6	196	55
Koskela et al. 2005 [500]	Stereotactic guidance automated gun 14G	82	2	1	117	4	3	33	7
Han et al. 2003 [512]	Stereotactic guidance automated gun 14G	44	8	11	33	8	0	39	4
Verkooijen et al. COBRA 2002 [526]	Stereotactic guidance automated gun 14G	480	20	15	307	26	6	190	32
Becker et al. 2001 [527]	Stereotactic guidance automated gun 14G	43	6	2	101	14	8	36	NR
Brenner et al. 2001 [528]	Stereotactic guidance automated gun 14G	230	0	24	234	NR	NR	NR	NR
Dahlstrom and Jain 2001 [530]	Stereotactic guidance automated gun 14G	56	4	11	219	15	11	NR	NR
Levin et al. 2001 [532]	Stereotactic guidance automated gun 14G	22	0	2	46	NR	NR	NR	NR
Kirwan et al. 2000 [540]	Stereotactic guidance automated gun 14G	23	6	0	34	11	5	3	0
Ward et al. 2000 [544]	Stereotactic guidance automated gun 14G	26	3	1	73	6	3	NR	NR
Jackman et al. 1999 [547]	Stereotactic guidance automated gun 14G	159	13	2	305	29	16	56	8
Soo et al. 1999 [550]	Stereotactic guidance automated gun 14G	12	0	0	48	1	1	0	0
Doyle et al. 1998 [552]	Stereotactic guidance automated gun 14G	51	4	0	77	4	4	21	NR
Vega-Bolivar et al. 1998 [558]	Stereotactic guidance Surecut 15G	74	5	0	44	11	6	18	6

Study	Type of Core Biopsy	TP	FP	FN	TN	N Atypia	N Atypia Underestimated	N DCIS	N DCIS Underestimated
Whitman et al. 1998 [559]	Stereotactic guidance automated gun 16G	6	2	0	3	2	0	4	3
Zannis and AliaNo 1998 [560]	Stereotactic guidance automated gun 14G	31	6	0	77	7	1	3	2
Bauer et al. 1997 [561]	Stereotactic guidance automated gun 14G	85	12	1	697	20	8	32	8
Liberman et al. 1997 [565]	Stereotactic guidance automated gun 14G	144	34	7	162	55	21	NR	NR
Pitre et al. 1997 [566]	Stereotactic guidance automated gun	10	2	1	100	3	1	NR	NR
Sutton, et al. 1997 [568]	Stereotactic guidance automated gun 14G	58	1	1	80	8	7	NR	NR
Walker et al. 1997 [569]	Stereotactic guidance automated gun 14G	95	9	14	60	14	5	43	6
Frazee et al. 1996 [570]	Stereotactic guidance automated gun	6	0	0	45	0	0	2	0
Fuhrman et al. 1996 [571]	Stereotactic guidance automated gun 14G	48	12	1	268	21	9	NR	NR
Head and Haynes 1996 [572]	Stereotactic guidance automated gun 18G	12	6	0	84	12	6	NR	NR
Mainiero et al. 1996 [573]	Stereotactic guidance automated gun 14G	23	10	3	79	14	4	13	6
Meyer et al. 1996 [574]	Stereotactic guidance automated gun 14G	60	1	0	210	2	1	2	2
Pettine et al. 1996 [576]	Stereotactic guidance automated gun 14G	6	0	1	17	NR	NR	1	0
Rosenblatt et al. 1996 [577]	Stereotactic guidance automated gun 14G	15	0	0	6	NR	NR	2	2
Cross et al. 1995 [579]	Stereotactic guidance automated gun 14G	44	0	0	172	NR	NR	NR	NR

Table F 25. (Continued).

Study	Type of Core Biopsy	TP	FP	FN	TN	N Atypia	N Atypia Underestimated	N DCIS	N DCIS Underestimated
Gisvold et al. 1994 [583]	Stereotactic guidance automated gun 14G	60	1	6	93	4	3	NR	NR
Smyth and Ceder-bom 1994 [585]	Stereotactic guidance automated gun 14G	14	0	0	44	NR	NR	NR	NR
Elvecrog et al. 1993 [586]	Stereotactic guidance automated gun 14G	31	8	0	64	8	0	NR	NR
Parker et al. 1990 [591]	Stereotactic guidance automated gun	15	0	1	80	NR	NR	NR	NR

Table F 26. Accuracy data ultrasound-guided vacuum-assisted core-needle biopsies.

Study	Type of Core Biopsy	TP	FP	FN	TN	N Atypia	N Atypia Underestimated	N DCIS	N DCIS Underestimated
Vag et al. 2007 [493]	US guidance vacuum-assisted 10G	28	0	1	41	NR	NR	NR	NR
Wu et al. 2005 [503]	US guidance vacuum-assisted 11G	0	0	1	112	0	0	0	0
Alonso-Bartolome et al. 2004 [504]	US guidance vacuum-assisted 1 1G	1	1	0	100	1	0	NR	NR
March et al. 2003 [514]	US guidance vacuum-assisted 11G	8	2	0	21	2	0	1	0
Philpotts et al. 2003 [516]	US guidance vacuum-assisted 1 1G	19	2	1	37	2	0	1	1
Johnson et al. 2002 [521]	US guidance vacuum-assisted 11 or 8G	3	2	0	70	2	0	0	0
Perez-Fuentes et al. 2001 [534]	US guidance vacuum-assisted 1 1G	14	1	0	42	1	0	NR	NR

Table F 27. Accuracy Data Stereotactic Guidance Vacuum-Assisted Core-Needle Biopsy.

Study	Type of Core Biopsy	TP	FP	FN	TN	N Atypia	N Atypia Underestimated	N DCIS	N DCIS Underestimated
Jackman et al. 2009 [485]	Stereotactic guidance vacuum- assisted 11G or 14G	503	97	5	604	NR	NR	NR	NR
Sim and Kei 2008 [488]	Stereotactic guidance vacuum- assisted 11G	16	7	0	69	7	0	15	0
Tonegutti and Girardi 2008 [489]	Stereotactic guidance vacuum- assisted 11G	56	22	0	140	27	5	35	3
Uematsu et al. 2007 [492]	Stereotactic guidance vacuum- assisted 11G	34	7	0	59	8	1	31	4
Chapellier et al. 2006 [494]	Stereotactic guidance vacuum- assisted 11G	85	17	0	209	19	2	51	11
Dhillon et al. 2006 [496]	Stereotactic guidance vacuum- assisted 11G	46	16	0	88	18	2	34	4
Weber et al. 2005 [502]	Stereotactic guidance vacuum- assisted 11G	62	8	2	118	9	1	40	6
Kettritz et al. 2004 [507]	Stereotactic guidance vacuum- assisted 11G	669	103	1	1461	135	32	434	49
Lomoschitz et al. 2004 [508]	Stereotactic guidance vacuum- assisted 11G	45	2	2	22	4	2	12	2
Ambrogetti et al. 2003 [510]	Stereotactic guidance vacuum- assisted 11G	144	12	15	66	17	5	115	20
Apesteguia et al. 2002 [518]	Stereotactic guidance vacuum- assisted 11G	47	13	0	70	14	1	32	5
Georgian-Smith et al. 2002 [519]	Stereotactic guidance vacuum- assisted 11G	29	7	1	106	9	2	17	2
Liberman et al. 2002 [522]	Stereotactic guidance vacuum- assisted 11G	213	38	3	321	49	11	120	17
Meloni et al. 2002 [523]	Stereotactic guidance vacuum- assisted	40	1	0	64	2	1	22	1
Morris et al. 2002 [524]	Stereotactic guidance vacuum- assisted 14G	4	1	0	12	1	0	0	0
Pfarl et al. 2002 [525]	Stereotactic guidance vacuum- assisted 11G	207	11	7	93	17	6	91	11
Cangiarella et al. 2001 [529]	Stereotactic guidance vacuum- assisted 11G	15	8	0	92	10	2	12	1
Lai et al. 2001 [531]	Stereotactic guidance vacuum- assisted 11G	148	8	2	321	10	2	48	6
Beck et al. 2000 [539]	Stereotactic guidance vacuum- assisted 11G	105	13	0	477	13	0	74	0
Soo et al. 1999 [550]	Stereotactic guidance vacuum- assisted 14G	10	1	0	22	1	0	2	0
Heywang-Kobrunner et al.	Stereotactic guidance vacuum-	45	6	0	129	6	0	30	0
Jackman et al. 2009 [485]	Stereotactic guidance vacuum- assisted 11G or 14G	503	97	5	604	NR	NR	NR	NR
Sim and Kei 2008 [488] 1998 [554]	Stereotactic guidance vacuum- assisted 11G assisted 11 or 14G	16	7	0	69	7	0	15	0
Zannis and AliaNo 1998 [560]	Stereotactic guidance vacuum- assisted 11G	17	4	0	33	4	0	9	0

Table F28. Accuracy Data Miscellaneous Methods Of Biopsy.

Study	Type Core Biopsy	TP	FP	FN	TN	N Atypia	N Atypia Underestimates	N DCIS	N DCIS Underestimates
Pfleiderer et al. 2003 [515]	MRI guidance automated gun 14G	5	0	1	8	1	1	NR	NR
Puglisi et al. 1999 [549]	Perforated compression grid automated gun 14G	32	2	3	63	4	1	7	2

Table F29. Accuracy Data Mixed Methods of Biopsy Not Reported Separately.

Study	Type Core Biopsy	TP	FP	FN	TN	N Atypia	N Atypia Underestimated	N DCIS	N DCIS Underestimated
Ciatto et al. 2007 [490]	Multiple methods	1,158	207	71	1,532	NR	NR	NR	NR
Cipolla et al. 2006 [495]	Multiple methods	182	11	1	232	16	6	8	3
Dillon et al. 2005 [499]	Multiple methods	1,299	120	85	461	181	71	NR	NR
Fajardo et al. 2004 [506]	Multiple methods	358	31	17	1,025	54	23	NR	NR
Abdsaleh et al. 2003 [509]	Multiple methods	104	1	16	18	NR	NR	7	2
Kirshenbaum et al. 2003 [513]	Multiple methods	117	20	2	253	24	6	NR	NR
Jackman and Lamm 2002 [520]	Multiple methods	11	3	0	17	3	0	5	0
Margolin et al. 2001 [533]	Multiple methods	158	14	0	1,120	26	12	NR	NR
White et al. 2001 [536]	Multiple methods	231	31	7	464	39	10	65	18
Latosinsky et al. 2000 [541]	Multiple methods	85	13	6	246	21	8	30	8
Liberman et al. 2000 [542]	Multiple methods	62	4	1	36	4	2	4	2
Makoske et al. 2000 [543]	Multiple methods	139	28	0	377	38	10	39	19
Welle et al. 2000 [545]	Multiple methods	36	15	0	122	13	4	7	3
Meyer et al. 1999 [548]	Multiple methods	493	63	0	855	88	25	133	20
Caruso et al. 1998 [551]	Multiple methods	67	0	0	7	NR	NR	2	2
Fuhrman et al. 1998 [553]	Multiple methods	295	31	3	852	67	36	84	30

Study	Type Core Biopsy	TP	FP	FN	TN	N Atypia	N Atypia Underestimated	N DCIS	N DCIS Underestimated
Loffe et al. 1998 [555]	Multiple methods	50	7	0	125	10	3	NR	NR
Britton et al. 1997 [562]	Multiple methods	94	2	7	95	NR	NR	NR	NR
Helbich et al. 1997 [563]	Multiple methods	100	2	3	105	4	2	12	0
Stolier et al. 1997 [567]	Multiple methods	30	6	2	170	12	3	10	0
Nguyen et al. 1996 [575]	Multiple methods	183	9	4	217	NR	NR	NR	NR
Doyle et al. 1995 [580]	Multiple methods	23	2	0	119	6	4	NR	NR
Burbank et al. 1994 [582]	Multiple methods	14	3	0	88	3	1	6	0
Parker et al. 1994 [584]	Multiple methods	967	129	15	2,654	186	57	148	18

Table F30. Miscellaneous Accuracy Data.

Study	Accuracy by Breast Lesion Factors	Accuracy by Patient Characteristics	Accuracy by Biopsy Methods	Accuracy by Clinician and Facility Factors
Ciatto et al. 2007 [490]	Palpable lesions: 400 true positives, 63 false positives, 27 false negatives, 493 true negatives Non-palpable lesions: 758 true positives, 144 false positives, 44 false negatives, 1038 true negative Masses on mammography: 540 true positives, 103 false positives, 36 false negatives, 839 true negatives Distortions on mammography: 17 true positives, 27 false positives, 1 false negative, 29 true negatives Microcalcifications: 601 true positives, 77 false positives, 34 false negatives, 663 true negatives	NR	NR	Overall sensitivity improved over the course of the study, 88% first year, 96% final year.
de Lucena et al. 2007[491]	NR	NR	The rate of false negatives decreased from 9.9% with only one core to 5.9% with two cores. Adding additional cores beyond 2 didn't improve the accuracy of the biopsy.	NR
Cipolla et al. 2006 [495]	Correspondence between the core-biopsy and surgical specimen was	NR	NR	NR

Table F 30. (Continued).

Study	Accuracy by Breast Lesion Factors	Accuracy by Patient Characteristics	Accuracy by Biopsy Methods	Accuracy by Clinician and Facility Factors
	100% in palpable lesions but only 88.6% in non-palpable lesions			
Koskela et al. 2005 [500]	Masses on mammography: 40 true positives, 1 false-negative, 55 true negatives Microcalcifications: 43 true positives, 0 false-negatives, 66 true negatives	NR	More than three samples are needed for a diagnosis of a mass lesion	NR
Fajardo et al. 2004 [506]	Nonpalpable lesions: Sensitivity 90.7% Masses on mammography: Sensitivity 97.4% Microcalcifications: 90.7%	NR	NR	NR
Lomoschitz et al. 2004 [508]	Masses on mammography: 25 true positives, 1 false-negative, 23 true negatives Microcalcifications: 18 true positives, 1 false-negative, 28 true negatives	NR	12 specimens were necessary to yield correct diagnoses in 96% of patients with masses and 92% of patients with microcalcifications, and addition of further cores did not improve accuracy.	NR
Abdsaleh et al. 2003 [509]	NR	34 of the 35 technical failures occurred in dense breasts	For one core there were 12 false- negatives out of 107 biopsies; for two cores there were 3 false-negatives out of 34 biopsies.	NR
Fishman et al. 2003 [511]	NR	NR	Cells indicating the final diagnosis were present in the first core in 51 cases, in the second core in 67 cases, in the third core in 70 cases, and in the fourth core in all 73 cases.	
Pfarl et al. 2002 [525]	Masses on mammography: 96 true positives, 3 false negatives, 52 true negatives Microcalcifications: 111 true positives, 4 false negatives, 42 true negatives	NR	NR	In six of the seven false- negative cases the biopsy was performed by an operator who had previously performed 15 or fewer stereotactic vacuum-assisted biopsies.
Doyle et al. 1998 [552]	NR	NR	Of 14 biopsies performed in the seated position, there were no technical failures and no false negatives	NR

Study	Accuracy by Breast Lesion Factors	Accuracy by Patient Characteristics	Accuracy by Biopsy Methods	Accuracy by Clinician and Facility Factors
			Of 137 biopsies performed in the decubuitus position, there were 2 technical failures and no false negatives	
Helbich et al. 1997 [563]	NR	NR	Patients were randomly assigned to supine, prone, sitting; authors comment they did not find patient position to impact the biopsy procedure.	NR
Walker et al. 1997 [569]	Masses on mammography: Sensitivity 93% Distortions on mammography: Sensitivity 89% Microcalcifications: Sensitivity 85%	NR	NR	NR
Barreto et al. 1991 [589]	Tumor size did not affect accuracy; however, patients with the lesion located in the right breast had a higher rate of false-negatives (right side, 45% were false negative, left side, 27% were false negative).	Age of patients did not affect accuracy	NR	Accuracy improved over time- first 25% of biopsies performed there were 50% true positives; second and third 25% of biopsies performed there were 63% true positives; last 25% of biopsies performed there were 83% true positives.
Cusick et al. 1990 [590]	24% of lesions smaller than 2 cm had false-negative findings compared to only 7% of larger lesions having false-negative findings	NR	NR	NR

Table F31. Harms Data.

Study	Number of Lesions Enrolled	Type of Biopsy	Hematomas	Bleeding	Vasovagal Reactions	Infections	Other	Time to Recovery or Time to Return to Work	Use of Pain Medications	Patient Satisfaction, Quality of Life Data	Impact of Biopsy Procedure on Accuracy of Subsequent Mammography Procedures
Peters et al. 2008 [486]	948	Stereotactic guidance automated gun 14G	NR	NR	NR	NR	NR	NR	NR	NR	NR
Sim and Kei 2008 [488]	105	Stereotactic guidance vacuum-assisted 11 G	9 had small hematomas that did not require treatment	NR	2	NR	NR	NR	NR	NR	NR
Tonegutti and Girardi 2008 [489]	268	Stereotactic guidance vacuum-assisted 11 G	3 had large hematomas that did not require treatment	2, but did not require treatment	1	NR	3 had acute localized infl-ammation, and one large abscess that required surgery	NR	NR	NR	NR
Youk et al. 200824	4,359	US guidance automated gun 14G	NR	NR	NR	NR	NR	NR	NR	NR	NR
Ciatto et al. 2007 [490]	4,035	Multiple methods	NR	NR	NR	NR	NR	NR	NR	NR	NR
de Lucena et al. 2007 [491]	150	US guidance automated gun 14G	NR	NR	NR	NR	NR	NR	NR	NR	NR
Uematsu et al. 2007 [492]	100	Stereotactic guidance vacuum-assisted 11 G	NR	NR	NR	NR	NR	NR	NR	NR	NR

Study	Number of Lesions Enrolled	Type of Biopsy	Hematomas	Bleeding	Vasovagal Reactions	Infections	Other	Time to Recovery or Time to Return to Work	Use of Pain Medications	Patient Satisfaction, Quality of Life Data	Impact of Biopsy Procedure on Accuracy of Subsequent Mammography Procedures
Chapellier et al. 2006 [494]	318	Stereotactic guidance vacuum-assisted 11 G	123 subclinical	NR	NR	NR	No abscesses occurred	NR	NR	269 found procedure had good tolerability and 49 rep-orted it was acceptable or poor. Of these 49, 17 complained of intense pain, 23 of pain that didn't resp-ond to the local anest-hetic, and 12 reported the procedure was stressful	NR
Cipolla et al. 2006 [495]	426	Multiple methods	NR	NR	NR	NR	NR	NR	NR	NR	NR
Dhillon et al. 2006 [496]	150	Stereotactic guidance vacuum-assisted 11 G	NR	NR	NR	NR	NR	NR	NR	NR	NR
Bolivar et al. 2005 [497]	214	US guidance automated gun 14G	NR	NR	NR	NR	NR	NR	NR	NR	NR

Table F 31. (Continued).

Study	Number of Lesions Enrolled	Type of Biopsy	Hematomas	Bleeding	Vasovagal Reactions	Infections	Other	Time to Recovery or Time to Return to Work	Use of Pain Medications	Patient Satisfaction, Quality of Life Data	Impact of Biopsy Procedure on Accuracy of Subsequent Mammography Procedures
Crystal et al. 2005 [498]	715	US guidance automated gun 14G	NR	NR	NR	NR	No major complications occurred	NR	NR	NR	NR
Dillon et al. 2005 [499]	2,427	Multiple methods	NR	NR	NR	NR	NR	NR	NR	NR	NR
Koskela et al. 2005 [500]	213	Stereotactic guidance automated gun 14G	No hematomas that required treatment occurred	NR	2	No infections that required treatment occurred	NR	NR	NR	NR	NR
Sauer et al. 2005 [501]	962	US guidance automated gun 14G	NR	Some cases of minor bleeding that did not require treatment	NR	1 that required surgery and antibiotics	NR	NR	NR	NR	NR
Weber et al. 2005 [502]	225	Stereotactic guidance vacuum- assisted 11 G	NR	NR	NR	2	1 biopsy was terminated after compla-ints of severe pain by the pat-ient, 5 patients had severe bruising and 2 complained of persistent pain	NR	NR	2 patients were not satisified with the cosmetic result	NR
Wu et al. 2005 [503]	113	US guidan-ce vacuum-assisted 11 G	NR	NR	NR	NR	2 cases pneum-othorax that resolved with-out treatment,	NR	NR	NR	NR

Study	Number of Lesions Enrolled	Type of Biopsy	Hematomas	Bleeding	Vasovagal Reactions	Infections	Other	Time to Recovery or Time to Return to Work	Use of Pain Medications	Patient Satisfaction, Quality of Life Data	Impact of Biopsy Procedure on Accuracy of Subsequent Mammography Procedures
							13 cases of severe ecc-hymosis that also resolved without treat-ment; All complications occurred during the first year of the study, no complications occurred during the second and third years				
Alonso-Bartolome et al. 2004 [504]	102	US guidance vacuum-assisted 11G	37 that did not require treatment	3, only one required treatment	NR	NR	1 patient complained of pain.	NR	NR	NR	NR
Delle and Terinde 2004 [505]	169	US guidance automated gun 14G	NR	NR	NR	NR	NR	NR	NR	NR	NR
Fajardo et al. 2004506	2,403	Multiple methods	NR	NR	NR	NR	NR	NR	NR	NR	NR
Kettritz et al. 2004 [507]	2,893	Stereotactic guidance vacuum-assisted 11 G	25 hemato-mas of which 3 were hosp-italized	4 patients were hospi-talized for persistent bleeding, of	5	5 that require d antibi-otics	1 seizure	NR	NR	NR	In 196 patie-nts a slight mammograp-hic density was observed.

Table F 31. (Continued).

Study	Number of Lesions Enrolled	Type of Biopsy	Hematomas	Bleeding	Vasovagal Reactions	Infections	Other	Time to Recovery or Time to Return to Work	Use of Pain Medications	Patient Satisfaction, Quality of Life Data	Impact of Biopsy Procedure on Accuracy of Subsequent Mammography Procedures
			overnight and 1 required surgery	which 3 needed surgery							In 4 patients a scar that might cause diagno-stic difficulty was observed.
Lomoschitz et al. 2004 [508]	100	Stereotactic guidance vacuum-assisted 11 G	NR	NR	NR	NR	NR	NR	NR	NR	NR
Abdsaleh et al. 2003 [509]	180	Multiple methods	NR	Mild bleeding occurred in all cases	NR	NR	No significant complications occurred	NR	NR	NR	NR
Ambrogetti et al. 2003 [510]	364	Stereotactic guidance vacuum-assisted 11 G	NR	NR	NR	NR	NR	NR	NR	NR	NR
Fishman et al. 2003 [511]	73	US guidance automated gun 14G	NR	NR	NR	NR	NR	NR	NR	NR	NR
Han et al. 2003 [512]	271	Stereotactic guidance automated gun 14G	NR	NR	NR	NR	NR	NR	NR	NR	NR
Kirshenbaum et al. 2003 [513]	506	Multiple methods	NR	Three cases of minor bleeding	5 vasovagal reactions; the most	NR	NR	NR	NR	NR	NR

Study	Number of Lesions Enrolled	Type of Biopsy	Hematomas	Bleeding	Vasovagal Reactions	Infecti ons	Other	Time to Recovery or Time to Return to Work	Use of Pain Medications	Patient Satisfaction, Quality of Life Data	Impact of Biopsy Procedure on Accuracy of Subsequent Mammograph y Procedures
				and one case of ma-jor bleeding that requir-ed surgery	experienced radiologist had 3 reacti-ons in 409 procedures while the two more inexperie-nced radiol-ogists had 1 reaction out of 47 proc-edures and 1 reaction out of 53 procedures						
March et al. 2003 [514]	34	US guidance vacuum-assisted 11 G	9 hematomas that did not require treatment	NR	NR	NR	19 reported no pain, 13 reported mild pain, 2 repor-ted moderate pain. 24 patients had ecchymosis 2-4 days after the procedure	16 repo-rted the procedu re had not interferr ed with usual activity at all, 14 a little, 4 somewh at	20 took acetamino-phen	NR	NR
Pfleiderer et al. 2003 [515]	14	MRI guidance automated gun 14G	NR	NR	NR	NR	No severe side effects were observed	NR	None used	NR	NR

Table F 31. (Continued).

Study	Number of Lesions Enrolled	Type of Biopsy	Hematomas	Bleeding	Vasovagal Reactions	Infections	Other	Time to Recovery or Time to Return to Work	Use of Pain Medications	Patient Satisfaction, Quality of Life Data	Impact of Biopsy Procedure on Accuracy of Subsequent Mammography Procedures
Philpotts et al. 2003 [516]	281	Multiple methods	3 hematomas in 11 G no surg-ery required	3 cases of bleeding with 14G	NR	NR	NR	NR	NR	NR	NR
Wong and Hisham 2003 [517]	150	Freehand automated gun 14G/16G	NR	1 patient in 14G group experien-ced trouble-some bleeding	NR	3 patients from 14G group develope d infections	There was no difference in the amount of pain experie-nced between 14G and 16G as meausured on a VAS, $p > 0.05$	NR	NR	NR	NR
Apesteguia et al. 2002 [518]	132	Stereotactic guidance vacuum-assisted 11 G	Some hematomas that did not require treatment	8 cases of bleeding which cau-sed premat-ure termina-tion of the procedure in 3 of the 8 cases	NR	NR	2 cases of severe pain	NR	NR	NR	NR
Georgian-Smith et al. 2002 [519]	185	Stereotactic guidance vacuum-assisted 11 G	3, one case of which it became infected and required antibiotics to treat	5, 2 of which were severe eno-ugh to requ-ire termina-tion of the biopsy	10, 2 of which were severe eno-ugh to requ-ire termina-tion of the biopsy procedure	NR	1 patient vomited	NR	NR	NR	NR

Study	Number of Lesions Enrolled	Type of Biopsy	Hematomas	Bleeding	Vasovagal Reactions	Infections	Other	Time to Recovery or Time to Return to Work	Use of Pain Medications	Patient Satisfaction, Quality of Life Data	Impact of Biopsy Procedure on Accuracy of Subsequent Mammography Procedures
Jackman and Lamm 2002 [520]	31	Multiple methods	NR	2 serious bleeding	NR	NR	NR	NR	NR	NR	NR
Johnson et al. 2002 [521]	101	US guidance vacuum-assisted 11 or 8G	1 large hematoma requiring narcotics	1 significant bleeding requiring surgery; less than 5% of cases had bleeding requiring treatment	NR	2 infections requiring antibiotics and surgical drainage	NR	NR	1 case required narcotics	NR	NR
Liberman et al. 2002 [522]	800	Stereotactic guidance vacuum-assisted 11 G	2 that required treatment	12	2	NR	1 patient was in such severe pain that the procedure was terminated	NR	NR	NR	NR
Meloni et al. 2002 [523]	129	Stereotactic guidance vacuum-assisted	2 that did not require treatment	1	5	NR	NR	NR	NR	NR	NR
Morris et al. 2002 [524]	21	Stereotactic guidance vacuum-assisted 14G	NR	NR	NR	NR	NR	NR	NR	NR	NR

Table F 31. (Continued).

Study	Number of Lesions Enrolled	Type of Biopsy	Hematomas	Bleeding	Vasovagal Reactions	Infections	Other	Time to Recovery or Time to Return to Work	Use of Pain Medications	Patient Satisfaction, Quality of Life Data	Impact of Biopsy Procedure on Accuracy of Subsequent Mammography Procedures
Pfarl et al. 2002 [525]	332	Stereotactic guidance vacuum-assisted 11G	NR	NR	NR	NR	NR	NR	NR	NR	NR
Verkooijen et al. COBRA 2002 [526]	984	Stereotactic guidance automated gun 14G	NR	NR	NR	NR	NR	NR	NR	NR	NR
Becker et al. 2001 [527]	232	Stereotactic guidance automated gun 14G	NR	3 minor	2	NR	NR	NR	NR	NR	NR
Brenner et al. 2001 [528]	1,003	Stereotactic guidance automated gun 14G	NR	NR	NR	NR	NR	NR	NR	NR	NR
Cangiarella et al. 2001 [529]	160	Stereotactic guidance vacuum-assisted 11 G	NR	NR	NR	NR	NR	NR	NR	NR	NR
Dahlstrom and Jain 2001 [530]	310	Stereotactic guidance automated gun 14G	NR	NR	NR	NR	NR	NR	NR	NR	NR
Lai et al. 2001 [531]	673	Stereotactic guidance vacuum-assisted 11 G	NR	NR	NR	NR	NR	NR	NR	NR	NR

Study	Number of Lesions Enrolled	Type of Biopsy	Hematomas	Bleeding	Vasovagal Reactions	Infections	Other	Time to Recovery or Time to Return to Work	Use of Pain Medications	Patient Satisfaction, Quality of Life Data	Impact of Biopsy Procedure on Accuracy of Subsequent Mammography Procedures
Levin et al. 2001 [532]	70	Stereotactic guidance automated gun 14G	NR	NR	3	NR	NR	NR	NR	NR	NR
Margolin et al. 2001 [533]	1,333	Multiple methods	NR	NR	NR	2 that required antibiotics	NR	NR	NR	NR	NR
Perez-Fuentes et al. 2001 [534]	88	US guidance vacuum-assisted 11G	NR	1 patient with implants experienced severe bleeding that required surgical treatment	NR	NR	NR	NR	NR	NR	NR
Smith et al. 2001 [535]	500	US guidance automated gun 14G	0	NR	NR	0	26 had large areas of ecchymosis; one patient had a small pneumothorax that resolved without treatment	NR	NR	NR	NR
White et al. 2001 [536]	1,042	Multiple methods	NR	NR	NR	NR	NR	NR	NR	NR	NR

Table F 31. (Continued).

Study	Number of Lesions Enrolled	Type of Biopsy	Hematomas	Bleeding	Vasovagal Reactions	Infectio ns	Other	Time to Recover y or Time to Return to Work	Use of Pain Medications	Patient Satisfaction, Quality of Life Data	Impact of Biopsy Procedure on Accuracy of Subsequent Mammography Procedures
Wunderbaldin ger et al. 2001 [537]	45	US guidance automated gun 14G	NR	NR	4	NR	NR	NR	NR	NR	NR
Yeow et al. 2001 [538]	98	US guidan-ce automa-ted gun 14 or 1 6G	0	NR	NR	0	1 patient had a puncture site ecchymosis	NR	NR	NR	NR
Beck et al. 2000 [539]	594	Stereota-ctic guidance vacuum-assisted 11 G	1 that required surgical treatment	NR	NR	NR	1 patient had a seizure	NR	NR	NR	In 90% of patie-nts no scarring was seen on subsequent mammo-graphy ; in 10% a faint density could be seen at the biopsy site; 1 patient had a diagnostically confusing scar that was evidentally benign on MRI
Kirwan et al. 2000 [540]	72	Stereotactic guidance automated gun 14G	NR	NR	NR	NR	NR	NR	NR	NR	NR
Latosinsky et al. 2000 [541]	692	Multiple methods	NR	NR	NR	NR	There were no significant complications of bleeding or infection	NR	NR	NR	NR

Study	Number of Lesions Enrolled	Type of Biopsy	Hematomas	Bleeding	Vasovagal Reactions	Infecti ons	Other	Time to Recover y or Time to Return to Work	Use of Pain Medications	Patient Satisfaction, Quality of Life Data	Impact of Biopsy Procedure on Accuracy of Subsequent Mammograph y Procedures
Liberman et al. 2000542	155	Multiple methods	NR	NR	NR	NR	NR	NR	NR	NR	NR
Makoske et al. 2000 [543]	887	Multiple methods	NR	NR	NR	NR	NR	NR	NR	NR	NR
Ward et al. 2000 [544]	121	Stereotactic guidance automated gun 14G	NR	NR	NR	NR	NR	NR	NR	NR	NR
Welle et al. 2000 [545]	225	Multiple methods	1 did not require treatment	1 did not require treatment	4 (in seated patients)	NR	NR	NR	NR	NR	NR
Helbich et al. 1999 [546]	44	Stereotactic guidance automated gun 14G	NR	NR	NR	NR	NR	NR	NR	NR	NR
Jackman et al. 1999 [547]	483	Multiple methods	NR	NR	NR	NR	NR	NR	NR	NR	NR
Meyer et al. 1 999 [548]	1,836	Perforated compress-ion grid automated gun 14G	0 that required treatment	NR	NR	1 that requir ed antibi o-tics	Complications were minor And infreq-uent. 1 pneumothorax requiring no treatment occurred	NR	NR	NR	NR
Puglisi et al. 1 999 [549]	106	Stereotactic guidance automated gun 14G	NRb	NR	NR	NR	No complications resulted from this technique	NR	NR	NR	NR

Table F 31. (Continued).

Study	Number of Lesions Enrolled	Type of Biopsy	Hematomas	Bleeding	Vasovagal Reactions	Infections	Other	Time to Recovery or Time to Return to Work	Use of Pain Medications	Patient Satisfaction, Quality of Life Data	Impact of Biopsy Procedure on Accuracy of Subsequent Mammography Procedures
Soo et al. 1999 [550]	116	Stereotactic guidance vacuum-assisted 14G	NR	NR	NR	NR	One patient was in such severe pain that the pro-cedure was terminated	NR	NR	NR	NR
Caruso et al. 1998 [551]	92	Multiple methods	NR	NR	NR	NR	NR	NR	NR	NR	NR
Doyle et al. 1 998 [552]	151	Stereotactic guidance automated gun 14G	NR	NR	4 (in seated patients)	1 minor	No serious complication-ns occurred	NR	NR	Most of our patients found that decubitus position was reasonably comfortable and that discomfort was mostly related to prolonged breast compression	NR
Fuhrman et al. 1998 [553]	1,440	Multiple methods	NR	NR	NR	NR	Hospitalizat-ion was not required for any subjects. The only com-plication enc-ountered was minor breast ecchymosis, which	NR	NR	NR	NR

Study	Number of Lesions Enrolled	Type of Biopsy	Hematomas	Bleeding	Vasovagal Reactions	Infecti ons	Other	Time to Recover y or Time to Return to Work	Use of Pain Medications	Patient Satisfaction, Quality of Life Data	Impact of Biopsy Procedure on Accuracy of Subsequent Mammograph y Procedures
							resol-ved uneven-fully in all cases				
Heywang-Kobrunner et al. 1998 [554]	261	Stereotactic guidance vacuum-assisted 11 or 14G	NR	1	NR	NR	No side effe-cts occurred. No patients complained about pain.	NR	NR	NR	117 of 129 patients had no scarring visible at 6-month mammo-graphy. Very slight sca-rring occurred in ten patients, and mammo-graphically vis-ible scarring in 2 patients, one of whom was sent for MRI to verify it was a scar and not a tumor.
Ioffe et al. 1998 [555]	224	US guidance automated gun 14G	NR	NR	NR	NR	NR	NR	NR	NR	NR
Liberman et al. 1998 [556]	151	Multiple methods	NR	NR	NR	NR	NR	NR	NR	NR	NR
Schulz-Wendtland et al. 1 998 [557]	2,307	US guidance automated gun 14G	NR	NR	NR	NR	NR	NR	NR	NR	NR

Table F 31. (Continued).

Study	Number of Lesions Enrolled	Type of Biopsy	Hematomas	Bleeding	Vasovagal Reactions	Infecti ons	Other	Time to Recover y or Time to Return to Work	Use of Pain Medications	Patient Satisfaction, Quality of Life Data	Impact of Biopsy Procedure on Accuracy of Subsequent Mammograph y Procedures
Vega-Bolivar et al. 1 998 [558]	182	Stereotactic guidance Surecut 1 5G	NR	NR	12	NR	NR	NR	NR	NR	NR
Whitman et al. 1998 [559]	12	Stereotactic guidance automated gun 1 6G	NR	NR	1	NR	NR	NR	NR	NR	NR
Zannis and AliaNo 1998 [560]	424	Multiple methods	NR	Bleeding requiring operative interventio n was not required in any group	NR	NR	Open biopsy: 12 cases cellulitis and 4 abscesses out of 190 procedures; zero cases of cellulitis and abscesses out of 234 core- needle biopsy procedures	NR	Open bio-psy: all 190 were sent home with oral narcotic analgesia; zero patients out of 157 SCNB and 77 VAB procedures required oral narco-tic analgesia	NR	NR
Bauer et al. 1997 [561]	799	Stereotactic guidance automated gun 14G	10 that did not require treatment	NR	NR	0	NR	NR	NR	NR	NR
Britton et al. 1 997 [562]	202	Multiple methods	0	NR	7		No complica-tions that req-uired treatm-ent occurred	NR	NR	NR	NR

Study	Number of Lesions Enrolled	Type of Biopsy	Hematomas	Bleeding	Vasovagal Reactions	Infecti ons	Other	Time to Recover y or Time to Return to Work	Use of Pain Medications	Patient Satisfaction, Quality of Life Data	Impact of Biopsy Procedure on Accuracy of Subsequent Mammograph y Procedures
Helbich et al. 1 997 [563]	210	Multiple methods	NR	NR	4 (in seated patients)	NR	No serious complications, patients toler-ated it well	NR	NR	NR	NR
Khattar et al. 1 997 [564]	106	US guida-nce autom-ated gun	NR	NR	NR	NR	NR	NR	NR	NR	NR
Liberman et al. 1997 [565]	442	Stereotactic guidance automated gun 1 4G	NR	NR	NR	NR	NR	NR	NR	NR	NR
Pitre et al. 1997 [566]	128	Stereotactic guidance automated gun	NR	NR	NR	NR	NR	NR	NR	NR	NR
Stolier et al. 1997 [567]	244	Multiple methods	NR	NR	NR	NR	NR	NR	NR	NR	NR
Sutton, et al. 1 997 [568]	206	Stereotactic guidance automated gun 14G	NR	NR	NR	NR	There were no cases of long-term morbidity and only 3 patients (1.5%) had a biopsy-related problem 3 days after their core-needle biopsy	NR	NR	Pain: 36% none, 27.6% uncomfortab-le, 12.3% slight, 7% quite, 0% very Discomfort: 50% none, 40% uncom-fortable, 6% slight, 4% quite, 0% very	NR

Table F 31. (Continued).

Study	Number of Lesions Enrolled	Type of Biopsy	Hematomas	Bleeding	Vasovagal Reactions	Infections	Other	Time to Recovery or Time to Return to Work	Use of Pain Medications	Patient Satisfaction, Quality of Life Data	Impact of Biopsy Procedure on Accuracy of Subsequent Mammograph y Procedures
Walker et al. 1 997 [569]	200	Stereotactic guidance automated gun 14G	NR	0	1	0	A few pati-ents compla-ined of pain; bruising was not infrequent	NR	NR	NR	NR
Frazee et al. 1996 [570]	103	Stereotactic guidance automated gun	NR	NR	NR	NR	Patients rating of post- operative pain was evaluated using a Pain Analog Scale. The mean score for open biopsy was 2.5 and for stereotactic biopsy was 2.8 (P = NS)	The inter-val of retu-rning to normal ac-tivies was measured . This aver-aged 3.8 days for open biop-sy and 1.5 days for Stererota c-tic biopsy (P = NS)	NR	Overall pati-ent satisfac-tion was evaluated. No signify-cant differ-ences were seen in ove-rall patient satisfaction between the two biopsy techniques	NR
Fuhrman et al. 1996 [571]	451	Stereotactic guidance automated gun 14G	NR	NR	NR	NR	NR	NR	NR	NR	NR
Head and Haynes 1996 [572]	115	Stereotactic guidance automated gun 1 8G	NR	NR	NR	NR	NR	NR	NR	NR	NR

Study	Number of Lesions Enrolled	Type of Biopsy	Hematomas	Bleeding	Vasovagal Reactions	Infections	Other	Time to Recovery or Time to Return to Work	Use of Pain Medications	Patient Satisfaction, Quality of Life Data	Impact of Biopsy Procedure on Accuracy of Subsequent Mammography Procedures
Mainiero et al. 1996 [573]	138	Stereotactic guidance automated gun 14G	NR	NR	NR	NR	NR	NR	NR	NR	NR
Meyer et al.1996 [574]	388	Stereotactic guidance automated gun 14G	3	NR	NR	NR	Ecchymosis at the biopsy site occured in 48% of patients	NR	NR	NR	NR
Nguyen et al. 1 996 [575]	431	Multiple methods	A few small superficial ones that required no treatment	NR	NR	NR	There were no serious comp-lications. Sev-eral patients complained of pain related to lying on the biopsy table for a prolon-ged period of time	NR	NR	NR	NR
Pettine et al. 1996 [576]	25	Stereotactic guidance automated gun 14G	NR	NR	NR	NR	NR	NR	NR	NR	NR
Rosenblatt et al. 1996 [577]	58	Stereotactic guidance automated gun 14G	NR	NR	NR	NR	NR	NR	NR	NR	NR
Scopa et al. 1996 [578]	120	Freehand TruCut	NR	NR	NR	NR	NR	NR	NR	NR	NR
Cross et al. 1995 [579]	250	Stereotactic guidance automated gun 14G	NR	NR	NR	0	Pain was reported to be minimal	NR	NR	NR	NR

Table F 31. (Continued).

Study	Number of Lesions Enrolled	Type of Biopsy	Hematomas	Bleeding	Vasovagal Reactions	Infections	Other	Time to Recovery or Time to Return to Work	Use of Pain Medications	Patient Satisfaction, Quality of Life Data	Impact of Biopsy Procedure on Accuracy of Subsequent Mammography Procedures
Doyle et al. 1995 [580]	365	Multiple methods	NR	NR	NR	NR	NR	NR	NR	NR	NR
Burbank et al. 1994 [582]	105	Multiple methods	NR	NR	NR	NR	NR	NR	NR	NR	NR
Gisvold et al. 1 994 [583]	160	Stereotactic guidance automated gun 14G	Hemotoma formation was infrequent	NR	0	1 serious systemic infection	Two patients had significant pain	NR	NR	NR	NR
Parker et al. 1 994 [584]	6,152	Multiple methods	3 that required surgery	NR	NR	3 that required antibiotic s	NR	NR	NR	NR	NR
Smyth and Cederbom 1 994 [585]	58	Stereotactic guidance automated gun 14G	NR	NR	NR	NR	NR	NR	NR	NR	NR
Elvecrog et al. 1 993 [586]	100	Stereotactic guidance automated gun 14G	1 that required surgical treatment	NR	NR	NR	NR	NR	NR	Some pati-ents compl-ained of pain from biopsy, but usually with only 1 or 2 needle pas-ses.	NR

Study	Number of Lesions Enrolled	Type of Biopsy	Hematomas	Bleeding	Vasovagal Reactions	Infections	Other	Time to Recovery or Time to Return to Work	Use of Pain Medications	Patient Satisfaction, Quality of Life Data	Impact of Biopsy Procedure on Accuracy of Subsequent Mammography Procedures
										frequent co-mplaints of neck, sho-ulder, and arm discom-fort from patients lyi-ng in the same posit-ion for an extended period of time	
Parker et al. 1 993 [587]	181	US guidance automated gun 1 4G	NR	NR	NR	NR	NR	NR	NR	NR	NR
McMahon et al. 1992 [588]	151	Freehand 14/1618G	NR	Troublesome bleeding occurred in 3 patients in Bioptycut 14G, 2 patients in Bioptycut 18G, and 1 in Trucut	NR	NR	There were no major com-plications. Mi-nor bruising was common. No patients developed pneumothorax	NR	NR	Pain scores on a 0 to 3 scale were recorded after the procedure: Trucut 40% had a 0, 40% a 1, 15% a 2, 5% a 3. Biopty 14G 70% had a 0, 12% a 1,	NR

Table F 31. (Continued).

Study	Number of Lesions Enrolled	Type of Biopsy	Hematomas	Bleeding	Vasovagal Reactions	Infections	Other	Time to Recovery or Time to Return to Work	Use of Pain Medications	Patient Satisfaction, Quality of Life Data	Impact of Biopsy Procedure on Accuracy of Subsequent Mammography Procedures
										15% a 2, 3% a 3. Biopty 18G 60% had a 0, 30% a 1, 10% a 2, 0% a 3. B18 was reported to have signify-cantly p = 0.01 less pain thanTrucut	
Barreto et al. 1991 [589]	107	Freehand automated gun 18G	NR	NR	NR	NR	NR	NR	NR	NR	NR
Cusick et al. 1990 [590]	96	Freehand	NR	NR	NR	NR	NR	NR	NR	NR	NR
Parker et al. 1990 [591]	103	Stereo-tactic guidance automated gun	NR	No signific-ant bleeding occured, even with use of the 14-gauge needle	2 (in seated patients)	Three that required treatment with antibiotics	None of the patients suffe-red immediate significant complications.	NR	NR	NR	NR

NR = Not Reported.

Table F32. Data for Women Diagnosed With Cancer By Biopsy.

Reference	Number who were able to be treated with only one surgical procedure	
	Core-needle diagnosis	Open biopsy diagnosis
Friese et al. 2009 [592]	Odds ratio 2.9 (2.7 to 2.9)	
Verkooijen et al. 2001 [593]	63 out of 84	13 out of 80
Morrow et al. 2000 [305]	222 out of 264	47 out of 142
Kaufman et al. 1998 [396]	52 out of 66	10 out of 47
Lind et al. 1998 [402]	47 out of 48	35 out of 69
Fenoglio et al. 1997 [419]	20 out of 20	1 out of 20
Liberman et al. 1997 [428]	76 out of 90	31 out of 107

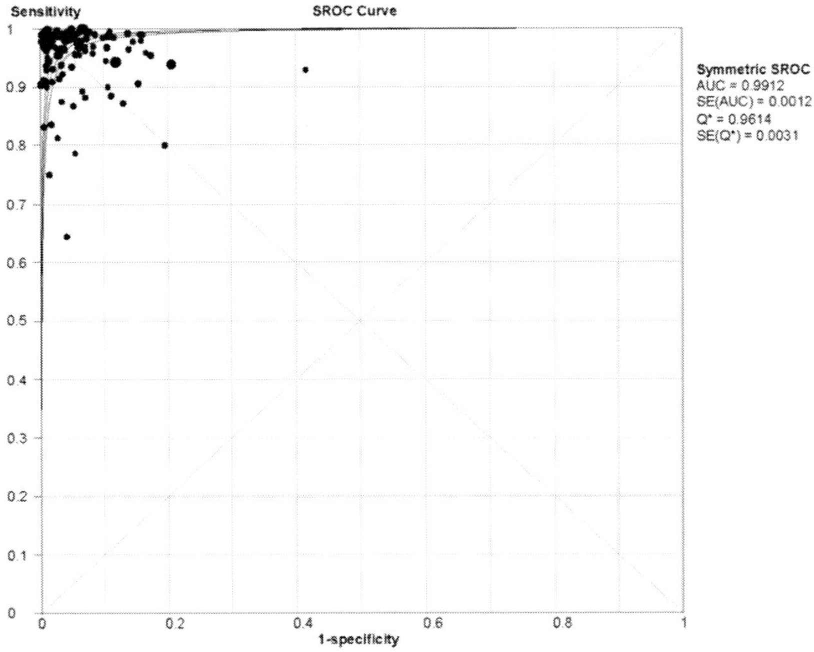

META-ANALYTIC INTEGRATION OF DIAGNOSTIC TEST ACCURACY STUDIES
Freehand biopsies
SUMMARY DATA AND PERFORMANCE ESTIMATES
Bivariate Binomial Mixed Model Number of studies = 5
Reference-positive Subjects = 419 Reference-negative Subjects = 191 Pretest Prob of Disease = 0.687
Between-study variance (varlogitSEN) = 0.438, 95% CI = [0.096-1.994]
Between-study variance (varlogitSPE) = 0.562, 95% CI = [0.001-309.743]
Correlation (Mixed Model) = -1.000 ROC Area, AUROC = 0.99 [0.98 - 1.00]
Heterogeneity (Chi-square): LRT_Q = 2.149, df = 2.00, LRT_p = 0.171
Inconsistency (I-square): LRT_I2 = 6.95, 95% CI = [0.00-100.00]

Parameter	Estimate 95% CI	
Sensitivity	0.858 [0.758,	0.921]
Specificity	0.993 [0.939,	0.999]

Positive Likelihood Ratio 121.004 [13.764, 1063.749]
Negative Likelihood Ratio 0.143 [0.082, 0.250] Diagnostic Score 6.738 [4.613, 8.863]
Diagnostic Odds Ratio 844.025 [100.826, 7065.427]

Figure F1. Summary ROC of all core-needle biopsy studies.

Meta-Analytic Integration Of Diagnostic Test Accuracy Studies All Biopsies

Could not fit a bivariate binomial model

Random-effects model:

Summary sensitivity: 96.4% (96.1% to 96.7%), I2 = 83.2%
Summary negative likelihood ratio: 0.03 8 (0.030 to 0.050), I2 = 86.6%

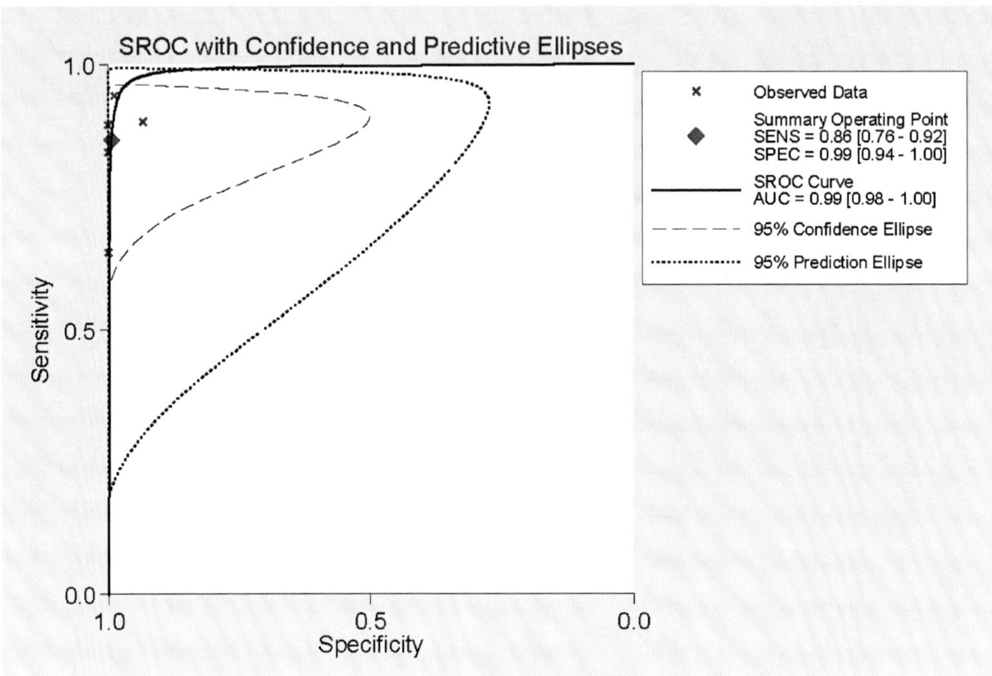

META-ANALYTIC INTEGRATION OF DIAGNOSTIC TEST ACCURACY STUDIES Ultrasound-guided automated gun biopsies
Could not fit a bivariate binomial model

Random-effects model :	to 98.2%) I2 =	39.9%	
Summary sensitivity: 97.7% (97.2			
Summary negative likelihood ratio:	0.030 (0.022 to 0.040)	I2 =	32.7%
Summary atypia underestimation rate:	0.292 (0.234 to 0.359)	I2 =	0.0%
Summary DCIS underestimation rate:	0.3 55 (0.27 1 to 0.450)	I2 =	17.9%
Meta-regression results :			
Country study conducted in p = 0.25			

Open surgery to verify all results vs. surgery + patient followup p = 0.79 19
Open surgery + at least 2 years followup to verify results vs. open surgery + some patients had less than 2 years followup p = 0.341

Figure F2. Summary ROC of freehand core-needle biopsies.

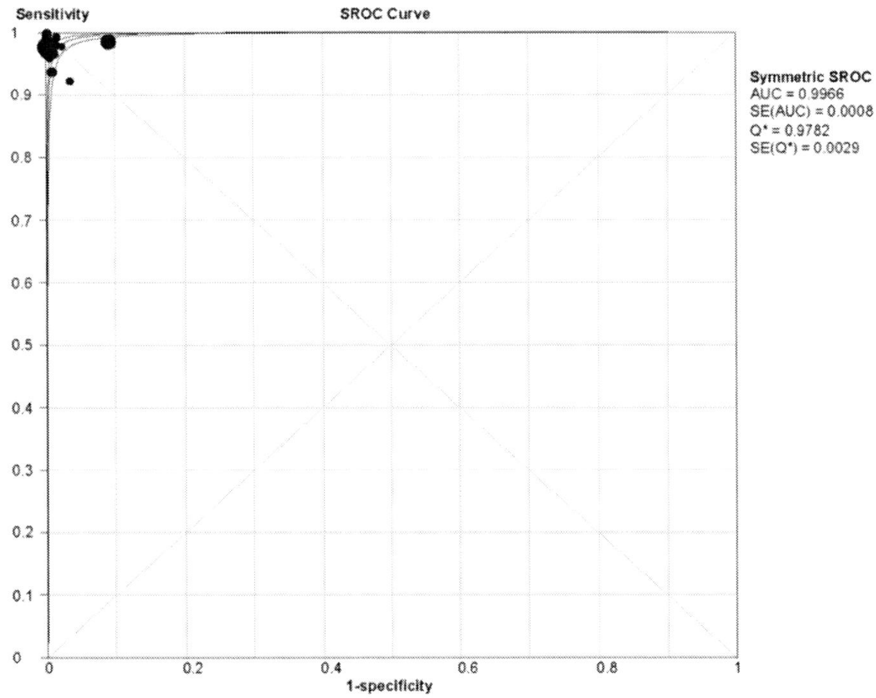

META-ANALYTIC INTEGRATION OF DIAGNOSTIC TEST ACCURACY STUDIES Stereotactic-guided automated gun biopsies
SUMMARY DATA AND PERFORMANCE ESTIMATES
Bivariate Binomial Mixed Model
Number of studies = 33
Reference-positive Subjects = 2,653
Reference-negative Subjects = 4,482
Pretest Prob of Disease = 0.372
Between-study variance (varlogitSEN) = 1.836, 95% CI = [0.777-4.339]
Between-study variance (varlogitSPE) = 1.592, 95% CI = [0.724-3.501]
Correlation (Mixed Model) = 0.062
ROC Area, AUROC = 1.00 [0.98 - 1.00]
Heterogeneity (Chi-square): LRT_Q = 76.75 1, df = 2.00, LRT_p = 0.000
Inconsistency (I-square): LRT_I2 = 97.39, 95% CI = [95.65-99.14]

Parameter	Estimate 95% CI	
Sensitivity	0.978 [0.958,	0.989]
Specificity	0.970 [0.950,	0.982]

Positive Likelihood Ratio 32.208 [19.313, 53.711]
Negative Likelihood Ratio 0.022 [0.012, 0.043] Diagnostic Score 7.269 [6.398, 8.140]
Diagnostic Odds Ratio 1435.328 [600.670, 3429.782]
Atypia underestimation rate = 0.435 (0.357 to 0.5 17) I2 = 35.7%
DCIS underestimation rate = 0.244 (0.18 to 0.321) I2 = 57.0%
Meta-regression results:
Gauge of needle p = 0.423
Number of centers p = 0.235
Type of facility p = 0.685
Country conducted in p = 0.543
Open surgery to verify all results vs. surgery + patient followup p = 0.459
Open surgery + at least 2 years followup to verify results vs. open surgery + some patients had less than 2 years followup p = 0.681

Figure F3. Summary ROC of ultrasound-guided automated gun core-needle biopsies.

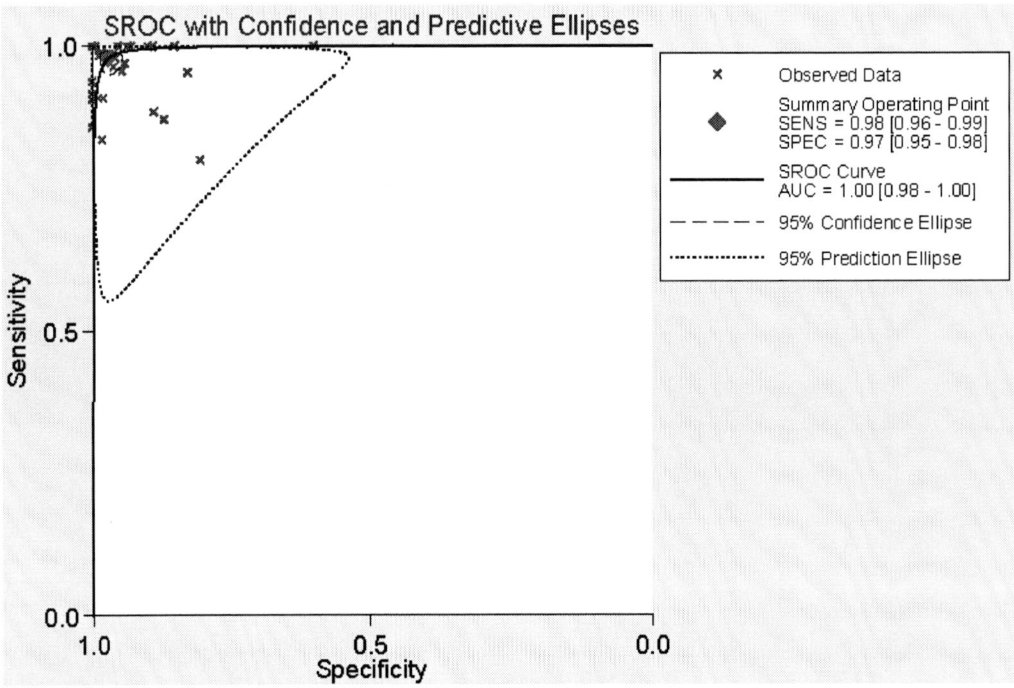

META-ANALYTIC INTEGRATION OF DIAGNOSTIC TEST ACCURACY STUDIES Ultrasound-guided vacuum-assisted biopsies

SUMMARY DATA AND PERFORMANCE ESTIMATES

Bivariate Binomial Mixed Model

Number of studies = 7

Reference-positive Subjects = 76

Reference-negative Subjects = 431

Pretest Prob of Disease = 0.150

Between-study variance (varlogitSEN) = 1.928, 95% CI = [0.014-270.021]

Between-study variance (varlogitSPE) = 0.574, 95% CI = [0.031-10.757]

Correlation (Mixed Model) = -1.000

ROC Area, AUROC = 0.99 [0.98 - 1.00]

Heterogeneity (Chi-square): LRT_Q = 1.085, df = 2.00, LRT_p = 0.291

Inconsistency (I-square): LRT_I2 = 0.00, 95% CI = [0.00-100.00]

Parameter	Estimate 95% CI
Sensitivity	0.965 [0.8 12, 0.994]
Specificity	0.982 [0.954, 0.993]
Positive Likelihood Ratio	53.843 [21.308, 136.059]
Negative Likelihood Ratio	0.036 [0.006, 0.212] Diagnostic Score 7.319 [5.502, 9.136]
Diagnostic Odds Ratio	1509.018 [245.261, 9284.523]

Figure F4. Summary ROC of stereotactic-guided automated gun core-needle biopsies.

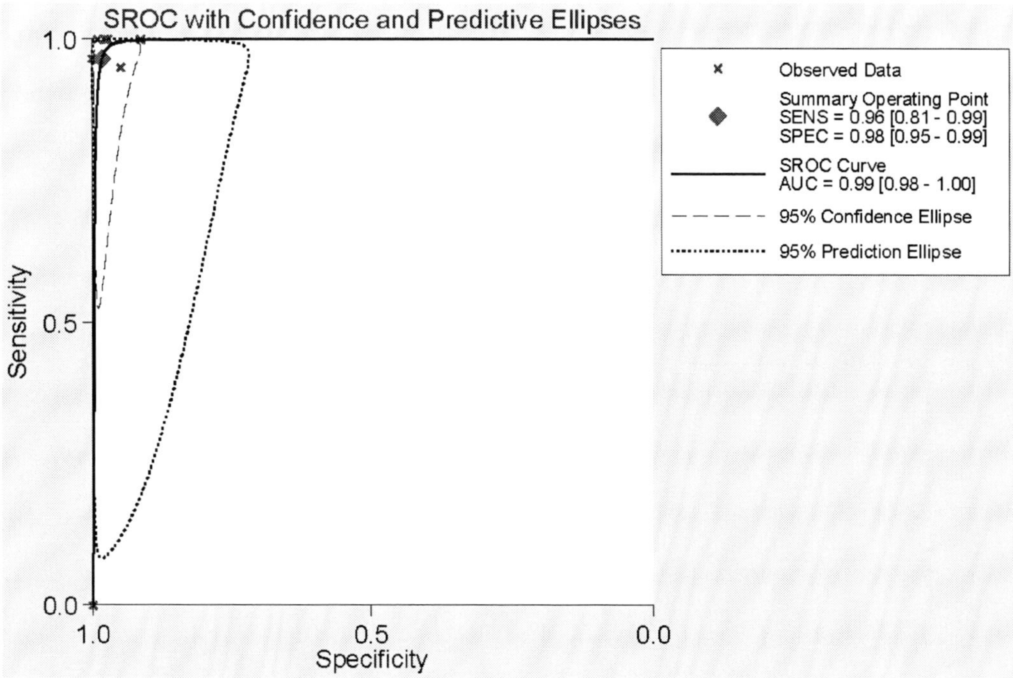

META-ANALYTIC INTEGRATION OF DIAGNOSTIC TEST ACCURACY STUDIES Stereotactic-guided vacuum-assisted biopsies
SUMMARY DATA AND PERFORMANCE ESTIMATES
Bivariate Binomial Mixed Model
Number of studies = 22
Reference-positive Subjects = 2,578
Reference-negative Subjects = 5,049
Pretest Prob of Disease = 0.326
Between-study variance (varlogitSEN) = 1.458, 95% CI = [0.416-5.116]
Between-study variance (varlogitSPE) = 0.271, 95% CI = [0.112-0.657]
Correlation (Mixed Model) = 0.429
ROC Area, AUROC = 0.99 [0.97 - 0.99]
Heterogeneity (Chi-square): LRT_Q = 13.534, df = 2.00, LRT_p = 0.001
Inconsistency (I-square): LRT_I2 = 85.22, 95% CI = [69.26-100.00]
Parameter Estimate 95% CI
Sensitivity 0.992 [0.981, 0.996]
Specificity 0.921 [0.899, 0.939]
Positive Likelihood Ratio 13.057 [10.069, 16.93 0]
Negative Likelihood Ratio 0.009 [0.004, 0.021]
Diagnostic Score 7.3 17 [6.262, 8.372]
Diagnostic Odds Ratio 1505.306 [524.041, 4323.988]
Atypia underestimation rate 0.217 (0.177 to 0.264) I2 = 0.0% DCIS underestimation rate 0.129 (0.111 to 0.151) I2 = 0.0% Meta-regression results :
Type of facility study conducted in p = 0.787
Country study was conducted in p = 0.1034
Open surgery + at least 2 years followup to verify results vs. open surgery + some patients had less than 2 years followup p = 0.456

Figure F5. Summary ROC of ultrasound-guided vacuum-assisted core-needle biopsies.

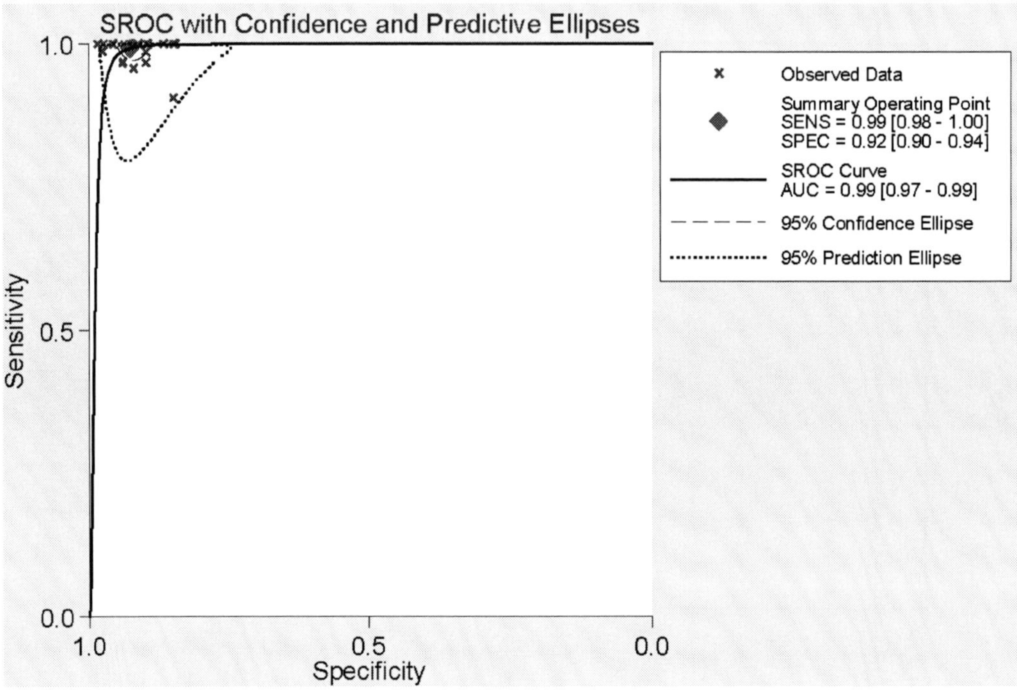

Figure F6. Summary ROC of stereotactic vacuum-assisted core-needle biopsies

Study name	Odds ratio	Lower limit	Upper limit	Z-Value	p-Value
	Statistics for each study				
Verkooijen et al. 2001	15.462	7.141	33.476	6.948	0.000
Morrow et al. 2000	10.684	6.607	17.276	9.661	0.000
Kaufman et al. 1998	13.743	5.507	34.294	5.617	0.000
Lind et al. 1998	45.657	5.960	349.784	3.678	0.000
Fenoglio et al. 1997	533.000	20.459	13885.844	3.775	0.000
Liberman et al. 1997	13.309	6.565	26.980	7.179	0.000
	13.285	9.611	18.364	15.658	0.000

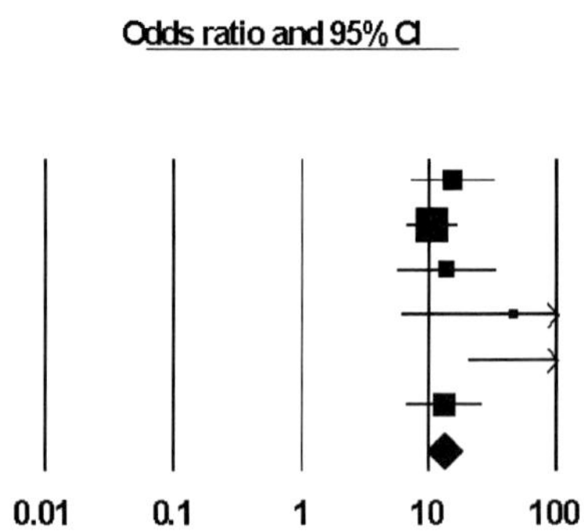

Figure F7. Meta-analysis of surgeries avoided.

Figure shows the odds of women to require only one surgical procedure for treatment of their cancer, after being diagnosed with cancer by either a core-needle biopsy procedure or an open biopsy procedure. j2 = 3 1.3%.

Appendix G. Grading the Strength of Evidence

Ideally, the body of evidence to support a conclusion would be strong. Often, however, the evidence suffers from various limitations concerning the possible risk of bias in available studies, small numbers of studies and patients, and/or inconsistent effects. These limitations often mean that the strength of the evidence is only moderate, weak, or even insufficient to permit any conclusion. In order to gauge the impact of these possible limitations, we applied a formal rating system that conforms with the CER Methods Guide Manual recommendations on grading the strength of evidence.

The strength of evidence supporting each major conclusion was graded as High, Moderate, Low, or Insufficient. The grade was developed by considering four important domains: the quality (risk of potential bias) of the evidence base, the size of the evidence base, the consistency (agreement across studies) of the findings, and the robustness of the findings (as determined by sensitivity analysis). The grading system moves stepwise to consider each important domain. These steps are described below.

Step 1. What is the quality of individual studies?

We used an internal validity rating scale for diagnostic studies to grade the internal validity of the evidence base. This scale is based on a modification of the QUADAS instrument. [595] Each question in the instrument addresses an aspect of study design or conduct that can help to protect against bias. Each question can be answered "yes", "no", or "not reported," and each is phrased such that an answer of "yes" indicates that the study reported a protection against bias on that aspect. A summary score was computed with each "yes" given a +1, each "no" a -1, and each "not reported" a zero. As all of the factors captured by the questions on the quality instrument were thought to be of equal importance for this topic, no weighting was utilized in computing the summary score. This summary score was then normalized to a scale from 0 to 10, with the lower the score the greater the risk that the study was affected by biases.

Step 2. What is the overall quality of evidence?

To evaluate the overall quality of the evidence base for each conclusion, we computed the median quality score of the studies contributing to that conclusion. We used the median because it is the appropriate measure of central tendency to represent the "typical" quality score, and is less sensitive to outliers than the mean. An evidence base with a median score higher than 8.4 was considered to be of high quality; an evidence base with a median score 8.4 or less but greater than 6.7 was considered to be of moderate quality; an evidence base with a median score 6.7 or less but greater than 5.0 was considered to be of low quality; and an evidence base with a median score less than 5.0 was considered to be of insufficient quality. The quality rating was considered to be the "baseline" grade of strength of evidence.

Step 3. Is the evidence base large enough to be informative?

For this Step, we first count the number of included studies. If there are fewer than three studies, the evidence grade is automatically set to Insufficient. Next, we determined whether the precision of the evidence base was sufficient to permit a conclusion. Precision is to a large degree dependent on the size of the evidence base- in general, as the evidence base increases in size the confidence interval around the summary effect becomes tighter due to the increase in statistical power. If the effect is statistically or clinically significant we conclude the data are informative. For diagnostic test evaluations, we consider the precision of the primary measures of diagnostic test accuracy, sensitivity and specificity. If the confidence interval bounds are within 20% of the point estimate for these measures we conclude the data are informative. Other measures of diagnostic test accuracy, such as likelihood ratios and predictive values, are calculated from the same analysis and data used to calculate sensitivity and specificity and therefore are not rated separately. If the data are not sufficiently precise, we down-grade the evidence rating by one level, for example, a rating of High from Step 2 would be down-graded to Moderate.

Step 4. Are data consistent?

Consistency refers to the extent to which the study findings are similar. Quantitative consistency can be tested with the Higgins and Thompson's I2 statistic. For this report, we considered an evidence base to be quantitatively consistent when I2 <50%. The evidence base is considered to be qualitatively consistent when the studies all report the same qualitative conclusion. If the data are not sufficiently consistent, we down-grade the evidence rating by one level, for example, a rating of High from Steps 2 and 4 would be down-graded to Moderate.

Step 5. Are data robust?

In this step we determine whether the data are robust to minor alterations of the data. What types of robustness tests should be performed may vary. For example, if some data were imputed, the analysis should be re-done using reasonable variations in the value(s) of the imputed data. Other robustness tests may include removing one study at a time from the analysis, or performing cumulative meta-analyses. We considered findings to not be robust only if a robustness analysis significantly altered the conclusion (e.g., a statistically significant finding becomes non-significant as studies are added to the evidence base, or the point estimate changed by more 20% after removal of any single study from the analysis). If the data are not sufficiently robust, we down-grade the evidence rating by one level, for example, a rating of High from Steps 2, 4, and 5 would be down-graded to Moderate.

In addition to the conclusions about diagnostic accuracy, we also rated the strength of evidence for one conclusion about a patient-oriented outcome, surgeries avoided. The method of rating patient-oriented outcomes is similar to, but not identical to, the method of rating the conclusions about diagnostic accuracy. In addition to the four important domains used for rating conclusions about diagnostic accuracy we also considered the domain Strength of Association (magnitude of the size of the effect). If the size of the effect was determined to be very small, we down-graded the rating of the strength of evidence by one level; and if the size of effect was determined to be very large we up-graded the strength of evidence by one level.

References

[1] Bukhari, MH; Akhtar, ZM. Comparison of accuracy of diagnostic modalities for evaluation of breast cancer with review of literature. *Diagn Cytopathol,* 2009, Jun, 37(6), 416-424. PMID: 19217034.

[2] Eliahou, R; Sella, T; Allweis, T; et al. Magnetic resonance-guided interventional procedures of the breast: initial experience. *Isr Med Assoc J,* 2009, May;1 1(5), 275-279. PMID: 19637504.

[3] Peters, NH; Meeuwis, C; Bakker, CJ; et al. Feasibility of MRI-guided large-core-needle biopsy of suspiscious breast lesions at 3 T. *Eur Radiol,* 2009, Jul;19(7), 1639-1644. PMID: 19214520.

[4] Salem, C; Sakr R; Chopier J;et al. Accuracy of stereotactic vacuum-assisted breast biopsy with a 10-gauge hand-held system. *Breast*, 2009, Jun;18(3), 178-182. PMID: 19364652.

[5] Tozaki, M; Yamashiro, N; Suzuki, T; et al. MR-guided vacuum-assisted breast biopsy: is it an essential technique? *Breast Cancer*, 2009, 16(2), 121-125. PMID: 18807122.

[6] Bernik, SF; Troob, S; Ying, BL; et al. Papillary lesions of the breast diagnosed by core needle biopsy: 71 cases with surgical follow-up. *Am J Surg,* 2008, Apr;197(4), 473-478. PMID: 18723154.

[7] Brem, RF; Lechner, MC; Jackman, RJ; et al. Lobular neoplasia at percutaneous breast biopsy: variables associated with carcinoma at surgical excision. *AJR Am J Roentgenol,* 2008, Mar; 190(3), 637-641. PMID: 18287433.

[8] Carder, PJ; Khan, T; Burrows, P; et al. Large volume "mammotome" biopsy may reduce the need for diagnostic surgery in papillary lesions of the breast. *J Clin Pathol,* 2008, Aug;61(8), 928-933. PMID: 18495791.

[9] Cheung, KL; Wong, AW; Parker, H; et al. Pathological features of primary breast cancer in the elderly based on needle core biopsies-A large series from a single centre. *Crit Rev Oncol Hematol,* 2008, Sep;67(3), 263-267.

[10] Choo, KS; Kwak, HS; Tae Bae, Y; et al. The value of a combination of wire localization and ultrasound-guided vacuum-assisted breast biopsy for clustered microcalcifications. *Breast*, 2008, Dec 1;17(6), 611-616. PMID: 18653339.

[11] Doren, E; Hulvat, M; Norton, J; et al. Predicting cancer on excision of atypical ductal hyperplasia. *Am J Surg,* 2008, Mar; 195(3), 358-362.

[12] Eby, PR; Ochsner, JE; Demartini, WB; et al. Is surgical excision necessary for focal atypical ductal hyperplasia found at stereotactic vacuum-assisted breast biopsy. *Ann Surg Oncol,* 2008, Nov; 15(1 1), 3232-3238. PMID: 18696163.

[13] Eun, YK; Bae, YA; Kim, MJ;et al. Factors affecting the efficacy of ultrasound- guided vacuum-assisted percutaneous excision for removal of benign breast lesions. *J Ultrasound Med,* 2008, Jan, 27(1), 65-73.

[14] Forgeard, C; Benchaib, M; Guerin, N; et al. Is surgical biopsy mandatory in case of atypical ductal hyperplasia on 11-gauge core needle biopsy? A retrospective study of 300 patients. *Am J Surg,* 2008, Sep;196(3), 339- 345. PMID: 18585676.

[15] Hahn, M; Okamgba, S; Scheler, P; et al. Vacuum-assisted breast biopsy: a comparison of 11-gauge and 8-gauge needles in benign breast disease. *World J Surg Oncol,* 2008, May 19, 6(1), 51. PMID: 18489771.

[16] Hauth, EA; Jaeger, HJ; Lubnau, J; et al. MR- guided vacuum-assisted breast biopsy with a handheld biopsy system: Clinical experience and results in postinterventional MR mammography after 24 h. *Eur Radiol,* 2008, Jan;18(1), 168-176. PMID: 17609959.

[17] He, Q; Fan, X; Guan, Y; et al. Percutaneous excisional biopsy of impalpable breast lesions under ultrasound visualization. *Breast*, 2008, Dec; 17(6), 666-670. PMID: 18835778.

[18] Hertl, K; Marolt-Music, M; Kocijancic, I; et al. Haematomas After Percutaneus Vacuum- Assisted Breast Biopsy. *Ultraschall Med*, 2009, Feb; 30(1), 33-36. PMID: 18773386.

[19] Hemmer, JM; Kelder, JC; van Heesewijk, HP. Stereotactic large-core needle breast biopsy: Analysis of pain and discomfort related to the biopsy procedure. *Eur Radiol,* 2008, Feb;18(2), 351-354. PMID: 17909818.

[20] Hukkinen, K; Kivisaari, L; Heikkila, PS; et al. Unsuccessful preoperative biopsies; fine needle aspiration cytology or core needle biopsy; lead to increased costs in the diagnostic workup in breast cancer. *Acta Oncol,* 2008, 47(6), 1037-1045. PMID: 18607862

[21] Hwang, H; Barke, LD; Mendelson, EB; et al. Atypical lobular hyperplasia and classic lobular carcinoma in situ in core biopsy specimens: Routine excision is not necessary. *Mod Pathol,* 2008, Oct, 21(10), 1208-1216.

[22] Jang, M; Cho, N; Moon, WK; et al. Underestimation of atypical ductal hyperplasia at sonographically guided core biopsy of the breast. *AJR Am J Roentgenol,* 2008, Nov;191(5), 1347-1351. PMID: 18941067.

[23] Ji, HY; Kim, EK; Min, JK;et al. Sonographically guided 14-gauge core needle biopsy of breast masses: A review of 2;420 cases with long-term follow-up. *AJR Am J Roentgenol,* 2008, Jan;190(1), 202-207.

[24] Youk, JH; Kim, EK; Kim, MJ; et al. Sonographically guided 14-gauge core needle biopsy of breast masses: a review of 2;420 cases with long-term follow-up. *AJR Am J Roentgenol,* 2008, Jan, 190(1), 202-207. PMID: 18094312.

[25] Kil, WH; Cho, EY; Kim, JH; et al. Is surgical excision necessary in benign papillary lesions initially diagnosed at core biopsy? *Breast*, 2008, Jun;17(3), 258-262. PMID: 18054232.

[26] Kim, MJ; Kim, EK; Park, SY; et al. Imaging- histologic discordance at sonographically guided percutaneous biopsy of breast lesions. *Eur J Radiol*, 2008, Jan, 65(1), 163-169.

[27] Kim, MJ; Kim, EK; Kwak, JY; et al. Nonmalignant papillary lesions of the breast at US-guided directional vacuum-assisted removal: A preliminary report. *Eur Radiol,* 2008, 18(9), 1774-1783.

[28] Kumaroswamy, V; Liston, J; Shaaban, AM. Vacuum assisted stereotactic guided mammotome biopsies in the management of screen detected microcalcifications: experience of a large breast screening centre. *J Clin Pathol,* 2008, Jun;61(6), 766- 769. PMID: 18326021.

[29] Lee, JM; Kaplan, JB; Murray, MP; et al. Complete excision of the MRI target lesion at MRI-guided vacuum-assisted biopsy of breast cancer. *AJR Am J Roentgenol,* 2008, Oct;191(4), 1198-1202. PMID: 18806165.

[30] Londero, V; Zuiani, C; Linda, A; et al. Lobular neoplasia: Core needle breast biopsy underestimation of malignancy in relation to radiologic and pathologic features. *Breast*, 2008, Dec 1, 17(6), 623-630. PMID: 18619840.

[31] Mahoney, MC. Initial clinical experience with a new MRI vacuum-assisted breast biopsy device. *J Magn Reson Imaging,* 2008, Oct;28(4), 900-905. PMID: 18821610.

[32] Menon, S; Porter, GJ; Evans, AJ; et al. The significance of lobular neoplasia on needle core biopsy of the breast. Virchows Arch 2008, May;452(5), 473-479. PMID: 18389278.

[33] Michalopoulos, NV; Zagouri, F; Sergentanis, TN; et al. Needle tract seeding after vacuum-assisted breast biopsy. *Acta Radiol,* 2008, Apr;49(3), 267-270. PMID: 18365811.

[34] Perretta, T; Pistolese, CA; Bolacchi, F; et al. MR imaging-guided 10-gauge vacuum-assisted breast biopsy: histological characterisation. *Radiol Med,* 2008, Sep; 113(6), 830-840. PMID: 18633687.

[35] Peter, D; Grunhagen, J; Wenke, R; et al. False- negative results after stereotactically guided vacuum biopsy. *Eur Radiol,* 2008, Jan; 18(1), 177-182. PMID: 17637996.

[36] Resetkova, E; Edelweiss, M; Albarracin, CT; et al. Management of radial sclerosing lesions of the breast diagnosed using percutaneous vacuum-assisted core needle biopsy: recommendations for excision based on seven years' of experience at a single institution. *Breast Cancer Res Treat,* 2008, Jul 15;:Epub ahead of print. PMID: 18626769.

[37] Rizzo, M; Lund, MJ; Oprea, G; et al. Surgical follow-up and clinical presentation of 142 breast papillary lesions diagnosed by ultrasound-guided core-needle biopsy. *Ann Surg Oncol,* 2008, Apr; 15(4), 1040-1047. PMID: 18204989.

[38] Salem, C; Sakr, R; Chopier, J; et al. Pain and complications of directional vacuum-assisted stereotactic biopsy: Comparison of the Mammotome and Vacora techniques. Eur J Radiol 2008, Aug 26, Epub ahead of print. PMID: 18755562.

[39] Shin, HJ; Kim, HH; Kim, SM; et al. Papillary lesions of the breast diagnosed at percutaneous sonographically guided biopsy: comparison of sonographic features and biopsy methods. *AJR Am J Roentgenol,* 2008, Mar; 190(3), 630-636. PMID: 18287432.

[40] Sigal-Zafrani, B; Muller, K; El Khoury, C; et al. Vacuum-assisted large-core needle biopsy (VLNB) improves the management of patients with breast microcalcifications - Analysis of 1009 cases. *Eur J Surg Oncol*, 2008, Apr, 34(4), 377-381.

[41] Skandarajah, AR; Field, L; Yuen Larn Mou, A; et al. Benign papilloma on core biopsy requires surgical excision. *Ann Surg Oncol,* 2008, Aug, 15(8), 2272-2277. PMID: 18473143.

[42] Smetherman, D; Dydynski, P; Jackson, P. Effect of breast core needle biopsy technique on detection of lobular intraepithelial neoplasia. *Ochsner J*, 2007, Sep, 7(3), 121-124.

[43] Sohn, VY; Arthurs, ZM; Kim, FS; et al. Lobular neoplasia: Is surgical excision warranted? *Am Surg,* 2008, Feb, 74(2), 172- 177. PMID: 18306873.

[44] Somerville, P; Seifert, PJ; Destounis, SV; et al. Anticoagulation and bleeding risk after core needle biopsy. *AJR Am J Roentgenol,* 2008, Oct, 191(4), 1194-1197. PMID: 18806164.

[45] Tagaya, N; Nakagawa, A; Ishikawa, Y; et al. Experience with ultrasonographically guided vacuum-assisted resection of benign breast tumors. *Clin Radiol,* 2008, Apr, 63(4), 396- 400.

[46] Taourel, P; Hoa, D; Chaveron, C; et al. Stereotactic vacuum biopsy of calcifications with a handheld portable biopsy system: A validation study. *Eur Radiol,* 2008, Jul;18(7), 13 19-1325.

[47] Tozaki, M; Yamashiro, N; Suzuki, T; et al. MR-guided vacuum-assisted breast biopsy: is it an essential technique. *Breast Cancer,* 2008, Sep 20, Epub ahead of print. PMID: 18807122.

[48] Tseng, HS; Chen, YL; Chen, ST; et al. The management of papillary lesion of the breast by core needle biopsy. *Eur J Surg Oncol,* 2009, Jan;35(1), 2 1-24. PMID: 18640002.

[49] Zagouri, F; Sergentanis, TN; Gounaris, A; et al. Pain in different methods of breast biopsy: Emphasis on vacuum-assisted breast biopsy. *Breast*, 2008, Feb, 1 7(1), 7 1-75.

[50] Zografos, G; Zagouri, F; Sergentanis, TN; et al. Vacuum-assisted breast biopsy in nonpalpable solid breast lesions without microcalcifications: the Greek experience. *Diagn Interv Radiol*, 2008, Sep;14(3), 127-130. PMID: 18814132.

[51] Zografos, GC; Zagouri, F; Sergentanis, TN; et al. Minimizing underestimation rate of microcalcifications excised via vacuum- assisted breast biopsy: a blind study. *Breast Cancer Res Treat,* 2008, May, 109(2), 397-402. PMID: 17653855.

[52] Zografos, GC; Zagouri, F; Sergentanis, TN; et al. Pain during vacuum-assisted breast biopsy: Are there any predictors. *Breast*, 2008, Dec, 17(6), 592-595. Epub 2008, Jul 26. PMID: 18657974.

[53] Andreu, FJ; Saez, A; Sentis, M; et al. Breast core biopsy reporting categories—An internal validation in a series of 3054 consecutive lesions. *Breast*, 2007, Feb, 16(1), 94-101. PMID: 16982194.

[54] Arora, N; Hill, C; Hoda, SA; et al. Clinicopathologic features of papillary lesions on core needle biopsy of the breast predictive of malignancy. *Am J Surg,* 2007, Oct; 1 94(4), 444-449. PMID: 17826053.

[55] Ashkenazi, I; Ferrer, K; Sekosan, M; et al. Papillary lesions of the breast discovered on percutaneous large core and vacuum- assisted biopsies: reliability of clinical and pathological parameters in identifying benign lesions. *Am J Surg,* 2007, Aug, 194(2), 183-188. PMID: 17618801.

[56] Bode, MK; Rissanen, T; Apaja-Sarkkinen, M. Ultrasonography and core needle biopsy in the differential diagnosis of fibroadenoma and tumor phyllodes. *Acta Radiol,* 2007, Sep;48(7), 708-713. PMID: 17728999.

[57] Cassano, E; Urban, LA; Pizzamiglio, M; et al. Ultrasound-guided vacuum-assisted core breast biopsy: experience with 406 cases. *Breast Cancer Res Treat,* 2007, Mar, 102(1), 103-110. PMID: 16838109.

[58] Ciatto, S; Houssami, N. Breast imaging and needle biopsy in women with clinically evident breast cancer: does combined imaging change overall diagnostic sensitivity? *Breast*, 2007, Aug; 1 6(4), 382-386. PMID: 17350262.

[59] Dillon, MF; McDermott, EW; Hill, AD; et al. Predictive value of breast lesions of "uncertain malignant potential" and "suspicious for malignancy" determined by needle core biopsy. *Ann Surg Oncol,* 2007, Feb;14(2), 704-711.

[60] Douglas-Jones, AG; Denson, JL; Cox AC; et al. Radial scar lesions of the breast diagnosed by needle core biopsy: analysis of cases containing occult malignancy. *J Clin Pathol,* 2007, Mar, 60(3), 295-298. PMID: 16731590.

[61] Duchesne, N; Parker, SH; Lechner, MC; et al. Multicenter evaluation of a new ultrasound- guided biopsy device: Improved ergonomics; sampling and rebiopsy rates. *Breast J*, 2007, Jan-Feb;13(1), 36-43. PMID: 17214791.

[62] Duijm, LEM; Groenewoud JH; Roumen RMH; et al. A decade of breast cancer screening in the Netherlands: Trends in the preoperative diagnosis of breast cancer. *Breast Cancer Res Treat,* 2007, Nov;106(1), 1 13-119.

[63] Easley, S; Abdul-Karim, FW; Klein, N; et al. Segregation of radiographic calcifications in stereotactic core biopsies of breast: Is it necessary? *Breast J*, 2007, Sep;13(5), 486-489.

[64] Esserman, LE; Lamea, L; Tanev, S; et al. Should the extent of lobular neoplasia on core biopsy influence the decision for excision? *Breast J*, 2007, Jan, 13(1), 55-61.

[65] Foxcroft, LM; Evans, EB; Porter, AJ. Difficulties in the pre-operative diagnosis of phyllodes tumours of the breast: a study of 84 cases. *Breast*, 2007, Feb, 16(1), 27-37. PMID: 16876413.

[66] Garg, S; Mohan, H; Bal, A; et al. A comparative analysis of core needle biopsy and fine-needle aspiration cytology in the evaluation of palpable and mammographically detected suspicious breast lesions. *Diagn Cytopathol,* 2007, Nov, 35(11), 681-689. PMID: 17924407.

[67] Holloway, CMB; Saskin, R; Brackstone, M; et al. Variation in the use of percutaneous biopsy for diagnosis of breast abnormalities in Ontario. *Ann Surg Oncol,* 2007, Oct; 14(10), 2932-2939.

[68] Houssami, N; Ciatto, S; Bilous, M; et al. Borderline breast core needle histology: Predictive values for malignancy in lesions of uncertain malignant potential (B3). *Br J Cancer*, 2007, Apr 23, 96(8), 1253-1257.

[69] Karabakhtsian, RG; Johnson, R; Sumkin, J; et al. The clinical significance of lobular neoplasia on breast core biopsy. *Am J Surg,* Pathol 2007, May;31(5), 717-723. PMID: 17460455.

[70] Kikuchi, M; Tsunoda-Shimizu, H; Kawasaki, T; et al. Indications for stereotactically-guided vacuum-assisted breast biopsy for patients with category 3 microcalcifications. *Breast Cancer,* 2007, 14(3), 285-291. PMID: 17690506.

[71] Kim, MJ; Kim, EK; Lee, JY; et al. Breast lesions with imaging-histologic discordance during US-guided 14G automated core biopsy: can the directional vacuum-assisted removal replace the surgical excision? Initial findings. *Eur Radiol,* 2007, Sep;17(9), 2376-2383. PMID: 17361422.

[72] Ko, ES; Cho, N; Cha, JH; et al. Sonographically-guided 14-gauge core needle biopsy for papillary lesions of the breast. *Korean J Radiol*, 2007, MayJun, 8(3), 206-211. PMID: 17554187.

[73] Krainick-Strobel, U; Huber, B; Majer, I; et al. Complete extirpation of benign breast lesions with an ultrasound-guided vacuum biopsy system. *Ultrasound Obstet Gynecol,* 2007, Mar, 29(3), 342-346.

[74] Kumaraswamy, V; Carder, PJ. Examination of breast needle core biopsy specimens performed for screen-detected microcalcification. *J Clin Pathol,* 2007, Jun, 60(6), 681-684. PMID: 16882700.

[75] Kunju, LP; Kleer, CG. Significance of flat epithelial atypia on mammotome core needle biopsy: should it be excised? *Hum Pathol*, 2007, Jan, 38(1), 35-41.

[76] Lavoue, V; Graesslin, O; Classe, JM; et al. Management of lobular neoplasia diagnosed by core needle biopsy: study of 52 biopsies with follow-up surgical excision. *Breast*, 2007, Oct, 16(5), 533-539. PMID: 17629481.

[77] Lee, JM; Kaplan, JB; Murray, MP; et al. Underestimation of DCIS at MRI-guided vacuum-assisted breast biopsy. *AJR Am J Roentgenol,* 2007, Aug; 189(2), 468-474. PMID: 17646475.

[78] Lee, JM; Kaplan, JB; Murray, MP; et al. Imaging-histologic discordance at MRIguided 9-gauge vacuum-assisted breast biopsy. *AJR Am J Roentgenol,* 2007, Oct; 189(4), 852-859.

[79] Leikola, J; Heikkila, P; Pamilo, M; et al. Predicting invasion in patients with DCIS in the preoperative percutaneous biopsy. *Acta Oncol,* 2007, 46(6), 798-802.

[80] Liberman, L; Holland, AE; Marjan, D; et al. Underestimation of atypical ductal hyperplasia at MRI-guided 9-gauge vacuum- assisted breast biopsy. *AJR Am J Roentgenol,* 2007, Mar; 1 88(3), 684-690. PMID: 17312054.

[81] Londero, V; Zuiani, C; Furlan, A; et al. Role of ultrasound and sonographically guided core biopsy in the diagnostic evaluation of ductal carcinoma in situ (DCIS) of the breast. *Radiol Med,* 2007, Sep, 112(6), 863- 876.

[82] Lourenco, AP; Mainiero, MB; Lazarus, E; et al. Stereotactic breast biopsy: Comparison of histologic underestimation rates with 11- and 9-gauge vacuum-assisted breast biopsy. *AJR Am J Roentgenol,* 2007 Nov; 1 89(5), W275-W279. PMID: 17954625.

[83] Luczynska, E; Skotnicki, P; Kocurek, A; et al. Vacuum mammotomy under ultrasound guidance. *Pol Przegl Radiol*, 2007, Jul, 72(3), 15-18.

[84] Martel, M; Barron-Rodriguez, P; Tolgay Ocal, I; et al. Flat DIN 1 (flat epithelial atypia) on core needle biopsy: 63 Cases identified retrospectively among 1;751 core biopsies performed over an 8-year period (1992- 1999). *Virchows Arch*, 2007, Nov;451(5), 883-891.

[85] Mathew, J; Crawford, DJ; Lwin, M; et al. Ultrasound-guided; vacuum-assisted excision in the diagnosis and treatment of clinically benign breast lesions. *Ann R Coll Surg Engl*, 2007, Jul;89(5), 494-496. PMID: 17688722.

[86] Mendel, JB; Long, M; Slanetz, PJ. CT-guided core needle biopsy of breast lesions visible only on MRI. *AJR Am J Roentgenol,* 2007, Jul, 189(1), 152-154. PMID: 17579165.

[87] Murta De Lucena, CE; Dos Santos Jr, JL; De Lima Resende, CA; et al. Ultrasound-guided core needle biopsy of breast masses: How many cores are necessary to diagnose cancer? *J Clin Ultrasound*, 2007, Sep, 35(7), 363-366.

[88] Nakano, S; Sakamoto, H; Ohtsuka, M; et al. Evaluation and indications of ultrasound-guided vacuum-assisted core needle breast biopsy. *Breast Cancer,* 2007; 14(3), 292-296. PMID: 17690507.

[89] Popiela, TJ; Herman-Sucharska, I; Kleinrok, K; et al. Core breast biopsy under MR control - Preliminary results. *Pol Przegl Radiol*, 2007, Apr, 72(2), 15-24.

[90] Povoski, SP; Jimenez, RE. A comprehensive evaluation of the 8-gauge vacuum-assisted Mammotome system for ultrasound-guided diagnostic biopsy and selective excision of breast lesions. *World J Surg Oncol,* 2007, 5, Article 83.

[91] Rutstein, LA; Johnson, RR; Poller, WR; et al. Predictors of residual invasive disease after core needle biopsy diagnosis of ductal carcinoma in situ. *Breast J*, 2007, MayJun, 13(3), 251-257. PMID: 17461899.

[92] Schaefer, FK; Eden, I; Schaefer, PJ; et al. Factors associated with one step surgery in case of non-palpable breast cancer. *Eur J Radiol,* 2007, Dec, 64(3), 426-43 1.

[93] Smitt, MC; Horst, K. Association of clinical and pathologic variables with lumpectomy surgical margin status after preoperative diagnosis or excisional biopsy of invasive breast cancer. *Ann Surg Oncol,* 2007, Mar; 14(3), 1040-1044. PMID: 17203329.

[94] Sohn, V; Arthurs, Z; Herbert, G; et al. Atypical ductal hyperplasia: Improved accuracy with the 11-gauge vacuum-assisted versus the 14-gauge core biopsy needle. *Ann Surg Oncol,* 2007, Sep, 14(9), 2497-2501. PMID: 17564749.

[95] Sydnor, MK; Wilson, JD; Hijaz, TA; et al. Underestimation of the presence of breast carcinoma in papillary lesions initially diagnosed at core-needle biopsy. *Radiology*, 2007, Jan, 242(1), 58-62. PMID: 17090707.

[96] Uematsu, T; Kasami, M. Risk of needle tract seeding of breast cancer: cytological results derived from core wash material. *Breast Cancer Res Treat,* 2008, Jul;1 10(1), 51-55. PMID: 17674195.

[97] Uematsu, T; Kasami, M; Uchida, Y; et al. Ultrasonographically guided 18-gauge automated core needle breast biopsy with post-fire needle position verification (PNPV). *Breast Cancer,* 2007, 14(2), 2 19-228. PMID: 17485909.

[98] Usami, S; Moriya, T; Amari, M; et al. Reliability of prognostic factors in breast carcinoma determined by core needle biopsy. *Jpn J Clin Oncol*, 2007, Apr, 37(4), 250-255.

[99] Zagouri, F; Sergentanis, TN; Nonni, A; et al. Vacuum-assisted breast biopsy: The value and limitations of cores with microcalcifications. *Pathol Res Pract*, 2007, Aug 30 203(8), 563-566.

[100] Zografos, GC; Zagouri, F; Sergentanis, TN; et al. Is zero underestimation feasible? Extended Vacuum-assisted breast biopsy in solid lesions—A blind study. *World J Surg Oncol,* 2007, May 14, 5, Article Number:53.

[101] Zuiani, C; Mazzarella, F; Londero, V; et al. Stereotactic vacuum-assisted breast biopsy: results; follow-up and correlation with radiological suspicion. *Radiol Med,* 2007, Mar, 112(2), 304-317. PMID: 17361368.

[102] Al-Attar, MA; Michell, MJ; Ralleigh, G; et al. The impact of image guided needle biopsy on the outcome of mammographically detected indeterminate microcalcification. *Breast*, 2006, Oct; 15(5), 635-639. PMID: 16488148.

[103] Becker, L; Trop, I; David, J; et al. Management of radial scars found at percutaneous breast biopsy. *Can Assoc Radiol J*, 2006, Apr, 57(2), 72-78. PMID: 16944680.

[104] Bedei, L; Falcini, F; Sanna, PA; et al. Atypical ductal hyperplasia of the breast: The controversial management of a borderline lesion: Experience of 47 cases diagnosed at vacuum-assisted biopsy. *Breast*, 2006, Apr, 15(2), 196-202. PMID: 16055333.

[105] Chrzan, R; Rudnicka, L; Popiela, Jr T; et al. The problems with histopathological verification of breast microcalcification clusters in the stereotactic mammotome biopsy specimens. *Pol J Pathol*, 2006, 57(3), 133-135.

[106] Cox, D; Bradley, S; England, D. The significance of mammotome core biopsy specimens without radiographically identifiable microcalcification and their influence on surgical management-A retrospective review with histological correlation. *Breast*, 2006, Apr; 1 5(2), 21 0-218. PMID: 16081287.

[107] Dillon, MF; McDermott, EW; Quinn, CM; et al. Predictors of invasive disease in breast cancer when core biopsy demonstrates DCIS only. *J Surg Oncol,* 2006, Jun 1, 93(7), 559- 563.

[108] Dillon, MF; Quinn, CM; McDermott, EW; et al. Needle core biopsy in the diagnosis of phyllodes neoplasm. *Surgery*, 2006, Nov, 140(5), 779-784. PMID: 17084721.

[109] Fine, RE; Staren, ED. Percutaneous radiofrequency-assisted excision of fibroadenomas. *Am J Surg,* 2006, 192(4), 545-547. PMID: 16978972.

[110] Fitzal, F; Sporn, EP; Draxler, W; et al. Preoperative core needle biopsy does not increase local recurrence rate in breast cancer patients. *Breast Cancer Res Treat,* 2006, May, 97(1), 9-15. PMID: 16502019.

[111] Gebauer, B; Bostanjoglo, M; Moesta, KT; et al. Magnetic resonance-guided biopsy of suspicious breast lesions with a handheld vacuum biopsy device. *Acta Radiol,* 2006, Nov;47(9), 907-913. PMID: 17077039.

[112] Ghate, SV; Rosen, EL; Soo, MS; et al. MRIguided vacuum-assisted breast biopsy with a handheld portable biopsy system. *AJR Am J Roentgenol,* 2006, Jun; 186(6), 1733-1736. PMID: 16714667.

[113] Govindarajulu, S; Narreddy, S; Shere, MH; et al. Preoperative mammotome biopsy of ducts beneath the nipple areola complex. *Eur J Surg Oncol,* 2006, May, 32(4), 410-412. PMID: 16516432.

[114] Hanley, C; Kessaram, R. Quality of diagnosis and surgical management of breast lesions in a community hospital: room for improvement? *Can J Surg*, 2006, Jun, 49(3), 185-192. PMID: 16749979.

[115] Hoffmann, J. Analysis of surgical and diagnostic quality at a specialist breast unit. *Breast*, 2006, Aug; 15(4), 490-497.

[116] Huo, L; Sneige, N; Hunt, KK; et al. Predictors of invasion in patients with core-needle biopsy-diagnosed ductal carcinoma in situ and recommendations for a selective approach to sentinel lymph node biopsy in ductal carcinoma in situ. *Cancer*, 2006, Oct 15, 107(8), 1760-1768. PMID: 16977650.

[117] Jackman, RJ; Rodriguez-Soto, J. Breast microcalcifications: retrieval failure at prone stereotactic core and vacuum breast biopsy-- frequency; causes; and outcome. *Radiology*, 2006, Apr, 239(1), 61-70. PMID: 16567483.

[118] Jensen, A; Rank, F; Dyreborg, U; et al. Performance of combined clinical mammography and needle biopsy: a nationwide study from Denmark. *APMIS*, 2006, Dec, 114(12), 884-892. PMID, 17207089.

[119] Kamer, E; Unalp, HR; Akguner, T; et al. Thick-needle vacuum-assisted biopsy technique for inflammatory breast carcinoma diagnosis. *Acta Cir Bras*, 2006, Nov, 21 (6), 422-424.

[120] Killebrew, LK; Oneson, RH. Comparison of the diagnostic accuracy of a vacuum-assisted percutaneous intact specimen sampling device to a vacuum-assisted core needle sampling device for breast biopsy: Initial experience. *Breast J*, 2006, Jul, 12(4), 302-308. PMID: 16848839.

[121] Koskela, A; Berg, M; Sudah, M; et al. Learning curve for add-on stereotactic core needle breast biopsy. *Acta Radiol,* 2006, Jun, 47(5), 454-460. PMID: 16796305.

[122] Lam, WW; Chu, WC; Tse, GM; et al. Role of fine needle aspiration and tru cut biopsy in diagnosis of mucinous carcinoma of breast-- from a radiologist's perspective. *Clin Imaging*, 2006, Jan-Feb, 30(1), 6-10. PMID: 16377477.

[123] Lannin, DR; Ponn, T; Andrejeva, L; et al. Should all breast cancers be diagnosed by needle biopsy? *Am J Surg,* 2006, Oct, 192(4), 450-454. PMID: 16978947.

[124] Liberman, L; Tornos, C; Huzjan, R; et al. Is surgical excision warranted after benign; concordant diagnosis of papilloma at percutaneous breast biopsy? *AJR Am J Roentgenol,* 2006, May; 186(5), 1328-1334. PMID: 16632727.

[125] Lieske, B; Ravichandran, D; Wright, D. Role of fine-needle aspiration cytology and core biopsy in the preoperative diagnosis of screen-detected breast carcinoma. *Br J Cancer,* 2006, Jul 3, 95(1), 62-66.

[126] Lim, CN; Ho, BC; Bay, BH; et al. Nuclear morphometry in columnar cell lesions of the breast: is it useful? *J Clin Pathol,* 2006, Dec;59(12), 1283-1286. PMID: 16603646.

[127] Lopez-Medina, A; Cintora E; Mugica, B; et al. Radial scars diagnosed at stereotactic core-needle biopsy: Surgical biopsy findings. *Eur Radiol,* 2006, Aug, 16(8), 1803-1810. PMID: 16708220.

[128] Margenthaler, JA; Duke, D; Monsees, BS; et al. Correlation between core biopsy and excisional biopsy in breast high-risk lesions. *Am J Surg,* 2006, Oct, 192(4), 534-537. PMID: 16978969.

[129] Mercado, CL; Hamele-Bena, D; Oken, SM; et al. Papillary lesions of the breast at percutaneous core-needle biopsy. *Radiology*, 2006, Mar;238(3), 801 -808. PMID: 16424237.

[130] Newman, EL; Kahn, A; Diehl, KM; et al. Does the method of biopsy affect the incidence of sentinel lymph node metastases? *Breast J*, 2006, Jan, 12(1), 53-57. PMID: 16409587.

[131] Orel, SG; Rosen, M; Mies, C; et al. MR imaging-guided 9-gauge vacuum-assisted core-neddle breast biopsy: Initial experience. *Radiology*, 2006, Jan, 238(1), 54- 61. PMID: 16304093.

[132] Perlet, C; Heywang-Kobrunner, SH; Heinig, A; et al. Magnetic resonance-guided; vacuum-assisted breast biopsy: Results from a European multicenter study of 538 lesions. *Cancer*, 2006, Mar, 1, 106(5), 982-990. PMID: 16456807.

[133] Popiela, TJ; Tabor, J; Chrzan, R; PosiadloKleinrok, B; Urbanik, A. Mammotome biopsy in the diagnostic management of non- palpable breast pathologies. *Pol Przegl Radiol*, 2006, Jul, 71(3), 48-56.

[134] Renshaw, AA; Gould, EW. Comparison of disagreement and amendment rates by tissue type and diagnosis: identifying cases for directed blinded review. *Am J Clin Pathol,* 2006, Nov;126(5), 736-739. PMID: 17050070.

[135] Renshaw, AA; Derhagopian, RP; Martinez, P; et al. Lobular neoplasia in breast core needle biopsy specimens is associated with a low risk of ductal carcinoma in situ or invasive carcinoma on subsequent excision. *Am J Clin Pathol,* 2006, Aug; 126(2), 3 10-313. PMID: 16891208.

[136] Senn Bahls, E; Dupont Lampert, V; Oelschlegel, C; et al. Multitarget stereotactic core-needle breast biopsy (MSBB)-an effective and safe diagnostic intervention for non-palpable breast lesions: A large prospective single institution study. *Breast*, 2006, Jun; 1 5(3), 339-346.

[137] Shin, S; Schneider, HB; Cole, Jr FJ; et al. Follow-up recommendations for benign breast biopsies. *Breast J*, 2006, Sep, 12(5), 413-417.

[138] Sie, A; Bryan, DC; Gaines, V; et al. Multicenter evaluation of the breast lesion excision system; a percutaneous; vacuum- assisted; intact-specimen breast biopsy device. *Cancer*, 2006, Sep 1, 107(5), 945-949. PMID: 16874817.

[139] Uriburu, JL; Vuoto, HD; Cogorno, L; et al. Local recurrence of breast cancer after skin-sparing mastectomy following core needle biopsy: Case reports and review of the literature. *Breast J*, 2006, May, 12(3), 194-198. PMID: 16684314.

[140] Valdes, EK; Tartter, PI; Genelus-Dominique, E; et al. Significance of papillary lesions at percutaneous breast biopsy. *Ann Surg Oncol,* 2006, Apr, 13(4), 480-482.

[141] Vargas, HI; Vargas, MP; Gonzalez, K; et al. Percutaneous excisional biopsy of palpable breast masses under ultrasound visualization. *Breast J*, 2006, Sep, 12(Suppl 2), S218-S222. PMID: 16959005.

[142] Viehweg, P; Bernerth, T; Kiechle, M; et al. MR-guided intervention in women with a family history of breast cancer. *Eur J Radiol*, 2006, Jan;57(1), 81-89. PMID: 16364583.

[143] Wu, YC; Chen, DR; Kuo, SJ. Personal experience of ultrasound-guided 14-gauge core biopsy of breast tumor. *Eur J Surg Oncol,* 2006, Sep;32(7), 71 5-718. PMID: 16769196.

[144] Yazici, B; Sever, AR; Mills, P; et al. Scar formation after stereotactic vacuum-assisted core biopsy of benign breast lesions. *Clin Radiol,* 2006, Jul, 61(7), 619-624. PMID: 16784949.

[145] Altomare, V; Guerriero, G; Giacomelli, L; et al. Management of nonpalpable breast lesions in a modern functional breast unit. *Breast Cancer Res Treat,* 2005, Sep, 93(1), 85- 89. PMID: 16184463

[146] Badoual, C; Maruani, A; Ghorra, C; et al. Pathological prognostic factors of invasive breast carcinoma in ultrasound-guided large core biopsies - Correlation with subsequent surgical excisions. *Breast*, 2005, Feb;14(1), 22-27. PMID: 15695077.

[147] Bonifacino, A; Petrocelli, V; Pisani, T; et al. Accuracy rates of US-guided vacuum-assisted breast biopsy. *Anticancer Res*, 2005, May, 25(3 C), 2465-2470. PMID: 16080477.

[148] Brem, RF; Tran, K; Rapelyea, J; et al. Percutaneous biopsy of papillary lesions of the breast: Accuracy of pathologic diagnosis. *J Womens Imaging*, 2005, Dec, 7(4), 157-162.

[149] Caines, JS; Schaller, GH; Iles, SE; et al. Ten years of breast screening in the Nova Scotia Breast Screening Program; 1991-2001. Experience: Use of an adaptable stereotactic device in the diagnosis of screening-detected abnormalities. *Can Assoc Radiol J*, 2005, Apr, 56(2), 82-93.

[150] Cho, N; Moon, WK; Cha, JH; et al. Sonographically guided core biopsy of the breast: comparison of 14-gauge automated gun and 11-gauge directional vacuum- assisted biopsy methods. *Korean J Radiol*, 2005, Apr-Jun;6(2), 102-109. PMID: 15968149.

[151] Costantini, R; Sardellone, A; Marino, C; et al. Vacuum-assisted core biopsy (mammotome) for the diagnosis of non-palpable breast lesions: Four-year experience in an Italian center. *Tumori*, 2005, Jul;91(4), 351-354. PMID: 16277103.

[152] Diebold, T; Hahn, T; Solbach, C; et al. Evaluation of the stereotactic 8G vacuum-assisted breast biopsy in the histologic evaluation of suspicious mammography findings (BI-RADS IV). *Invest Radiol*, 2005, Jul;40(7), 465-47 1. PMID: 15973139.

[153] Doridot, V; Meunier, M; El Khoury, C; et al. Stereotactic radioguided surgery by siteSelect for subclinical mammographic lesions. *Ann Surg Oncol,* 2005, Feb;12(2), 181-188. PMID: 15827800.

[154] Doyle, JM; O'Doherty, A; Coffey, L; et al. Can the radiologist accurately predict the adequacy of sampling when performing ultrasound-guided core biopsy of BI-RADS

category 4 and 5 lesions detected on screening mammography? *Clin Radiol,* 2005, Sep, 60(9), 999-1 005. PMID: 16124982.

[155] Elsheikh, TM; Silverman, JF. Follow-up surgical excision is indicated when breast core needle biopsies show atypical lobular hyperplasia or lobular carcinoma in situ: a correlative study of 33 patients with review of the literature. *Am J Surg Pathol*, 2005, Apr, 29(4), 534-543. PMID: 15767810.

[156] Gambos, EC; Godinez, J; Poppiti Jr, RJ. Significance of extent of lobular neoplasia on breast core biopsy. *J Womens Imaging,* 2005, Dec;7(4), 150-156.

[157] Grady, I; Gorsuch, H; Wilburn-Bailey, S. Ultrasound-guided; vacuum-assisted; percutaneous excision of breast lesions: an accurate technique in the diagnosis of atypical ductal hyperplasia. *J Am Coll Surg,* 2005, Jul, 201(1), 14-17. PMID: 15978438

[158] Hanna, WC; Demyttenaere, SV; Ferri, LE; et al. The use of stereotactic excisional biopsy in the management of invasive breast cancer. *World J Surg*, 2005, Nov, 29(1 1), 1490-1494. PMID: 16240063.

[159] Homesh, NA; Issa, MA; El-Sofiani, HA. The diagnostic accuracy of fine needle aspiration cytology versus core needle biopsy for palpable breast lump(s). *Saudi Med J*, 2005, Jan, 26(1), 42-46. PMID: 15756351.

[160] Lehman, CD; DePeri, ER; Peacock, S; et al. Clinical experience with MRI-guided vacuum-assisted breast biopsy. *AJR Am J Roentgenol,* 2005, Jun; 184(6), 1782-1787. PMID: 15908530.

[161] Monticciolo, DL. Histologic grading at breast core needle biopsy: Comparison with results from the excised breast specimen. *Breast J*, 2005, Jan, 11(1), 9-14. PMID: 15647072.

[162] Pilgrim, S; Ravichandran, D. Fine needle aspiration cytology as an adjunct to core biopsy in the assessment of symptomatic breast carcinoma. *Breast*, 2005, Oct, 14(5), 41 1-414.

[163] Qazi, DES; Mohayuddin, N. Role of fine needle aspiration cytology and core biopsy in the diagnosis of breast lumps. *J Postgrad Med Inst,* 2005, Jan;19(1), 67-70.

[164] Riedl, CC; Pfarl, G; Memarsadeghi, M; et al. Lesion miss rates and false-negative rates for 1115 consecutive cases of stereotactically guided needle-localized open breast biopsy with long-term follow- up. *Radiology*, 2005, Dec;237(3), 847-853. PMID: 16237133.

[165] Rulli, A; Lauro, A; Bisacci, C; et al. Non- palpable breast lesion-biopsy by ABBI system: A diagnostic tool. *Chirurgia*, 2005, Aug, 18(4), 175-179.

[166] Satchithananda, K; Fernando, RA; Ralleigh, G; et al. An audit of pain/discomfort experienced during image-guided breast biopsy procedures. *Breast J*, 2005, Nov-Dec;1 1(6), 398-402. PMID: 16297083.

[167] Schneider, J; Lucas, R; Tejerina, A. Predicting complete removal of impalpable breast carcinomas using stereotactic radiologically guided surgery. *Br J Surg*, 2005, May;92(5), 563-564. PMID: 15739212.

[168] Soo, MS; Kliewer, MA; Ghate, S; et al. Stereotactic breast biopsy of noncalcified lesions: A cost-minimization analysis comparing 14-gauge multipass automated core biopsy to 14- and 11-gauge vacuum- assisted biopsy. *Clin Imaging*, 2005, Jan, 29(1), 26-33.

[169] Wahner-Roedler, DL; Whaley, DH; Brandt, KR; et al. Vacuum-assisted breast biopsy device (Mammotome) malfunction simulating microcalcifications. *Breast J*, 2005, Nov; 11(6), 474-475.

[170] Wiratkapun, C; Wibulpholprasert, B; Wongwaisayawan, S; et al. Nondiagnostic core needle biopsy of the breast under imaging guidance: result of rebiopsy. *J Med Assoc Thai*, 2005, Mar, 88(3), 350-357. PMID: 15962643.

[171] Wong, TT; Cheung, PS; Ma, MK; et al. Experience of stereotactic breast biopsy using the vacuum-assisted core needle biopsy device and the advanced breast biopsy instrumentation system in Hong Kong women. *Asian J Surg*, 2005, Jan, 28(1), 18-23.

[172] You, JK; Kim, EK; Kwak, JY; et al. Focal fibrosis of the breast diagnosed by a sonographically guided core biopsy of nonpalpable lesions: imaging findings and clinical relevance. *J Ultrasound Med,* 2005, Oct, 24(10), 1377-1384. PMID: 16179621.

[173] Zuiani, C; Londero, V; Bestagno, A; et al. Proliferative high-risk lesions of the breast: Contribution and limits of US-guided core biopsy. *Radiol Med,* 2005, Nov; 110(5-6), 589-602. PMID: 16437044.

[174] Agoff, SN; Lawton, TJ. Papillary lesions of the breast with and without atypical ductal hyperplasia: Can we accurately predict benign behavior from core needle biopsy. Am *J Clin Pathol,* 2004, Sep;122(3), 440-443.

[175] Arpino, G; Allred, DC; Mohsin, SK; et al. Lobular neoplasia on core-needle biopsy--clinical significance. Cancer 2004, Jul 15;101(2), 242-250. PMID: 15241819.

[176] Carmon, M; Rivkin, L; Abu-Dalo, R; et al. Increased mammographic screening and use of percutaneous image-guided core biopsy in non-palpable breast cancer: Impact on surgical treatment. *Isr Med Assoc J,* 2004, Jun, 6(6), 326-328. PMID: 15214456.

[177] Chagpar, AB; Martin II RCG; Hagendoorn, LJ; et al. Lumpectomy margins are affected by tumor size and histologic subtype but not by biopsy technique. *Am J Surg,* 2004, Oct, 188(4 Spec issue), 399-402.

[178] Chen, X; Lehman, CD; Dee, KE. MRI-guided breast biopsy: clinical experience with 14- gauge stainless steel core biopsy needle. *AJR Am J Roentgenol,* 2004, Apr, 182(4), 1075-1080. PMID: 15039191.

[179] Collins, LC; Connolly, JL; Page, DL; et al. Diagnostic agreement in the evaluation of image-guided breast core needle biopsies: results from a randomized clinical trial. *Am J Surg Pathol*, 2004, Jan, 28(1), 126-131. PMID: 14707874.

[180] Docktor, BJ; MacGregor, JH; Burrowes, PW. Ultrasonographic findings 6 months after 11-gauge vacuum-assisted large-core breast biopsy. *Can Assoc Radiol J*, 2004, Jun;55(3), 151-156. PMID: 15237775.

[181] Foster, MC; Helvie, MA; Gregory, NE; et al. Lobular carcinoma in situ or atypical lobular hyperplasia at core-needle biopsy: is excisional biopsy necessary? *Radiology*, 2004, Jun, 231(3), 813-819. PMID: 15105449.

[182] Gan, FY; Wettlaufer, JR; Lundell, AL. Breast imaging in a military setting: a comparison with civilian breast imaging. Mil *Med*, 2004, May;169(5), 361-367. PMID: 15186000.

[183] Geller, BM; Oppenheimer, RG; Mickey, RM; et al.. Patient perceptions of breast biopsy procedures for screen-detected lesions. *Am J Obstet Gynecol*, 2004, Apr; 190(4), 1063-1069. PMID: 15118643.

[184] Gendler, LS; Feldman, SM; Balassanian, R; et al. Association of breast cancer with papillary lesions identified at percutaneous image-guided breast biopsy. *Am J Surg,* 2004, Oct, 188(4), 365-370. PMID: 15474427.

[185] Georgian-Smith, D; Kricun, B; et al. The mammary hamartoma: appreciation of additional imaging characteristics. *J Ultrasound Med,* 2004, Oct, 23(10), 1267-1273. PMID: 15448315.

[186] Golshan, M; Fung, BB; Wiley, E; et al. Prediction of breast cancer size by ultrasound; mammography and core biopsy. *Breast*, 2004, Aug, 13(4), 265-271. PMID: 15325659.

[187] Golub, RM; Bennett, CL; Stinson, T; et al. Cost minimization study of image-guided core biopsy versus surgical excisional biopsy for women with abnormal mammograms. *J Clin Oncol*, 2004, 22(12), 2430-2437.

[188] Hansen, NM; Ye, X; Grube, BJ; et al. Manipulation of the primary breast tumor and the incidence of sentinel node metastases from invasive breast cancer. *Arch Surg*, 2004, Jun, 139(6), 634-640.

[189] Hoorntje, LE; Peeters, PH; Mali, WP; et al. Is stereotactic large-core needle biopsy beneficial prior to surgical treatment in BIRADS 5 lesions? *Breast Cancer Res Treat,* 2004, Jul, 86(2), 165-170. PMID: 15319568.

[190] Hoorntje, LE; Schipper, MEI; et al. Tumour cell displacement after 14G breast biopsy. *Eur J Surg Oncol,* 2004, Jun, 30(5), 520-525.

[191] Ivan, D; Selinko, V; Sahin, AA; et al. Accuracy of core needle biopsy diagnosis in assessing papillary breast lesions: histologic predictors of malignancy. *Mod Pathol,* 2004, Feb, 17(2), 165-171. PMID: 14631369.

[192] Margolin, FR; Kaufman, L; Jacobs, RP; et al. Stereotactic core breast biopsy of malignant calcifications: Diagnostic yield of cores with and cores without calcifications on specimen radiographs. Radiology 2004, Oct;233(1), 251-254. PMID: 15333764.

[193] Mendez, A; Cabanillas, F; Echenique, M; et al. Evaluation of Breast Imaging Reporting and Data System Category 3 mammograms and the use of stereotactic vacuum-assisted breast biopsy in a nonacademic community practice. *Cancer*, 2004, Feb 15; 100(4), 7 10- 714. PMID: 14770425.

[194] O'Leary, R; Hawkins, K; Beazley, JCS; et al. Agreement between preoperative core needle biopsy and postoperative invasive breast cancer histopathology is not dependent on the amount of clinical material obtained. *J Clin Pathol,* 2004, Feb, 57(2), 193.

[195] Peters-Engl, C; Konstantiniuk, P; Tausch, C; et al. The impact of preoperative breast biopsy on the risk of sentinel lymph node metastases: Analysis of 2502 cases from the Austrian sentinel node biopsy study group. *Br J Cancer*, 2004, Nov 15, 91(10), 1782-1786.

[196] Piana De Andrade, V; Gobbi, H. Accuracy of typing and grading invasive mammary carcinomas on core needle biopsy compared with the excisional specimen. *Virchows Arch*, 2004, Dec, 445(6), 597-602.

[197] Pijnappel, RM; van den Donk, M; Holland, R; et al. Diagnostic accuracy for different strategies of image-guided breast intervention in cases of nonpalpable breast lesions. *Br J Cancer*, 2004, Feb 9;90(3), 595-600. PMID: 14760370.

[198] Renshaw, AA. Minimal (< or =0.1 cm) invasive carcinoma in breast core needle biopsies. Incidence; sampling; associated findings; and follow-up. *Arch Pathol Lab Med*, 2004, Sep;128(9), 996-999. PMID: 15335264.

[199] Renshaw, AA; Derhagopian, RP; TizolBlanco, DM; et al. Papillomas and atypical papillomas in breast core needle biopsy specimens: Risk of carcinoma in subsequent excision. Am *J Clin Pathol,* 2004, Aug, 122(2), 21 7-221.

[200] Rotenberg, L; Verhille, R; Schulz-Wendtland, R; et al. Multicenter clinical experience with large core soft tissue biopsy without vacuum assistance. *Eur J Cancer Prev*, 2004, Dec;13(6), 491-498. PMID: 15548942.

[201] Agarwal, T; Patel, B; Rajan, P; et al. Core biopsy versus FNAC for palpable breast cancers. Is image guidance necessary? *Eur J Cancer*, 2003, Jan, 39(1), 52-56. PMID: 12504658.

[202] Baez, E; Huber, A; Vetter, M; et al. Minimal invasive complete excision of benign breast tumors using a three-dimensional ultrasound-guided mammotome vacuum device. *Ultrasound Obstet Gynecol*, 2003, Mar;2 1(3), 267-272. PMID: 12666222.

[203] Bauer, VP; Ditkoff, BA; Schnabel, F; et al. The management of lobular neoplasia identified on percutaneous core breast biopsy. *Breast J*, 2003, Jan;9(1), 4-9. PMID: 12558663.

[204] Berg, WA; Campassi, CI; Ioffe, OB. Cystic lesions of the breast: sonographic-pathologic correlation. *Radiology*, 2003, Apr;227(1), 183-191. PMID: 12668745.

[205] Bonnett, M; Wallis, T; Rossmann, M; et al. Histopathologic analysis of atypical lesions in image-guided core breast biopsies. *Mod Pathol,* 2003, Feb 1;16(2), 154-160. PMID: 12591968.

[206] Brenner, RJ; Jackman, RJ; Parker, SH; et al. Percutaneous core needle biopsy of radial scars of the breast: when is excision necessary? *AJR Am J Roentgenol,* 2003, Jul;181(1), 275; author reply 275. PMID: 12388495.

[207] Carder, PJ; Liston, JC. Will the spectrum of lesions prompting a "B3" breast core biopsy increase the benign biopsy rate? *J Clin Pathol,* 2003, Feb, 56(2), 133-138. PMID: 12560393.

[208] Cawson, JN; Malara, F; Kavanagh, A; et al. Fourteen-gauge needle core biopsy of mammographically evident radial scars: Is excision necessary? Cancer 2003, Jan 15;97(2), 345-351. PMID: 12518358.

[209] Charles, M; Edge, SB; Winston, JS; et al. Effect of stereotactic core needle biopsy on pathologic measurement of tumor size of T1 invasive breast carcinomas presenting as mammographic masses. Cancer, 2003, May 1;97(9), 2137-2141.

[210] Chen, SC; Yang, HR; Hwang, TL; et al. Intraoperative ultrasonographically guided excisional biopsy or vacuum-assisted core needle biopsy for nonpalpable breast lesions. *Ann Surg*, 2003, Nov;238(5), 738-742. PMID: 14578737.

[211] Corn, CC. Review of 125 SiteSelect stereotactic large-core breast biopsy procedures. *Breast J*, 2003, MayJun;9(3), 147-152. PMID: 12752621.

[212] Crisi, GM; Mandavilli, S; Cronin, E; et al. Invasive mammary carcinoma after immediate and short-term follow-up for lobular neoplasia on core biopsy. *Am J Surg Pathol*, 2003, Mar 1, 27(3), 325-333.

[213] Crowe, Jr JP; Rim, A; Patrick, RJ; et al. Does core needle breast biopsy accurately reflect breast pathology? *Surgery*, 2003, Oct; 134(4), 523-528.

[214] Dennison, G; Anand, R; Makar, SH; et al. A prospective study of the use of fine-needle aspiration cytology and core biopsy in the diagnosis of breast cancer. *Breast J*, 2003, Nov;9(6), 491-493. PMID: 14616944.

[215] Dmytrasz, K; Tartter, PI; Mizrachy, H; et al. The significance of atypical lobular hyperplasia at percutaneous breast biopsy. *Breast J*, 2003, Jan;9(1), 10-12.
[216] Farshid, G; Rush, G. The use of fine-needle aspiration cytology and core biopsy in the assessment of highly suspicious mammographic microcalcifications: analysis of outcome for 182 lesions detected in the setting of a population-based breast cancer screening program. *Cancer Cytol*, 2003, Dec 25;99(6), 357-364. PMID: 14681944.
[217] Fine, RE; Whitworth, PW; Kim, JA; et al. Low-risk palpable breast masses removed using a vacuum-assisted hand-held device. *Am J Surg,* 2003, Oct, 186(4), 362-367. PMID: 14553851.
[218] Fures, R; Bukovic, D; Lez, C; et al. Large- gauge needle biopsy in diagnosing malignant breast neoplasia. *Coll Antropol*, 2003, Jun;27(1), 259-262. PMID: 12974154
[219] Harris, GC; Denley, HE; Pinder, SE; et al. Correlation of histologic prognostic factors in core biopsies and therapeutic excisions of invasive breast carcinoma. *Am J Surg Pathol*, 2003, Jan 1, 27(1), 11-15.
[220] Hoorntje, LE; Schipper, MEI; Peeters, PHM; et al. The finding of invasive cancer after a preoperative diagnosis of ductal carcinomain-situ: Causes of ductal carcinoma-in-situ underestimates with stereotactic 14-gauge needle biopsy. *Ann Surg Oncol,* 2003; 10(7), 748-753.
[221] Jackman, RJ; Marzoni, Jr FA. Stereotactic histologic biopsy with patients prone: technical feasibility in 98% of mammographically detected lesions. *AJR Am J Roentgenol,* 2003, Mar;180(3), 785-794. PMID: 12591697.
[222] Kneeshaw, PJ; Turnbull, LW; Smith, A; et al. Dynamic contrast enhanced magnetic resonance imaging aids the surgical management of invasive lobular breast cancer. *Eur J Surg Oncol,* 2003, Feb, 29(1), 32-37. PMID: 12559074.
[223] Komenaka, IK; El-Tamer, M; Pile-Spellman, E; et al. Core needle biopsy as a diagnostic tool to differentiate phyllodes tumor from fibroadenoma. *Arch Surg*, 2003, Sep, 1, 1 38(9), 987-990.
[224] Lee, AHS; Denley, HE; Pinder, SE; et al. Excision biopsy findings of patients with breast needle core biopsies reported as suspicious of malignancy (B4) or lesion of uncertain malignant potential (B3). *Histopathology*, 2003, Apr 1, 42(4), 331-336.
[225] Leifland, K; Lagerstedt, U; Svane, G. Comparison of stereotactic fine needle aspiration cytology and core needle biopsy in 522 non-palpable breast lesions. *Acta Radiol,* 2003, Jul;44(4), 387-391. PMID: 12846688.
[226] Leifland, K; Lundquist, H; Lagerstedt, U; et al. Comparison of preoperative simultaneous stereotactic fine needle aspiration biopsy and stereotactic core needle biopsy in ductal carcinoma in situ of the breast. *Acta Radiol,* 2003, Mar;44(2), 213-217. PMID: 12694110.
[227] Liberman, L; Morris, EA; Dershaw, DD; et al. Fast MRI-guided vacuum-assisted breast biopsy: initial experience. *AJR Am J Roentgenol,* 2003, Nov; 181(5), 1283-1293. PMID: 14573421.
[228] Mariotti, C; Feliciotti, F; Baldarelli, M; et al. Digital stereotactic biopsies for nonpalpable breast lesion. Surg Endosc 2003, Jun;17(6), 911-917. PMID: 12632135.
[229] Masood, S; Loya, A; Khalbuss, W. Is core needle biopsy superior to fine-needle aspiration biopsy in the diagnosis of papillary breast lesions? *Diagn Cytopathol,* 2003, Jun, 28(6), 329-334. PMID: 12768640.

[230] Middleton, LP; Grant, S; Stephens, T; et al. Lobular carcinoma in situ diagnosed by core needle biopsy: When should it be excised? *Mod Pathol,* 2003, Feb 1;16(2), 120-129. PMID: 12591964.

[231] Miller, KL; Marks, LB; Barrier Jr, RC; et al. Increased sectioning of pathologic specimens with ductal carcinoma in situ of the breast: are there clinical consequences? *Clin Breast Cancer*, 2003, Aug;4(3), 198-202. PMID: 14499013.

[232] Puglisi, F; Zuiani, C; Bazzocchi, M; et al. Role of mammography; ultrasound and large core biopsy in the diagnostic evaluation of papillary breast lesions. *Oncology*, 2003, 65(4), 311-315. PMID: 14707450.

[233] Shah, VI; Raju, U; Chitale, D; et al. False- negative core needle biopsies of the breast: An analysis of clinical; radiologic; and pathologic findings in 27 consecutive cases of missed breast cancer. *Cancer*, 2003, Apr 15, 97(8), 1824-1831. PMID: 12673707.

[234] Sneige, N; Lim, SC; Whitman, GJ; et al. Atypical ductal hyperplasia diagnosis by directional vacuum-assisted stereotactic biopsy of breast microcalcifications. Considerations for surgical excision. Am *J Clin Pathol,* 2003, Feb, 119(2), 248-253. PMID: 12579995.

[235] Sperber, F; Blank, A; Metser, U; et al. Diagnosis and treatment of breast fibroadenomas by ultrasound-guided vacuum-assisted biopsy. *Arch Surg*, 2003, Jul, 138(7), 796-800. PMID: 12860764.

[236] Tsang, FHF; Lo, JJ; Wong, JLN; et al. Application of image-guided biopsy for impalpable breast lesions in Chinese women. *ANZ J Surg*, 2003, Jan;73(1-2), 23-25.

[237] Verkooijen, HM; Peterse, JL; Schipper, MEI; et al. Interobserver variability between general and expert pathologists during the histopathological assessment of large-core needle and open biopsies of non-palpable breast lesions. *Eur J Cancer*, 2003, Oct, 39(1 5), 21 87-2191.

[238] Winchester, DJ; Bernstein, JR; Jeske, JM; et al. Upstaging of atypical ductal hyperplasia after vacuum-assisted 11-gauge stereotactic core needle biopsy. *Arch Surg*, 2003, Jun, 138(6), 619-22; discussion, 622-623. PMID: 12799332.

[239] Witt, A; Yavuz, D; Walchetseder, C; et al. Preoperative core needle biopsy as an independent risk factor for wound infection after breast surgery. *Obstet Gynecol*, 2003, Apr 1;101(4), 745-750. PMID: 12681880.

[240] Yeh, IT; Dimitrov, D; Otto, P; et al. Pathologic review of atypical hyperplasia identified by image-guided breast needle core biopsy: Correlation with excision specimen. Arch *Pathol Lab Med*, 2003, Jan;127(1), 49-54.

[241] Zhao, L; Freimanis, R; Bergman, S; et al. Biopsy needle technique and the accuracy of diagnosis of atypical ductal hyperplasia for mammographic abnormalities. *Am Surg,* 2003, Sep;69(9), 757-762; discussion, 762. PMID: 14509322.

[242] Acheson, MB; Patton, RG; Howisey, RL; et al. Three- to six-year followup for 379 benign image-guided large-core needle biopsies of nonpalpable breast abnormalities. *J Am Coll Surg*, 2002, Oct; 1 95(4), 462-466. PMID: 12375750.

[243] Bonnett, M; Wallis, T; Rossmann, M; et al. Histologic and radiographic analysis of ductal carcinoma in situ diagnosed using stereotactic incisional core breast biopsy. *Mod Pathol,* 2002, 15(2), 95-101.

[244] Chen, AM; Haffty, BG; Lee, CH. Local recurrence of breast cancer after breast conservation therapy in patients examined by means of stereotactic core-needle biopsy. *Radiology*, 2002, Dec, 225(3), 707-712. PMID: 12461249.

[245] Chun, K; Velanovich, V. Patient-perceived cosmesis and satisfaction after breast biopsy: Comparison of stereotactic incisional; excisional; and wire-localized biopsy techniques. *Surgery*, 2002, 131(5), 497-501. PMID: 12019401.

[246] Fine, RE; Boyd, BA; Whitworth, PW; et al. Percutaneous removal of benign breast masses using a vacuum-assisted hand-held device with ultrasound. *Am J Surg,* 2002, Oct 1, 184(4), 332-336. PMID: 12383895.

[247] Gal-Gombos, EC; Esserman, LE; Recine, MA; et al. Large-needle core biopsy in atypical intraductal epithelial hyperplasia including immunohistochemical expression of high molecular weight cytokeratin: analysis of results of a single institution. *Breast J*, 2002, Sep-Oct, 8(5), 269-274. PMID: 12199753.

[248] Giardina, C; Guerrieri, AM; Ingravallo, G; et al. [Mammary stereotaxic core-biopsy by Mammotome: An alternative to frozen section examination]. *Pathologica*, 2002, Aug;94(4), 182-189. (Ita).

[249] Haj, M; Kniaz, D; Eitan, A; et al. Three years of experience with advanced breast biopsy instrumentation (ABBI). *Breast J*, 2002, Sep;8(5), 275-280. PMID: 12199754.

[250] Harvey, JM; Sterrett, GF; Frost, FA. Atypical ductal hyperplasia and atypia of uncertain significance in core biopsies from mammographically detected lesions: correlation with excision diagnosis. *Pathology*, 2002, Oct, 34(5), 410-416. PMID: 12408338.

[251] Hoorntje, LE; Peeters, PHM; Borel Rinkes, IHM; et al. Stereotactic large core needle biopsy for all nonpalpable breast lesions? *Breast Cancer Res Treat,* 2002, 73(2), 177-182.

[252] Hui, JY; Chan, LK; Chan, RL; et al. Prone table stereotactic breast biopsy. *Hong Kong Med J*, 2002, Dec, 8(6), 447-451. PMID: 12459602.

[253] Insausti, LP; Alberro, JA; Regueira, FM; et al. An experience with the Advanced Breast Biopsy Instrumentation (ABBI) system in the management of non-palpable breast lesions. *Eur Radiol,* 2002, Jul 1, 12(7), 1703- 1710.

[254] Jackman, RJ; Birdwell, RL; Ikeda, DM. Atypical ductal hyperplasia: can some lesions be defined as probably benign after stereotactic 11-gauge vacuum-assisted biopsy; eliminating the recommendation for surgical excision. *Radiology*, 2002, Aug, 224(2), 548-554. PMID: 12147855.

[255] Jan, WA; Zada, N; Samieullah; et al. Comparison of FNAC and core biopsy for evaluating breast lumps. *Med Forum Mon*, 2002, Dec 1, 13(12), 26-28.

[256] Knight, R; Horiuchi, K; Parker, SH; et al. Risk of needle-track seeding after diagnostic image-guided core needle biopsy in breast cancer. *J Soc Laparoendosc Surg*, 2002, Jul-Sep;6(3), 207-209. PMID: 12166757.

[257] Liberman, L; Goodstine, SL; Dershaw, DD; et al. One operation after percutaneous diagnosis of nonpalpable breast cancer: Frequency and associated factors. *AJR Am J Roentgenol,* 2002, 178(3), 673-679. PMID: 11856696.

[258] Lifrange, E; Dondelinger, RF; Foidart, JM; et al. Percutaneous stereotactic en bloc excision of nonpalpable breast carcinoma: A step in the direction of supraconservative surgery. *Breast*, 2002, Dec;1 1(6), 501-508.

[259] Mainiero, MB; Gareen, IF; Bird, CE; et al. Preferential use of sonographically guided biopsy to minimize patient discomfort and procedure time in a percutaneous image-guided breast biopsy program. *J Ultrasound Med,* 2002, Nov, 21(11), 1221-1226. PMID: 12418763.

[260] McKee, MD; Cropp, MD; Hyland, A; et al. Provider case volume and outcome in the evaluation and treatment of patients with mammogram-detected breast carcinoma. *Cancer*, 2002, Aug, 15, 95(4), 704-712.

[261] Perlet, C; Schneider, P; Amaya, B; et al. MR- Guided vacuum biopsy of 206 contrast-enhancing breast lesions. *Rofo Fortschr Geb Rontgenstr Neuen Bildgeb Verfahr*, 2002, Jan, 174(1), 88-95. PMID: 11793291.

[262] Pijnappel, RM; Peeters, PH; van den Donk, M; et al. Diagnostic strategies in non-palpable breast lesions. *Eur J Cancer*, 2002, Mar, 38(4), 550-555. PMID: 11872348.

[263] Popiela, TJ; Tabor, J; Nowak, W; et al. Detectability of pre-clinical breast pathologies in own experience. *Pol Przegl Chir*, 2002, 74(1), 36-43.

[264] Rao, A; Parker, S; Ratzer, E; et al. Atypical ductal hyperplasia of the breast diagnosed by 11-gauge directional vacuum-assisted biopsy. *Am J Surg,* 2002, Dec, 184(6), 534-537; discussion 537. PMID: 12488158.

[265] Renshaw, AA. Can mucinous lesions of the breast be reliably diagnosed by core needle biopsy? Am *J Clin Pathol,* 2002, 118(1), 82- 84. PMID: 12109860.

[266] Renshaw, AA; Cartagena, N; Derhagopian, RP; et al. Lobular neoplasia in breast core needle biopsy specimens is not associated with an increased risk of ductal carcinoma in situ or invasive carcinoma. Am *J Clin Pathol,* 2002, 11 7(5), 797-799.

[267] Rosen, EL; Bentley, RC; Baker, JA; et al. Imaging-guided core needle biopsy of papillary lesions of the breast. *AJR Am J Roentgenol,* 2002, Nov, 179(5), 1185-1192. PMID: 12388496.

[268] Schneider, JP; Schulz, T; Horn, LC; et al. MR- guided percutaneous core biopsy of small breast lesions: first experience with a vertically open 0.5T scanner. *J Magn Reson Imaging,* 2002, Apr; 15(4), 374-385. PMID: 11948826.

[269] Shin, SJ; Rosen, PP. Excisional biopsy should be performed if lobular carcinoma in situ is seen on needle core biopsy. *Arch Pathol Lab Med*, 2002, 126(6), 697-701.

[270] Smyczek-Gargya, B; Krainick, U; MullerSchimpfle, M; et al. Large-core needle biopsy for diagnosis and treatment of breast lesions. *Arch Gynecol Obstet*, 2002, Aug;266(4), 198-200. PMID: 12192478.

[271] Soo, MS; Baker, JA; Rosen, EL; et al. Sonographically guided biopsy of suspicious microcalcifications of the breast: A pilot study. *AJR Am J Roentgenol,* 2002, 178(4), 1007-1015. PMID, 11906892.

[272] Tan, SM; Behranwala, KA; Trott, PA; et al. A retrospective study comparing the individual modalities of triple assessment in the preoperative diagnosis of invasive lobular breast carcinoma. *Eur J Surg Oncol,* 2002, Apr;28(3), 203-208. PMID: 11944950.

[273] Tse, GM; Law, BK; Ma, TK; et al. Hamartoma of the breast: a clinicopathological review. *J Clin Pathol,* 2002, Dec;55(12), 951-954. PMID: 12461066.

[274] Verkooijen, HM; Peeters, PHM. Diagnostic accuracy of stereotactic large-core needle biopsy for nonpalpable breast disease: Results of a multicenter prospective study with 95% surgical confirmation. *Int J Cancer*, 2002, Jun 20, 99(6), 853-859.

[275] Verkooijen, HM; Buskens, E; Peeters, PH; et al. Diagnosing non-palpable breast disease: short-term impact on quality of life of large- core needle biopsy versus open breast biopsy. *Surg Oncol*, 2002, May;10(4), 177- 181. PMID: 12020672.

[276] Watermann, DO; Einert, A; Ehritt-Braun, C; et al. Experience with the Advanced Breast Biopsy Instrumentation (ABBI) System. *Anticancer Res*, 2002, Sep, 22(5), 3067-3070.

[277] Wunderbaldinger, P; Wolf, G; Turetschek, K; et al. Comparison of sitting versus prone position for stereotactic large-core breast biopsy in surgically proven lesions. *AJR Am J Roentgenol,* 2002, 178(5), 1221-1225. PMID: 11959735.

[278] Bagnall, MJC; Evans, AJ; Wilson, ARM; et al. Predicting invasion in mammographically detected microcalcification. *Clin Radiol,* 2001, Oct;56(10), 828-832.

[279] Berg, WA; Arnoldus, CL; Teferra, E; et al. Biopsy of amorphous breast calcifications: Pathologic outcome and yield at stereotactic biopsy. *Radiology*, 2001, 221(2), 495-503. PMID: 11687695.

[280] Berg, WA; Mrose, HE; Ioffe, OB. Atypical lobular hyperplasia or lobular carcinoma in situ at core-needle breast biopsy. *Radiology*, 2001, 218(2), 503-509. PMID: 11161169.

[281] Brem, RF; Schoonjans, JM; Goodman, SN; et al. Nonpalpable breast cancer: Percutaneous diagnosis with 11- and 8-gauge stereotactic vacuum-assisted biopsy devices. *Radiology*, 2001, Jun;219(3), 793-796.

[282] Chao, C; Torosian, MH; Boraas, MC; et al. Local recurrence of breast cancer in the stereotactic core needle biopsy site: case reports and review of the literature. *Breast J*, 2001, Mar-Apr, 7(2), 124-127. PMID: 11328321.

[283] Clarke, D; Sudhakaran, N; Gateley, CA. Replace fine needle aspiration cytology with automated core biopsy in the triple assessment of breast cancer. *Ann R Coll Surg Engl*, 2001, Mar, 83(2), 1 10-112. PMID: 11320918.

[284] Daniel, BL; Birdwell, RL; Butts, K; et al. Freehand iMRI-guided large-gauge core needle biopsy: A new minimally invasive technique for diagnosis of enhancing breast lesions. *J Magn Reson Imaging,* 2001, Jun; 13(6), 896-902.

[285] Deurloo, EE; Gilhuijs, KGA; Schultze Kool, LJ; et al. Displacement of breast tissue and needle deviations during stereotactic procedures. *Invest Radiol*, 2001, 36(6), 347- 353.

[286] Ely, KA; Carter, BA; Jensen, RA; et al. Core biopsy of the breast with atypical ductal hyperplasia: a probabilistic approach to reporting. *Am J Surg Pathol*, 2001, Aug, 25(8), 1017-1021. PMID: 11474285.

[287] Fine, RE; Israel, PZ; Walker, LC; et al. A prospective study of the removal rate of imaged breast lesions by an 11-gauge vacuum-assisted biopsy probe system. *Am J Surg,* 2001, Oct; 182(4), 335-340. PMID: 11720666.

[288] Grimes, MM; Karageorge, LS; Hogge, JP. Does exhaustive search for microcalcifications improve diagnostic yield in stereotactic core needle breast biopsies? *Mod Pathol,* 2001, 14(4), 350-353. PMID: 11301352.

[289] Hung, WK; Lam, HS; Lau, Y; et al. Diagnostic accuracy of vacuum-assisted biopsy device for image-detected breast lesions. *Aust N Z J Surg*, 2001, Aug, 71(8), 457-460. PMID: 11504288.

[290] Ibrahim, AEK; Bateman, AC; Theaker, JM; et al. The role and histological classification of needle core biopsy in comparison with fine needle aspiration cytology in the preoperative assessment of impalpable breast lesions. *J Clin Pathol,* 2001, 54(2), 121-125.

[291] Jackman, RJ; Burbank, F; Parker, SH; et al. Stereotactic breast biopsy of nonpalpable lesions: Determinants of ductal carcinoma in situ underestimation rates. *Radiology*, 2001, 218(2), 497-502.

[292] Jacobs, IA; Chevinsky, AH; Diehl, W; et al. Advanced breast biopsy instrumentataion (ABBI) and management of nonpalpable breast abnormalities: A community hospital experience. *Breast*, 2001, 10(5), 421-426.

[293] Joshi, M; Duva-Frissora, A; Padmanabhan, R; et al. Atypical ductal hyperplasia in stereotactic breast biopsies: enhanced accuracy of diagnosis with the mammotome. *Breast J*, 2001, Jul-Aug, 7(4), 207-213. PMID: 11678796.

[294] Kaufman, HJ; Witherspoon, LE; Gwin Jr, JL; et al. Stereotactic breast biopsy: a study of first core samples. *Am Surg,* 2001, Jun, 67(6), 572-575; discussion 575-576. PMID: 11409806.

[295] King, TA; Hayes, DH; Cederbom, GJ; et al. Biopsy technique has no impact on local recurrence after breast-conserving therapy. *Breast J*, 2001, Jan-Feb;7(1), 19-24. PMID: 11348411.

[296] Kuhl, CK; Morakkabati, N; Leutner, CC; et al. MR imaging--guided large-core (14-gauge) needle biopsy of small lesions visible at breast MR imaging alone. *Radiology*, 2001, Jul, 220(1), 31-39. PMID: 11425969.

[297] Liberman, L; Benton, CL; Dershaw, DD; et al. Learning curve for stereotactic breast biopsy: how many cases are enough? *AJR Am J Roentgenol,* 2001, Mar, 176(3), 721-727. PMID: 11222213.

[298] Liberman, L; Gougoutas, CA; Zakowski, MF; et al. Calcifications highly suggestive of malignancy: comparison of breast biopsy methods. *AJR Am J Roentgenol,* 2001, Jul;177(1), 165-172. PMID: 11418420.

[299] Lifrange, E; Dondelinger, RF; Fridman, V; et al. En bloc excision of nonpalpable breast lesions using the advanced breast biopsy instrumentation system: An alternative to needle guided surgery? *Eur Radiol,* 2001, 11(5), 796-801. PMID: 11372610.

[300] Maganini, RO; Klem, DA; Huston, BJ; et al. Upgrade rate of core biopsy-determined atypical ductal hyperplasia by open excisional biopsy. *Am J Surg,* 2001, Oct, 182(4), 355-358. PMID: 11720670.

[301] Marti, WR; Zuber, M; Oertli, D; et al. Advanced breast biopsy instrumentation for the evaluation of impalpable lesions: A reliable diagnostic tool with little therapeutic potential. *Eur J Surg*, 2001, 167(1), 15-18.

[302] Meloni, GB; Dessol, S; Becchere, MP; et al. Ultrasound-guided mammotome vacuum biopsy for the diagnosis of impalpable breast lesions. Ultrasound Obstet Gynecol 2001, 18(5), 520-524.

[303] Mendez, I; Andreu, FJ; Saez, E; et al. Ductal carcinoma in situ and atypical ductal hyperplasia of the breast diagnosed at stereotactic core biopsy. *Breast J*, 2001, 7(1), 14-18. PMID: 11348410.

[304] Mercado, CL; Hamele-Bena, D; Singer, C; et al. Papillary lesions of the breast: evaluation with stereotactic directional vacuum-assisted biopsy. *Radiology*, 2001, Dec;221(3), 650- 655. PMID: 11719659.

[305] Morrow, M; Venta, L; Stinson, T; et al. Prospective comparison of stereotactic core biopsy and surgical excision as diagnostic procedures for breast cancer patients. *Ann Surg*, 2001, Apr, 233(4), 537-541. PMID: 11303136.

[306] O'Driscoll, D; Britton, P; Bobrow, L; et al. Lobular carcinoma in situ on core biopsy - What is the clinical significance? *Clin Radiol,* 2001, Mar 1, 56(3), 216-220.
[307] Parker, SH; Klaus, AJ; McWey, PJ; et al. Sonographically guided directional vacuum-assisted breast biopsy using a handheld device. *AJR Am J Roentgenol,* 2001, Aug, 177(2), 405-408. PMID: 11461871.
[308] Parker, SJ; Wheaton, M; Wallis, MG; et al. Why should diagnostic benign breast biopsies weight less than twenty grams? *Ann R Coll Surg Engl*, 2001, Mar, 83(2), 113-116. PMID: 11320919.
[309] Renshaw, AA. Adequate histologic sampling of breast core needle biopsies. *Arch Pathol Lab Med*, 2001, 125(8), 1055-1057.
[310] Renshaw, AA; Cartagena, N; Schenkman, RH; et al. Atypical ductal hyperplasia in breast core needle biopsies. Correlation of size of the lesion; complete removal of the lesion; and the incidence of carcinoma in follow-up biopsies. Am *J Clin Pathol,* 2001, Jul, 116(1), 92-96. PMID: 11447758.
[311] Saarenmaa, I; Salminen, T; Geiger, U; et al. Validity of radiological examinations of patients with breast cancer in different age groups in a population based study. *Breast,* 2001, 10(1), 78-81.
[312] Schneider, E; Rohling, KW; Schnall, MD; et al. An apparatus for MR-guided breast lesion localization and core biopsy: Design and preliminary results. *J Magn Reson Imaging,* 2001, 14(3), 243-253.
[313] Schoonjans, JM; Brem, RF. Fourteen-gauge ultrasonographically guided large-core needle biopsy of breast masses. *J Ultrasound Med,* 2001, 20(9), 967-972. PMID: 11549157.
[314] Shannon, J; Douglas-Jones, AG; Dallimore, NS. Conversion to core biopsy in preoperative diagnosis of breast lesions: is it justified by results? *J Clin Pathol,* 2001, Oct, 54(10), 762-765. PMID: 11577122.
[315] Sklair-Levy, M; Samuels, TH; Catzavelos, C; et al. Stromal fibrosis of the breast. *AJR Am J Roentgenol,* 2001, 177(3), 573-577. PMID, 11517049.
[316] Smith, LF; Henry-Tillman, R; Mancino, AT; et al. Magnetic resonance imaging-guided core needle biopsy and needle localized excision of occult breast lesions. *Am J Surg,* 2001, Oct;182(4), 414-418. PMID: 11720683.
[317] Sun, W; Li, A; Abreo, F; et al. Comparison of fine-needle aspiration cytology and core biopsy for diagnosis of breast cancer. *Diagn Cytopathol,* 2001, 24(6), 42 1-425. PMID: 11391825.
[318] Verkooijen, HM; Borel Rinkes, IH; Peeters, PH; et al. Impact of stereotactic large-core needle biopsy on diagnosis and surgical treatment of nonpalpable breast cancer. *Eur J Surg Oncol,* 2001, Apr;27(3), 244-249. PMID: 11393185.
[319] Westenend, PJ; Sever, AR; Beekman-de Volder, HJC; et al. A comparison of aspiration cytology and core needle biopsy in the evaluation of breast lesions. *Cancer*, 2001, 93(2), 146-150.
[320] Adrales, G; Turk, P; Wallace, T; et al. Is surgical excision necessary for atypical ductal hyperplasia of the breast diagnosed by Mammotome? *Am J Surg,* 2000, Oct, 180(4), 313-315. PMID: 11113443.
[321] Bagnall, MJ; Evans, AJ; Wilson, AR; et al. When have mammographic calcifications been adequately sampled at needle core biopsy? *Clin Radiol,* 2000, Jul;55(7), 548-553. PMID: 10924380.

[322] Burns, RP; Brown, JP; Roe, SM; et al. Stereotactic core-needle breast biopsy by surgeons: Minimum 2-year follow-up of benign lesions. *Ann Surg*, 2000, 232(4), 542-548.

[323] Darling, ML; Smith, DN; Lester, SC; et al. Atypical ductal hyperplasia and ductal carcinoma in situ as revealed by large-core needle breast biopsy: results of surgical excision. *AJR Am J Roentgenol,* 2000, Nov, 175(5), 1341-1346. PMID: 11044038.

[324] Cangiarella, JF; Waisman, J; Weg, N; et al. The use of stereotaxic core biopsy and stereotaxic aspiration biopsy as diagnostic tools in the evaluation of mammary calcification. *Breast J*, 2000, 6(6), 366-372.

[325] Cangiarella, J; Gross, J; Symmans, WF; et al. The incidence of positive margins with breast conserving therapy following mammotome biopsy for microcalcification. *J Surg Oncol,* 2000, Aug, 74(4), 263-266. PMID: 10962457.

[326] Gukas, ID; Nwana, EJ; Ihezue, CH; et al. Trucut biopsy of palpable breast lesions: a practical option for pre-operative diagnosis in developing countries. *Cent Afr J Med 2000*, May, 46(5), 127-130. PMID: 11210334.

[327] Hatada, T; Ishii, H; Ichii, S; et al. Diagnostic value of ultrasound-guided fine-needle aspiration biopsy; core-needle biopsy; and evaluation of combined use in the diagnosis of breast lesions. *J Am Coll Surg*, 2000, Mar, 190(3), 299-303. PMID: 10703854.

[328] Lamm, RL; Jackman, RJ. Mammographic abnormalities caused by percutaneous stereotactic biopsy of histologically benign lesions evident on follow-up mammograms. *AJR Am J Roentgenol,* 2000, Mar, 174(3), 753-756. PMID: 10701620.

[329] Lee, CH; Carter, D; Philpotts, LE; et al. Ductal carcinoma in situ diagnosed with stereotactic core needle biopsy: can invasion be predicted? *Radiology*, 2000, Nov;217(2), 466-470. PMID: 11058647.

[330] Liberman, L; Drotman, M; Morris, EA; et al. Imaging-histologic discordance at percutaneous breast biopsy: an indicator of missed cancer. *Cancer*, 2000, Dec 15, 89(12), 2538-2546.

[331] Melotti, MK; Berg, WA. Core needle breast biopsy in patients undergoing anticoagulation therapy: preliminary results. *AJR Am J Roentgenol,* 2000, Jan, 174(1), 245- 249. PMID: 10628487.

[332] Mok, PM; Keepin, Y. Stereotactic breast biopsies for lesions discovered on routine mammography: experience at the North Shore Hospital. *N Z Med J*, 2000, Jul 14, 113(1113), 273-274. PMID: 10935565.

[333] Moritz, JD; Mertens, C; Westerhof, JP; et al. Role of high magnification specimen radiography in surgical and core biopsies of the breast. *Br J Radiol*, 2000, 73(875), 1170- 1177.

[334] Nisbet, AP; Borthwick-Clarke, A; Scott, N. 11-gauge vacuum assisted directional biopsy of breast calcifications; using upright stereotactic guidance. *Eur J Radiol*, 2000, Dec;36(3), 144-146.

[335] O'hea, BJ; Tornos, C. Mild ductal atypia after large-core needle biopsy of the breast: is surgical excision always necessary? *Surgery*, 2000, Oct, 128(4), 738-743. PMID: 11015109.

[336] Philpotts, LE; Lee, CH; Horvath, LJ; et al. Underestimation of breast cancer with II-gauge vacuum suction biopsy. *AJR Am J Roentgenol,* 2000, Oct; 175(4), 1047-1050. PMID: 11000162.

[337] Philpotts, LE; Shaheen, NA; Jain, KS; et al. Uncommon high-risk lesions of the breast diagnosed at stereotactic core-needle biopsy: Clinical importance. *Radiology*, 2000, 216(3), 831-837. PMID: 10966718.

[338] Portincasa, G; Lucci, E; Navarra, GG; et al. Initial experience with breast biopsy utilizing the Advanced Breast Biopsy Instrumentation (ABBI). *J Surg Oncol*, 2000, 74(3), 201 -203.

[339] Schwartzberg, BS; Goates, JJ; Keeler, SA; et al. Use of advanced breast biopsy instrumentation while performing stereotactic breast biopsies: review of 150 consecutive biopsies. *J Am Coll Surg*, 2000, Jul, 191(1), 9-15. PMID: 10898178.

[340] Simon, JR; Kalbhen, CL; Cooper, RA; et al. Accuracy and complication rates of US guided vacuum-assisted core breast biopsy: Initial results. Radiology 2000, Jun;215(3), 694-697. PMID: 10831686.

[341] Sneige, N; Tulbah, A. Accuracy of cytologic diagnoses made from touch imprints of image-guided needle biopsy specimens of nonpalpable breast abnormalities. *Diagn Cytopathol,* 2000, Jul, 23(1), 29-34. PMID: 10907929.

[342] Stolier, A; Skinner, J; Levine, EA. A prospective study of seeding of the skin after core biopsy of the breast. *Am J Surg,* 2000, Aug;180(2), 104-107. PMID: 11044522.

[343] The, WL; Wilson, ARM; Evans, AJ; et al. Ultrasound guided core biopsy of suspicious mammographic calcifications using high frequency and power doppler ultrasound. *Clin Radiol,* 2000, 55(5), 390-394.

[344] Whitlock, JPL; Evans, AJ; Burrell, HC; et al. Digital imaging improves upright stereotactic core biopsy of mammographic microcalcifications. *Clin Radiol,* 2000, 55(5), 374-377.

[345] Yang, JH; Lee, SD; Nam, SJ. Diagnostic utility of ABBI (Advanced Breast Biopsy Instrumentation) for nonpalpable breast lesions in Korea. *Breast J*, 2000, 6(4), 257-262.

[346] Al-Sobhi, SS; Helvie, MA; Pass, HA; et al. Extent of lumpectomy for breast cancer after diagnosis by stereotactic core versus wire localization biopsy. *Ann Surg Oncol,* 1999, Jun;6(4), 330-335.

[347] Baker, JA; Soo, MS; Mengoni, P. Sonographically guided percutaneous interventions of the breast using a steerable ultrasound beam. *AJR Am J Roentgenol,* 1999, Jan, 172(1), 157-159.

[348] Bloomston, M; D'Angelo, P; Galliano, D; et al. One hundred consecutive advanced breast biopsy instrumentation procedures: complications; costs; and outcome. *Ann Surg Oncol,* 1999, Mar;6(2), 195-199. PMID: 10082046.

[349] Bokran, W; Reynolds, HE; Lazaridis, CL; et al. Stereotactic biopsy of ductal carcinoma in situ of the breast using an II-gauge vacuum-assisted device: Persistent underestimation of disease. *AJR Am J Roentgenol,* 1999, Jul; 173(1), 227-229.

[350] Brem, RF; Behrndt, VS; Sanow, L; et al. Atypical ductal hyperplasia: Histologic underestimation of carcinoma in tissue harvested from impalpable breast lesions using 11-gauge stereotactically guided directional vacuum-assisted biopsy. *AJR Am J Roentgenol,* 1999, May, 172(5), 1405- 1407.

[351] Britton, PD; McCann, J. Needle biopsy in the NHS breast screening programme 1996/97: How much and how accurate? *Breast*, 1999, Feb;8(1), 5-11.

[352] Damascelli, B; Frigerio, LF; Patelli, G; et al. Stereotactic breast biopsy: En bloc excision of microcalcifications with a large-bore cannula device. *AJR Am J Roentgenol,* 1999, Oct; 1 73(4), 895-900.

[353] Deschryver, K; Radford, DM; Schuh, ME. Pathology of large-caliber stereotactic biopsies in nonpalpable breast lesions. *Semin Diagn Pathol*, 1999, Aug, 16(3), 224-234. PMID: 10490199.

[354] Diaz, LK; Wiley, EL; Venta, LA. Are malignant cells displaced by large-gauge needle core biopsy of the breast. *AJR Am J Roentgenol,* 1999, Nov, 173(5), 1303-1313. PMID: 10541110.

[355] DiPiro, PJ; Meyer, JE; Denison, CM; et al. Image-guided core breast biopsy of ductal carcinoma in situ presenting as a non- calcified abnormality. *Eur J Radiol*, 1999, Jun;30(3), 231-236. PMID: 10452723.

[356] El-Tamer, M; Axiotis, C; Kim, E; et al. Accurate prediction of the amount of in situ tumor in palpable breast cancers by core needle biopsy: Implications for neoadjuvant therapy. *Ann Surg Oncol,* 1999, Jul, 6(5), 461-466.

[357] Evans, AJ; Whitlock, JP; Burrell, HC; et al. A comparison of 14 and 12 gauge needles for core biopsy of suspicious mammographic calcification. *Br J Radiol*, 1999, 72, 1152-1154.

[358] Ferzli, GS; Puza, T; VanVorst-Bilotti, S; et al. Breast biopsies with ABBI: Experience with 183 attempted biopsies. *Breast J*, 1999, 5(1), 26-28.

[359] Fraser Symmans, W; Weg, N; Gross, J; et al. A prospective comparison of stereotaxic fine-needle aspiration versus stereotaxic core needle biopsy for the diagnosis of mammographic abnormalities. *Cancer*, 1999, 85(5), 1119-1132.

[360] Gajdos, C; Levy, M; Herman, Z; et al. Complete removal of nonpalpable breast malignancies with a stereotactic percutaneous vacuum-assisted biopsy instrument. *J Am Coll Surg*, 1999, Sep, 1 89(3), 237-240. PMID: 10472922.

[361] Gentry, CL; Henry, CA. Stereotactic percutaneous breast biopsy: A comparative analysis between surgeon and radiologist. *Breast J*, 1999, 5(2), 101-104.

[362] Gray, RE; Benson, GW; Lustig, DD. Stereotactic breast biopsy: experience in a community setting. *J Miss State Med Assoc*, 1999, Jan, 40(1), 3-7. PMID: 9919043.

[363] Harlow, SP; Krag, DN; Ames, SE; et al. Intraoperative ultrasound localization to guide surgical excision of nonpalpable breast carcinoma. *J Am Coll Surg*, 1999, Sep; 189(3), 241 -246.

[364] Harvey, SC; Denison, CM; Lester, SC; et al. Fibrous nodules found at large-core needle biopsy of the breast: Imaging features. *Radiology*, 1999, May;211(2), 535-540. PMID: 10228539.

[365] Johnson, JM; Dalton, RR; Wester, SM; et al. Histological correlation of microcalcifications in breast biopsy specimens. *Arch Surg*, 1999, Jul, 134(7), 712-716. PMID: 10401820.

[366] Klem, D; Jacobs, HK; Jorgensen, R; et al. Stereotactic breast biopsy in a community hospital setting. *Am Surg,* 1999, Aug, 65(8), 737-740; discussion 740-741. PMID: 10432083.

[367] LaRaja, RD; Saber, AA; Sickles, A. Early experience in the use of the advanced breast biopsy instrumentation: A report of one hundred twenty-seven patients. *Surgery*, 1999, 125(4), 380-384. PMID: 10216528.

[368] Liberman, L; Bracero, N; Vuolo, MA; et al. Percutaneous large-core biopsy of papillary breast lesions. *AJR Am J Roentgenol,* 1999, Feb, 172(2), 331-337.
[369] Liberman, L; Sama, M; Susnik, B; et al. Lobular carcinoma in situ at percutaneous breast biopsy: Surgical biopsy findings. *AJR Am J Roentgenol,* 1999, Aug, 173(2), 291-299. PMID: 10430122.
[370] Liberman, L; Vuolo, M; Dershaw, DD; et al. Epithelial displacement after stereotactic 11- gauge directional vacuum-assisted breast biopsy. *AJR Am J Roentgenol,* 1999, Mar; 1 72(3), 677-68 1. PMID: 10063859.
[371] Matthews, BD; Williams, GB. Initial experience with the advanced breast biopsy instrumentation system. *Am J Surg,* 1999, Feb, 177(2), 97-101. PMID: 10204548.
[372] Mitnick, JS; Gianutsos, R; Pollack, AH; et al. Tubular carcinoma of the breast: sensitivity of diagnostic techniques and correlation with histopathology. *AJR Am J Roentgenol,* 1999, Feb; 172(2), 3 19-323. PMID: 9930775.
[373] Philpotts, LE; Shaheen, NA; Carter, D; et al. Comparison of rebiopsy rates after stereotactic core needle biopsy of the breast with 11-gauge vacuum suction probe versus 14-gauge needle and automatic gun. *AJR Am J Roentgenol,* 1999, Mar;172(3), 683-687. PMID: 10063860.
[374] Rebner, M; Chesbrough, R; Gregory, N. Initial experience with the advanced breast biopsy instrumentation device. *AJR Am J Roentgenol,* 1999, Jul; 173(1), 221-226.
[375] Rich, PM; Michell, MJ; Humphreys, S; et al. Stereotactic 14G core biopsy of non-palpable breast cancer: What is the relationship between the number of core samples taken and the sensitivity for detection of malignancy? *Clin Radiol,* 1999, Jun, 54(6), 384-389.
[376] Rosen, EL; Soo, MS; Bentley, RC. Focal fibrosis: A common breast lesion diagnosed at imaging-guided core biopsy. *AJR Am J Roentgenol,* 1999, Dec, 173(6), 1657-1662. PMID: 10584816.
[377] Roth, WD; von Smitten, K; Heikkila, P; et al. Automated stereotactic core needle biopsy of microcalcifications with correlation to surgical biopsy. *Acta Radiol,* 1999, Jul;40(4), 390-393. PMID: 10394866.
[378] Sharifi, S; Peterson, MK; Baum, JK; et al. Assessment of pathologic prognostic factors in breast core needle biopsies. *Mod Pathol,* 1999, Oct, 12(10), 941-945.
[379] Sheth, D; Wesen, CA; Schroder, D; et al. The Advanced Breast Biopsy Instrumentation (ABBI) experience at a community hospital. *Am Surg,* 1999, Aug;65(8), 726-730.
[380] Shin, HJC; Sneige, N; Staerkel, GA. Utility of punch biopsy for lesions that are hard to aspirate by conventional fine-needle aspiration. *Cancer*, 1999, Jun 25, 87(3), 149-154.
[381] Staren, ED; O'Neill, TP. Ultrasound-guided needle biopsy of the breast. Surgery 1999; 126(4), 629-635. PMID: 10520908.
[382] Tran, DQ; Wilkerson, DK; Namm, J; et al. Needle-localized breast biopsy for mammographic abnormalities: A community hospital experience. *Am Surg,* 1999, Mar, 65(3), 283-288. PMID: 10075310.
[383] Velanovich, V; Lewis Jr, FR; Nathanson, SD; et al. Comparison of mammographically guided breast biopsy techniques. *Ann Surg*, 1999, May;229(5), 625-630; discussion 630- 633. PMID: 10235520.
[384] Williams, AB; Roberts, JV; Michell, MJ; et al. Prone stereotactic breast core biopsy: The impact on surgical management of nonpalpable breast cancers. *Breast*, 1999, Feb;8(1), 12-15.

[385] Won, B; Reynolds, HE; Lazaridis, CL; et al. Stereotactic biopsy of ductal carcinoma in situ of the breast using an 11-gauge vacuum- assisted device: persistent underestimation of disease. *AJR Am J Roentgenol,* 1999, Jul, 173(1), 227-229. PMID: 10397131.
[386] Yong, WS; Chia, KH; Poh, WT; et al. A comparison of trucut biopsy with fine needle aspiration cytology in the diagnosis of breast cancer. *Singapore Med J,* 1999, Sep;40(9), 587-589. PMID: 10628249.
[387] Andreu, FJ; Sentis, M; Castaner, E; et al. The impact of stereotactic large-core needle biopsy in the treatment of patients with nonpalpable breast lesions: a study of diagnostic accuracy in 510 consecutive cases. *Eur Radiol,* 1998, 8(8), 1468-1474. PMID: 9853239.
[388] Antley, CM; Mooney, EE; Layfield, LJ. A comparison of accuracy rates between open biopsy; cutting-needle biopsy; and fine- needle aspiration biopsy of the breast: A 3-year experience. *Breast J*, 1998, 4(1), 3-8.
[389] Bleznak, AD; Magaram, D. Surgical biopsy techniques for mammographically detected abnormalities. *Breast J*, 1998, 4(6), 426-429.
[390] Damascelli, B; Frigerio, LF; Lanocita, R; et al. Stereotactic excisional breast biopsy performed by interventional radiologists using the advanced breast biopsy instrumentation system. *Br J Radiol*, 1998, Oct;71(850), 1003-1011. PMID: 10211058
[391] Doyle, AJ; King, AR; Miller, MV; et al. Implementation of image-guided large-core needle biopsy of the breast on a limited budget. *Australas Radiol*, 1998, 42(3), 199-203.
[392] Goodman, KA; Birdwell, RL; Ikeda, DM. Compliance with recommended follow-up after percutaneous breast core biopsy. *AJR Am J Roentgenol,* 1998, 170(1), 89-93.
[393] Helbich, TH; Rudas, M; Haitel, A; et al. Evaluation of needle size for breast biopsy: Comparison of 14-; 16-; and 18-gauge biopsy needles. *AJR Am J Roentgenol,* 1998, Jul, 171(1), 59-63. PMID: 9648764.
[394] Jackman, RJ; Marzoni Jr, FA; Nowels, KW. Percutaneous removal of benign mammographic lesions: Comparison of automated large-core and directional vacuum-assisted stereotactic biopsy techniques. *AJR Am J Roentgenol,* 1998, Nov, 171(5), 1325-1330.
[395] Johnson, JM; Dalton, RR; Landercasper, J; et al. Image-guided or needle-localized open biopsy of mammographic malignant- appearing microcalcifications? *J Am Coll Surg,* 1998, 187(6), 604-609. PMID: 9849733.
[396] Kaufman, CS; Delbecq, R; Jacobson, L. Excising the reexcision: stereotactic core-needle biopsy decreases need for reexcision of breast cancer. *World J Surg*, 1998, Oct, 22(10), 1023-1027. PMID: 9747160.
[397] Kelley Jr, WE; Bailey, R; Bertelsen, C; et al. Stereotactic automated surgical biopsy using the ABBI biopsy device: A multicenter study. *Breast J*, 1998, 4(5), 302-306.
[398] King, TA; Cederbom, GJ; Champaign, JL; et al. A core breast biopsy diagnosis of invasive carcinoma allows for definitive surgical treatment planning. *Am J Surg,* 1998, Dec;176(6), 497-501. PMID: 9926778.
[399] Liberman, L; Dershaw, DD; Rosen, PP; et al. Percutaneous removal of malignant mammographic lesions of stereotactic vaccum-assisted biopsy. *Radiology*, 1998, Mar;206(3), 711-715. PMID: 9494489.
[400] Liberman, L; Smolkin, JH; Dershaw, DD; et al. Calcification retrieval at stereotactic; 11- gauge; directional; vacuum- assisted breast biopsy. *Radiology*, 1998, Jul, 208(1), 251-260. PMID: 9646821.

[401] Lin, PH; Clyde, JC; Bates, DM; et al. Accuracy of stereotactic core-needle breast biopsy in atypical ductal hyperplasia. *Am J Surg,* 1998, May, 175(5), 380-382. PMID: 9600282.
[402] Lind, DS; Minter, R; Steinbach, B; et al. Stereotactic core biopsy reduces the reexcision rate and the cost of mammographically detected cancer. *J Surg Res*, 1998, Jul 15;78(1), 23-26.
[403] Meyer, JE; Smith, DN; Lester, SC; et al. Large-needle core biopsy: Nonmalignant breast abnormalities evaluated with surgical excision or repeat core biopsy. *Radiology*, 1998, Mar;206(3), 717-720.
[404] Mitnick, JS; Gianutsos, R; Pollack, AH; et al. Comparative value of mammography; fine- needle aspiration biopsy; and core biopsy in the diagnosis of invasive lobular carcinoma. *Breast J*, 1998, 4(2), 75-83.
[405] Seoudi, H; Mortier, J; Basile, R; et al. Stereotactic core needle biopsy of nonpalpable breast lesions: Initial experience with a promising technique. *Arch Surg*, 1998, Apr;133(4), 366-372. PMID: 9565115.
[406] Slanetz, PJ; Giardino, AA; McCarthy, KA; et al. Previous breast biopsy for benign disease rarely complicates or alters interpretation on screening mammography. *AJR Am J Roentgenol,* 1998, Jul, 170(6), 1539-1541.
[407] Soo, MS; Walsh, R; Patton, J. Prone table stereotactic breast biopsy: Facilitating biopsy of posterior lesions using the armthrough-the-hole technique. *AJR Am J Roentgenol,* 1998, Sep;171(3), 615-617.
[408] Woodcock, NP; Glaves, I; Morgan, DR; et al. Ultrasound-guided Tru-cut biopsy of the breast. *Ann R Coll Surg Engl*, 1998, 80(4), 253-256. PMID: 9771224.
[409] Zardawi, IM. Fine needle aspiration cytology vs. Core biopsy in a rural setting. *Acta Cytol*, 1998, 42(4), 883-887. PMID, 9684572.
[410] Zonderland, HM; Hermans, J; Van De Vijver, MJ; et al. Triple diagnostic approach versus ultrasound-guided 18 gauge core biopsy in suspicious breast masses. *Breast*, 1998, Jun, 7(3), 168-172.
[411] Acheson, MB; Patton, RG; Howisey, RL; et al. Histologic correlation of image-guided core biopsy with excisional biopsy of nonpalpable breast lesions. *Arch Surg*, 1997, Aug; 132(8), 81 5-818; discussion 819-821. PMID: 9267263.
[412] Anania, G; Bazzocchi, M; Di Loreto, C; et al. Percutaneous large core needle biopsy versus surgical biopsy in the diagnosis of breast lesions. *Int Surg*, 1997 Jan, 82(1), 52-55. PMID: 9189803.
[413] Burbank, F. Stereotactic breast biopsy of atypical ductal hyperplasia and ductal carcinoma in situ lesions: Improved accuracy with directional; vacuum- assisted biopsy. *Radiology*, 1997, Mar, 202(3), 843- 847.
[414] Burbank, F. Stereotactic breast biopsy: comparison of 14- and 11-gauge Mammotome probe performance and complication rates. *Am Surg,* 1997, Nov, 63(11), 988-995. PMID: 9358788.
[415] Burbank, F. Mammographic findings after 14-gauge automated needle and 14-gauge directional; vacuum-assisted stereotactic breast biopsies. *Radiology*, 1997, Jul, 204(1), 153-156. PMID: 9205238.
[416] Cerwenka, H; Hoff, M; Rosanelli, G; et al. Experience with a high speed biopsy gun in breast cancer diagnosis. *Eur J Surg Oncol,* 1997, 23(3), 206-207. PMID: 9236891.

[417] D'Angelo, PC; Galliano, DE; Rosemurgy, AS. Stereotactic excisional breast biopsies utilizing the advanced breast biopsy instrumentation system. *Am J Surg,* 1997, Sep; 174(3), 297-302. PMID: 9324141.

[418] Devia, A; Murray, KA; Nelson, EW. Stereotactic core needle biopsy and the workup of mammographic breast lesions. *Arch Surg*, 1997 May;132(5), 512-515; discussion 515-517. PMID: 9161394.

[419] Fenoglio, ME; Gallagher, JQ; Joy, N; et al. Stereotactic core breast biopsy versus needle localization breast biopsy—The effect of initial diagnostic modality on surgical therapy in patients with breast cancer. Minim Invasive Ther Allied Technol 1997, Jun, 6(3), 225-227.

[420] Ferzli, GS; Hurwitz, JB; Puza, T; et al. Advanced breast biopsy instrumentation: A critique. *J Am Coll Surg*, 1997, 185(2), 145- 151.

[421] Florentine, BD; Cobb, CJ; Frankel, K; et al. Core needle biopsy: A useful adjunct to fine-needle aspiration in select patients with palpable breast lesions. *Cancer*, 1997, Feb 25;81(1), 33-39.

[422] Gadzala, DE; Cederbom, GJ; Bolton, JS; et al. Appropriate management of atypical ductal hyperplasia diagnosed by stereotactic core needle breast biopsy. *Ann Surg Oncol,* 1997, Jun;4(4), 283-286. PMID: 9181225.

[423] Hirst, C; Davis, N. Core biopsy for microcalcifications in the breast. *Aust N Z J Surg*, 1997, 67(6), 320-324.

[424] Howisey, RL; Acheson, MB; Rowbotham, RK; et al. A comparison of Medicare reimbursement and results for various imaging- guided breast biopsy techniques. *Am J Surg,* 1997, May, 173(5), 395-398. PMID: 9168074.

[425] Jackman, RJ; Marzoni, Jr FA. Needle- localized breast biopsy: Why do we fail? *Radiology*, 1997, Sep, 204(3), 677-684.

[426] Jackman, RJ; Burbank, F; Parker, SH; et al. Atypical ductal hyperplasia diagnosed at stereotactic breast biopsy: Improved reliability with 14-gauge; directional; vacuum-assisted biopsy. *Radiology*, 1997, Aug, 204(2), 485-488.

[427] Liberman, L; Hann, LE; Dershaw, DD; et al. Mammographic findings after stereotactic 14-gauge vacuum biopsy. *Radiology*, 1997, May;203(2), 343-347. PMID: 9114086.

[428] Liberman, L; Latrenta, LR; Dershaw, DD; et al. Impact of core biopsy on the surgical management of impalpable breast cancer. *AJR Am J Roentgenol,* 1997, 168(2), 495-499.

[429] Lifrange, E; Kridelka, F; Colin, C. Stereotaxic needle-core biopsy and fine-needle aspiration biopsy in the diagnosis of nonpalpable breast lesions: controversies and future prospects. *Eur J Radiol*, 1997, Jan, 24(1), 39-47. PMID: 9056148.

[430] Meyer, JE; Smith, DN; DiPiro, PJ; et al. Stereotactic breast biopsy of clustered microcalcifications with a directional; vacuum-assisted device. *Radiology*, 1997, Aug, 204(2), 575-576. PMID: 9240556.

[431] Pijnappel, RM; van Dalen, A; Borel Rinkes, IH; et al. The diagnostic accuracy of core biopsy in palpable and non-palpable breast lesions. *Eur J Radiol*, 1997, Feb;24(2), 120-123. PMID: 9097053.

[432] Roe, SM; Mathews, JA; Burns, RP; et al. Stereotactic and ultrasound core needle breast biopsy performed by surgeons. *Am J Surg,* 1997, Dec, 174(6), 699-703; discussion 703-704. PMID: 9409600.

[433] Smith, DN; Christian, R; Meyer, JE. Large- core needle biopsy of nonpalpable breast cancers. The impact on subsequent surgical excisions. *Arch Surg*, 1997, Mar;132(3), 256-259; discussion, 260. PMID: 9125023.

[434] Stolier, AJ; Rupley, DG. The impact of image-directed core biopsy on the practice of breast surgery: A new algorithm for a changing technology. *Am Surg,* 1997, Sep;63(9), 827-830. PMID: 9290531.

[435] Whitten, TM; Wallace, TW; Bird, RE; et al. Image-guided core biopsy has advantages over needle localization biopsy for the diagnosis of nonpalpable breast cancer. *Am Surg,* 1997 Dec;63(12), 1072-1077; discussion 1077-1078. PMID: 9393255.

[436] Written, TM; Wallace, TW; Bird, RE; et al. Image-guided core biopsy has advantages over needle localization biopsy for the diagnosis of nonpalpable breast cancer. *Am Surg,* 1997, 63(12), 1072-1078.

[437] Ballo, MS; Sneige, N. Can core needle biopsy replace fine-needle aspiration cytology in the diagnosis of palpable breast carcinoma. A comparative study of 124 women. *Cancer*, 1996, Aug, 15, 78(4), 773-777. PMID: 8756371.

[438] Burbank, F; Parker, SH; Fogarty, TJ. Stereotactic breast biopsy: improved tissue harvesting with the Mammotome. *Am Surg,* 1996, Sep, 62(9), 738-744. PMID: 8751765.

[439] Caines, JS; Chantziantoniou, K; Wright, BA; et al. Nova Scotia Breast Screening Program experience: use of needle core biopsy in the diagnosis of screening-detected abnormalities. *Radiology*, 1996, Jan, 198(1), 125-130.

[440] Chare, MJB; Flowers, CI; O'Brien, CJ; et al. Image-guided core biopsy in patients with breast disease. *Br J Surg*, 1996, 83(10), 1415-1416.

[441] Crotch-Harvey, MA; Loughran, CF. Combined stereotactic wide-core needle biopsy and fine-needle aspiration cytology in the assessment of impalpable mammographic abnormalities detected in a breast-screening programme. *Breast*, 1996, 5(1), 48-49.

[442] Dershaw, DD; Morris, EA; Liberman, L; et al. Nondiagnostic stereotaxic core breast biopsy: results of rebiopsy. *Radiology*, 1996, Feb; 198(2), 323-325. PMID: 8596825.

[443] Di Loreto, C; Puglisi, F; Rimondi, G; et al. Large core biopsy for diagnostic and prognostic evaluation of invasive breast carcinomas. *Eur J Cancer*, 1996, Sep, 32A(10), 1693-1700. PMID: 8983276.

[444] Frayne, J; Sterrett, GF; Harvey, J; et al. Stereotactic 14 gauge core-biopsy of the breast: results from 101 patients. *Aust N Z J Surg*, 1996, Sep, 66(9), 585-591. PMID: 8859155.

[445] Handy, RB; Fajardo, LL; Innis, CA; et al. Patient perceptions of stereotaxic large-core breast biopsy. *Acad Radiol*, 1996, Dec, 3(12), 1007-1011. PMID: 9017015.

[446] Hillhouse, RA; Norvill, KA; Buchanan, SW; et al. Analysis of malignancy detected by needle-localized breast biopsy. *J Am Osteopath Assoc,* 1996, Jul;96(7), 398-400. PMID: 8758871.

[447] Hunter, TB; Roberts, CC; Hunt, KR; et al. Occurrence of fibroadenomas in postmenopausal women referred for breast biopsy. *J Am Geriatr Soc*, 1996, Jan, 44(1), 61-64.

[448] Liberman, L; Dershaw, DD; Rosen, PP; et al. Core needle biopsy of synchronous ipsilateral breast lesions: impact on treatment. *AJR Am J Roentgenol,* 1996, Jun, 166(6), 1429-1432.

[449] Pillsbury Jr, SG; Haugen, JA; Roux S. Reliability of multimodal evaluation of abnormal screening mammogram results. *Am J Obstet Gynecol*, 1996, Jun, 174(6), 1683-1686; discussion 1686- 1687. PMID: 8678127.

[450] Poole, GH; Willsher, PC; Pinder, SE; et al. Diagnosis of breast cancer with core-biopsy and fine needle aspiration cytology. Aust N Z J Surg 1996 Sep;66(9), 592-594. PMID: 8859156.

[451] Taft, R; Chao, K; Dear, P; et al. The role of core biopsy in the diagnosis of mammographically detected lesions. *Aust N Z J Surg*, 1996, Oct;66(10), 664-667. PMID: 8855919.

[452] Tocino, I; Garcia, BM; Carter, D. Surgical biopsy findings in patients with atypical hyperplasia diagnosed by stereotaxic core needle biopsy. *Ann Surg Oncol,* 1996, Sep;3(5), 483-488. PMID: 8876891.

[453] Wallace, JE; Sayler, C; McDowell, NG; et al. The role of stereotactic biopsy in assessment of nonpalpable breast lesions. *Am J Surg,* 1996, May, 171(5), 471-473. PMID: 8651387.

[454] Yim, JH; Barton, P; Weber, B; et al. Mammographically detected breast cancer. Benefits of stereotactic core versus wire localization biopsy. Ann Surg 1996 Jun;223(6), 688-697; discussion 697-670. PMID: 8645042.

[455] Hann, LE; Liberman, L; Dershaw, DD; et al. Mammography immediately after stereotaxic breast biopsy: is it necessary? *AJR Am J Roentgenol,* 1995, 165(1), 59-62.

[456] Israel, PZ; Fine, RE. Stereotactic needle biopsy for occult breast lesions: a minimally invasive alternative. *Am Surg,* 1995, Jan;61(1), 87-91. PMID: 7832390.

[457] Liberman, L; Cohen, MA; Dershaw, DD; et al. Atypical ductal hyperplasia diagnosed at stereotaxic core biopsy of breast lesions: an indication for surgical biopsy. *AJR Am J Roentgenol,* 1995, 164(5), 1111-1113.

[458] Liberman, L; Dershaw, DD; Rosen, PP; et al. Stereotaxic core biopsy of impalpable spiculated breast masses. *AJR Am J Roentgenol,* 1995;165(3), 551-554.

[459] Liberman, L; Dershaw, D; Durfee, S; et al. Recurrent carcinoma after breast conservation: diagnosis with stereotaxic core biopsy. *Radiology*, 1995, Dec, 197(3), 735- 738.

[460] McCombs, MM; Bassett, LW; Jahan, R; et al. Imaging-guided core biopsy of the breast. *Breast J*, 1995, Jan-Feb;1(1), 9-16.

[461] Nath, ME; Robinson, TM; Tobon, H; et al. Automated large-core needle biopsy of surgically removed breast lesions: comparison of samples obtained with 14-; 16-; and 18-gauge needles. *Radiology*, 1995, Dec, 197(3), 739-742. PMID: 7480748.

[462] Rubin, E; Dempsey, PJ; Pile, NS; et al. Needle-localization biopsy of the breast: impact of a selective core needle biopsy program on yield. *Radiology*, 1995, Jun;195(3), 627-631. PMID: 7753985.

[463] Strong, JW; Worsham, GF; Austin, RM; et al. Stereotactic core biopsy of nonpalpable breast lesions. *J S C Med Assoc*, 1995, Dec;9 1 (12), 489-496. PMID: 8587312

[464] Vega, A; Arrizabalaga, R; Garijo, F; et al. Nonpalpable breast lesion. Stereotaxic core needle aspiration biopsy with a single pass. *Acta Radiol,* 1995, Mar, 36(2), 117-121. PMID: 7710788.

[465] Vega, A; Garijo, F; Ortega, E. Core needle aspiration biopsy of palpable breast masses. *Acta Oncol,* 1995, 34(1), 31-34. PMID: 7865233.

[466] Youngson, BJ; Liberman, L; Rosen, PP. Displacement of carcinomatous epithelium in surgical breast specimens following stereotaxic core biopsy. *Am J Clin Pathol,* 1995, May, 103(5), 598-602. PMID: 7741106.

[467] Caines, JS; McPhee, MD; Konok, GP; et al. Stereotaxic needle core biopsy of breast lesions using a regular mammographic table with an adaptable stereotaxic device. *AJR Am J Roentgenol, 1994*, Aug, 163(2), 317-321. PMID: 8037022.

[468] Jackman, RJ; Nowels, KW; Shepard, MJ; et al. Stereotaxic large-core needle biopsy of 450 nonpalpable breast lesions with surgical correlation in lesions with cancer or atypical hyperplasia. *Radiology*, 1994, Oct; 193(1), 9 1-95. PMID: 8090927.

[469] Janes, RH; Bouton, MS. Initial 300 consecutive stereotactic core-needle breast biopsies by a surgical group. *Am J Surg,* 1994 Dec; 1 68(6), 533-536; discussion 536-537. PMID: 7977991.

[470] Kaye, MD; Vicinanza-Adami, CA; Sullivan, ML. Mammographic findings after stereotaxic biopsy of the breast performed with large-core needles. *Radiology*, 1994, Jul;192(1), 149-151. PMID: 8208927.

[471] Liberman, L; Dershaw, DD; Rosen, PP; et al. Stereotaxic 14-gauge breast biopsy: how many core biopsy specimens are needed? *Radiology*, 1994, Sep, 192(3), 793-795.

[472] Liberman, L; Evans III, WP; Dershaw, DD; et al. Radiography of microcalcifications in stereotaxic mammary core biopsy specimens. *Radiology*, 1994, 190(1), 223-225.

[473] Mikhail, RA; Nathan, RC; Weiss, M; et al. Stereotactic core needle biopsy of mammographic breast lesions as a viable alternative to surgical biopsy. *Ann Surg Oncol,* 1994, Sep, 1(5), 363-367. PMID: 7850536.

[474] Morrow, M; Schmidt, R; Cregger, B; et al. Preoperative evaluation of abnormal mammographic findings to avoid unnecessary breast biopsies. Arch Surg 1994 Oct, 129(10), 1091-1096. PMID: 7944941.

[475] Sadler, GP; McGee, S; Dallimore, NS; et al. Role of fine-needle aspiration cytology and needle-core biopsy in the diagnosis of lobular carcinoma of the breast. *Br J Surg*, 1994, 81(9), 13 15-13 17.

[476] Youngson, BJ; Cranor, M; Rosen, PP. Epithelial displacement in surgical breast specimens following needling procedures. *Am J Surg Pathol*, 1994, Sep, 18(9), 896-903. PMID: 8067510.

[477] Rotten, D; Levaillant, JM; Leridon, H; et al. Ultrasonographically guided fine needle aspiration cytology and core-needle biopsy in the diagnosis of breast tumors. *Eur J Obstet Gynecol Reprod Biol,* 1993 May;49(3), 175-186. PMID: 8405632.

[478] Dronkers, DJ. Stereotaxic core biopsy of breast lesions. *Radiology*, 1992, Jun; 1 83(3), 63 1-634. PMID: 1584909.

[479] Elliott, RL; Haynes, AE; Bolin, JA; et al. Stereotaxic needle localization and biopsy of occult breast lesions: first year's experience. *Am Surg,* 1992, Feb, 58(2), 126-131. PMID: 1550304.

[480] Harter, LP; Curtis, JS; Ponto, G; et al. Malignant seeding of the needle track during stereotaxic core needle breast biopsy. *Radiology*, 1992, Dec;185(3), 713-714. PMID: 1343569.

[481] Pezner, RD; Lorant, JA; Terz, J; et al. Wound- healing complications following biopsy of the irradiated breast. *Arch Surg*, 1992 Mar;127(3), 321-324. PMID: 1550480.

[482] Khanna, AK; Singh, MR; Khanna, S; et al. Fine needle aspiration cytology; imprint cytology and tru-cut needle biopsy in breast lumps: a comparative evaluation. *J Indian Med Assoc*, 1991, Jul, 89(7), 192-195. PMID: 1940411.

[483] Fahrbach, K; Sledge, I; Cella, C; et al. A comparison of the accuracy of two minimally invasive breast biopsy methods: a systematic literature review and meta- analysis. Arch Gynecol Obstet 2006, May;274(2), 63-73. PMID: 16598478 Verkooijen HM; Peeters PH; Buskens E; et al. Diagnostic accuracy of large-core needle biopsy for nonpalpable breast disease: a meta-analysis. Br J Cancer 2000, Mar;82(5), 1017-1021. PMID: 10737383.

[484] Verkooijen, HM; Peeters, PH; Buskens, E; et al. Diagnostic accuracy of large-core needle biopsy for nonpalpable breast disease: a meta-analysis. *Br J Cancer* 2000 Mar;82(5):1017-1021. PMID: 10737383

[485] Jackman, RJ; Marzoni Jr, FA; Rosenberg, J. False-negative diagnoses at stereotactic vacuum-assisted needle breast biopsy: longterm follow-up of 1;280 lesions and review of the literature. *AJR Am J Roentgenol,* 2009, Feb;192(2), 341-351. PMID: 19155393.

[486] Peters, N; Hoorntje, L; Mali, W; et al. Diagnostic performance of stereotactic large core needle biopsy for nonpalpable breast lesions in routine clinical practice. *Int J Cancer,* 2008, Jan, 15, 122(2), 468-47 1. PMID: 17935136.

[487] Schueller G; Jaromi, S; Ponhold, L; et al. US- guided 14-gauge core-needle breast biopsy: results of a validation study in 1352 cases. *Radiology*, 2008, Aug, 248(2), 406-413, PMID, 18641246.

[488] Sim, LS; Kei, PL. Upright stereotactic vacuum-assisted needle biopsy of suspicious breast microcalcifications. *J Med Imaging Radiat Oncol*, 2008, Aug, 52(4), 358-364. PMID: 18811759.

[489] Tonegutti, M; Girardi, V. Stereotactic vacuum-assisted breast biopsy in 268 nonpalpable lesions. *Radiol Med,* 2008, Feb;113(1), 65-75. PMID: 18338128.

[490] Ciatto, S; Houssami, N; Ambrogetti, D; et al. Accuracy and underestimation of malignancy of breast core needle biopsy: the Florence experience of over 4000 consecutive biopsies. *Breast Cancer Res Treat,* 2007, Mar; 101(3), 29 1-297. PMID: 16823506.

[491] de Lucena, CE; Dos Santos Junior, JL; de Lima Resende, CA; et al. Ultrasound-guided core needle biopsy of breast masses: How many cores are necessary to diagnose cancer? *J Clin Ultrasound*, 2007, Sep;35(7), 363-366. PMID: 17663457.

[492] Uematsu, T; Yuen, S; Kasami, M; et al. Dynamic contrast-enhanced MR imaging in screening detected microcalcification lesions of the breast: is there any value? *Breast Cancer Res Treat,* 2007, Jul, 103(3), 269-281. PMID: 17063274.

[493] Vag, T; Pfleiderer, SO; Bottcher, J; et al. Ultrasound-guided breast biopsy using a 10-gauge self-contained vacuum-assisted device. *Eur Radiol,* 2007, Dec;17(12), 3100- 3 102. PMID: 17639409.

[494] Chapellier, C; Balu-Maestro, C; Amoretti, N; et al. Vacuum-assisted breast biopsies: Experience at the Antoine Lacassagne Cancer Center (Nice; France). Clin Imaging 2006, Mar;30(2), 99-107. PMID: 16500540.

[495] Cipolla, C; Fricano, S; Vieni, S; et al. Validity of needle core biopsy in the histological characterisation of mammary lesions. Breast 2006, Feb;15(1), 76-80. PMID: 16473738

[496] Dhillon MS; Bradley SA; England DW. Mammotome biopsy: Impact on preoperative diagnosis rate. *Clin Radiol,* 2006, Mar;61(3), 276-281. PMID: 16488210.

[497] Bolivar, AV; Alonso-Bartolome, P; Garcia, EO; et al. Ultrasound-guided core needle biopsy of non-palpable breast lesions: a prospective analysis in 204 cases. *Acta Radiol,* 2005, Nov, 46(7), 690-695. PMID: 16372687.
[498] Crystal, P; Koretz, M; Shcharynsky, S; et al. Accuracy of sonographically guided 14-gauge core-needle biopsy: Results of 715 consecutive breast biopsies with at least two-year follow-up of benign lesions. *J Clin Ultrasound*, 2005, Feb, 33(2), 47-52. PMID: 15674836.
[499] Dillon, MF; Hill, AD; Quinn, CM; et al. The accuracy of ultrasound; stereotactic; and clinical core biopsies in the diagnosis of breast cancer; with an analysis of false-negative cases. *Ann Surg*, 2005, Nov, 242(5), 701-707. PMID: 16244544.
[500] Koskela, AK; Sudan, M; Berg, MH; et al. Add-on device for stereotactic core-needle breast biopsy: How many biopsy specimens are needed for a reliable diagnosis? Radiology 2005, Sep, 236(3), 801-809. PMID: 16020555.
[501] Sauer, G; Deissler, H; Strunz, K; et al. Ultrasound-guided large-core needle biopsies of breast lesions: Analysis of 962 cases to determine the number of samples for reliable tumour classification. *Br J Cancer*, 2005, Jan 31, 92(2), 231-235. PMID: 15611793.
[502] Weber, WP; Zanetti, R; Langer, I; et al. Mammotome: Less invasive than ABBI with similar accuracy for early breast cancer detection. *World J Surg*, 2005, Apr, 29(4), 495-499. PMID: 15770379.
[503] Wu, YK; Huang, YM; Chou, AS; et al. Management of breast fibroadenomas by ultrasound-guided vacuum-assisted biopsy - Three years experience. Tzu Chi Med J 2005, Dec; 1 7(6), 405-408; 52.
[504] Alonso-Bartolome, P; Vega-Bolivar, A; Torres-Tabanera, M; et al. Sonographically guided 11 -G directional vacuum-assisted breast biopsy as an alternative to surgical excision: utility and cost study in probably benign lesions. *Acta Radiol,* 2004, Jul, 45(4), 390-396. PMID: 15323390.
[505] Delle Chiaie, L; Terinde, R. Three- dimensional ultrasound-validated large-core needle biopsy: is it a reliable method for the histological assessment of breast lesions. *Ultrasound Obstet Gynecol*, 2004, Apr;23(4), 393-397. PMID: 15065192.
[506] Fajardo, LL; Pisano, ED; Caudry, DJ; et al. Stereotactic and sonographic large-core biopsy of nonpalpable breast lesions: results of the Radiologic Diagnostic Oncology Group V study. *Acad Radiol*, 2004, Mar;11(3), 293-308. PMID: 15035520.
[507] Kubota, K; Gomi, N; Wakita, T; et al. Magnetic resonance imaging of the metal clip in a breast: safety and its availability as a negative marker. *Breast Cancer*, 2004, 11(1), 55-59. PMID: 14718794.
[508] Lomoschitz, FM; Helbich, TH; Rudas, M; et al. Stereotactic 11-gauge vacuum-assisted breast biopsy: influence of number of specimens on diagnostic accuracy. Radiology 2004, Sep, 232(3), 897-903. PMID: 15273332.
[509] Abdsaleh, S; Azavedo, E; Lindgren, PG. Semiautomatic core biopsy. A modified biopsy technique in breast diseases. *Acta Radiol,* 2003, Jan;44(1), 47-51. PMID: 12630998.
[510] Ambrogetti D; Bianchi S; Ciatto S. Accuracy of percutaneous core biopsy of isolated breast microcalcifications identified by mammography. Experience with a vacuum-assisted large-core biopsy device. *Radiol Med,* 2003, Oct; 1 06(4), 3 13-319. PMID: 14612823.

[511] Fishman, JE; Milikowski, C; Ramsinghani, R; et al. US-guided core-needle biopsy of the breast: How many specimens are necessary? *Radiology*, 2003, Mar 1, 226(3), 779-782. PMID: 12601206.

[512] Han, BK; Choe, YH; Ko, YH; et al. Stereotactic core-needle biopsy of non-mass calcifications: outcome and accuracy at long-term follow-up. *Korean J Radiol*, 2003, Oct-Dec;4(4), 2 17-223. PMID: 14726638.

[513] Kirshenbaum, KJ; Voruganti, T; Overbeeke, C; et al. Stereotactic core needle biopsy of nonpalpable breast lesions using a conventional mammography unit with an add-on device. *AJR Am J Roentgenol,* 2003, Aug, 181(2), 527-531. PMID: 12876040.

[514] March, DE; Coughlin, BF; Barham, RB; et al. Breast masses: Removal of all US evidence during biopsy by using a handheld vacuum- assisted device—Initial experience. *Radiology*, 2003, May 1;227(2), 549-555. PMID: 12676972.

[515] Pfleiderer, SOR; Reichenbach, JR; Azhari, T; et al. A manipulator system for 14-gauge large core breast biopsies inside a high-field whole-body MR scanner. *J Magn Reson Imaging,* 2003, Apr 1, 17(4), 493-498.

[516] Philpotts, LE; Hooley, RJ; Lee, CH. Comparison of automated versus vacuum- assisted biopsy methods for sonographically guided core biopsy of the breast. *AJR Am J Roentgenol,* 2003, Feb; 180(2), 347-35 1. PMID: 12540431.

[517] Wong, TE; Hisham, AN. Core needle biopsy of palpable breast lump: the influence of needle size. *Med J Malaysia*, 2003, Aug;58(3), 399-404. PMID: 14750380.

[518] Apesteguia, L; Mellado, M; Saenz, J; et al. Vacuum-assisted breast biopsy on digital stereotaxic table of nonpalpable lesions non- recognisable by ultrasonography. *Eur Radiol,* 2002, Mar;12(3), 638-645. PMID: 11870480.

[519] Georgian-Smith, D; D'Orsi, C; Morris, E; et al. Stereotactic biopsy of the breast using an upright unit; a vacuum-suction needle; and a lateral arm-support system. *AJR Am J Roentgenol,* 2002, Apr;178(4), 1017-1024. Also available: http://www.ajronline.org. PMID: 11906893.

[520] Jackman, RJ; Lamm, RL. Stereotactic histologic biopsy in breasts with implants. Radiology 2002, Jan, 222(1), 157-164. PMID: 11756720.

[521] Johnson, AT; Henry-Tillman, RS; Smith, LF; et al. Percutaneous excisional breast biopsy. *Am J Surg,* 2002, Dec;184(6), 550-554; discussion 554. PMID: 12488164.

[522] Liberman, L; Kaplan, JB; Morris, EA; et al. To excise or to sample the mammographic target: what is the goal of stereotactic 11- gauge vacuum-assisted breast biopsy. *AJR Am J Roentgenol,* 2002, Sep;179(3), 679-683. PMID: 12185043.

[523] Meloni, GB; Becchere, MP; Soro D; et al. Percutaneous vacuum-assisted core breast biopsy with upright stereotactic equipment. Indications; limitations and results. *Acta Radiol,* 2002, Nov, 43(6), 575-578. PMID: 12485254.

[524] Morris, EA; Liberman, L; Trevisan, SG; et al. Histologic heterogeneity of masses at percutaneous breast biopsy. *Breast J*, 2002, Jul-Aug;8(4), 187-191. PMID: 12100109.

[525] Pfarl, G; Helbich, TH; Riedl, CC; et al. Stereotactic 11-gauge vacuum-assisted breast biopsy: a validation study. *AJR Am J Roentgenol,* 2002, Dec; 179(6), 1503-1507. PMID: 12438044.

[526] Verkooijen, HM; Core Biopsy After Radiological Localisation (COBRA) Study Group. Diagnostic accuracy of stereotactic large-core needle biopsy for nonpalpable breast disease: results of a multicenter prospective study with 95% surgical confirmation. *Int J Cancer,* 2002, Jun 20;99(6), 853-859. PMID: 12115488.

[527] Becker, L; Taves, D; McCurdy, L; et al. Stereotactic core biopsy of breast microcalcifications: comparison of film versus digital mammography; both using an add-on unit. *AJR Am J Roentgenol,* 2001, Dec;177(6), 1451-1457. PMID: 11717106.

[528] Brenner, RJ; Bassett, LW; Fajardo, LL; et al. Stereotactic core-needle breast biopsy: a multi-institutional prospective trial. *Radiology*, 2001, Mar;2 1 8(3), 866-872. PMID: 11230668.

[529] Cangiarella, J; Waisman, J; Symmans, WF; et al. Mammotome core biopsy for mammary microcalcification: analysis of 160 biopsies from 142 women with surgical and radiologic followup. *Cancer*, 2001, Jan 1, 91(1), 173-177. PMID: 11148574.

[530] Dahlstrom, JE; Jain, S. Histological correlation of mammographically detected microcalcifications in stereotactic core biopsies. *Pathology*, 2001, 33(4), 444-448. PMID: 11827410.

[531] Lai, JT; Burrowes, P; MacGregor, JH. Diagnostic accuracy of a stereotaxically guided vacuum-assisted large-core breast biopsy program in Canada. *Can Assoc Radiol J*, 2001, Aug, 52(4), 223-227. PMID: 11512293.

[532] Levin, MF; Papoff, WJ; Doan, L; et al. Stereotaxic percutaneous core biopsy versus surgical biopsy of nonpalpable breast lesions using a standard mammographic table with an add-on device. *Can Assoc Radiol J*, 2001, 52(1), 29-32. PMID: 11247262.

[533] Margolin, FR; Leung, JW; Jacobs, RP; et al. Percutaneous imaging-guided core breast biopsy: 5 years' experience in a community hospital. *AJR Am J Roentgenol,* 2001, Sep;177(3), 559-564. PMID: 11517047.

[534] Perez-Fuentes, JA; Longobardi, IR; Acosta, VF; et al. Sonographically guided directional vacuum-assisted breast biopsy: preliminary experience in Venezuela. *AJR Am J Roentgenol,* 2001, Dec, 177(6), 1459- 1463. PMID: 11717107.

[535] Smith, DN; Rosenfield Darling, ML; Meyer, JE; et al. The utility of ultrasonographically guided large-core needle biopsy: results from 500 consecutive breast biopsies. *J Ultrasound Med,* 2001, Jan;20(1), 43-49. PMID: 11149527.

[536] White, RR; Halperin, TJ; Olson Jr, JA; et al. Impact of core-needle breast biopsy on the surgical management of mammographic abnormalities. *Ann Surg*, 2001, Jun;233(6), 769-777. PMID: 11371735.

[537] Wunderbaldinger, P; Helbich, TH; Partik, B; et al. First experience with a new dedicated ultrasound system for computer-guided large-core breast biopsy. *Eur Radiol,* 2001, 11(12), 2460-2464. PMID: 11734940.

[538] Yeow, KM; Lo, YF; Wang, CS; et al. Ultrasound-guided core needle biopsy as an initial diagnostic test for palpable breast masses. *J Vasc Interv Radiol,* 2001, Nov;12(11), 1313-1317. PMID: 11698631.

[539] Beck, RM; Gotz, L; Heywang-Kobrunner, SH. Stereotaxic vacuum core breast biopsy—experience of 560 patients. Swiss Surg 2000;6(3), 108-110. PMID: 10894010.

[540] Kirwan, SE; Denton, ER; Nash, RM; et al. Multiple 14G stereotactic core biopsies in the diagnosis of mammographically detected stellate lesions of the breast. *Clin Radiol,* 2000, Oct, 55(10), 763-766. PMID: 11052877.

[541] Latosinsky, S; Cornell, D; Bear, HD; et al. Evaluation of stereotactic core needle biopsy (SCNB) of the breast at a single institution. *Breast Cancer Res Treat,* 2000, Apr;60(3), 277-283. PMID: 10930116.

[542] Liberman, L; Ernberg, LA; Heerdt, A; et al. Palpable breast masses: is there a role for percutaneous imaging-guided core biopsy. *AJR Am J Roentgenol,* 2000, Sep; 175(3), 779-787. PMID: 10954467.

[543] Makoske, T; Preletz, R; Riley, L; et al. Longterm outcomes of stereotactic breast biopsies. *Am Surg,* 2000, 66(12), 1104-1109.

[544] Ward, SE; Taves, DH; McCurdy, LI. Stereotaxic core needle biopsy of breast microcalcifications obtained using a standard mammography table with an add- on unit. *Can Assoc Radiol J*, 2000, Feb;51(1), 10-15. PMID: 10711288.

[545] Welle, GJ; Clark, M; Loos, S; et al. Stereotactic breast biopsy: recumbent biopsy using add-on upright equipment. *AJR Am J Roentgenol,* 2000, Jul; 175(1), 59-63. PMID: 10882246.

[546] Helbich, TH; Rudas, M; Bohm, G; et al. Randomized in vitro and in vivo evaluation of different biopsy needles and devices for breast biopsy. *Clin Radiol,* 1999, 54(1), 56-62. PMID: 9915512.

[547] Jackman, RJ; Nowels, KW; Rodriguez-Soto, J; et al. Stereotactic; automated; large-core needle biopsy of nonpalpable breast lesions: false-negative and histologic underestimation rates after long-term follow-up. *Radiology*, 1999, Mar, 2, 10(3), 799-805. PMID: 10207484.

[548] Meyer, JE; Smith, DN; Lester, SC; et al. Large-core needle biopsy of nonpalpable breast lesions. *JAMA*, 1999, May, 5, 281(17), 1638-1641. PMID: 10235159.

[549] Puglisi, F; Pertoldi, B; Ramello, M; et al. Diagnostic accuracy of perforated compression grid approach for mammographically guided core needle biopsy of breast lesions. *Cancer Lett*, 1999, Nov, 15, 146(2), 181-188. PMID: 10656624.

[550] Soo, MS; Ghate, S; Delong, D. Stereotactic biopsy of noncalcified breast lesions: utility of vacuum-assisted technique compared to multipass automated gun technique. *Clin Imaging*, 1999, Nov-Dec, 23(6), 347-352. PMID: 10899415.

[551] Caruso, ML; Gabrieli, G; Marzullo, G; et al. Core Biopsy as Alternative to Fine-Needle Aspiration Biopsy in Diagnosis of Breast Tumors. *Oncologist*, 1998, 3(1), 45-49. PMID: 10388083.

[552] Doyle, AJ; Collins, JP; Forkert, CD. Decubitus stereotactic core biopsy of the breast: technique and experience. *AJR Am J Roentgenol*, 1999, Mar; 1 72(3), 688-690. PMID: 10063861.

[553] Fuhrman, GM; Cederbom, GJ; Bolton, JS; et al. Image-guided core-needle breast biopsy is an accurate technique to evaluate patients with nonpalpable imaging abnormalities. *Ann Surg*, 1998, Jun, 227(6), 932-939. PMID: 9637557.

[554] Heywang-Kobrunner, SH; Schaumloffel, U; Viehweg, P; et al. Minimally invasive stereotaxic vacuum core breast biopsy. *Eur Radiol,* 1998;8(3), 377-385. PMID: 9510569.

[555] Ioffe, OB; Berg, WA; Silverberg, SG; et al. Mammographic-histopathologic correlation of large-core needle biopsies of the breast. *Mod Pathol,* 1998, Aug, 11(8), 721-727. PMID: 9720499.

[556] Liberman, L; Feng, TL; Dershaw, DD; et al. US-guided core breast biopsy: use and cost- effectiveness. *Radiology*, 1998, Sep, 208(3), 717-723. PMID: 9722851.

[557] Schulz-Wendtland, R; Kramer, S; Lang, N; et al. Ultrasonic guided microbiopsy in mammary diagnosis: indications; technique and results. Anticancer Res 1998 May- Jun; 1 8(3C), 2145-2146. PMID: 9703772.

[558] Vega Bolivar, A; Ortega Garcia, E; Garijo Ayensa, F. Stereotaxic core needle aspiration biopsy with multiple passes in nonpalpable breast lesions. *Acta Radiol,* 1998, Jul, 39(4), 389-394. PMID: 9685825.

[559] Whitman, GJ; Kopans, DB; McCarthy, KA; et al. Coaxial core needle biopsy under mammographic guidance: indications and applications. *AJR Am J Roentgenol,* 1998, 171(1), 67-70. PMID: 9648766.

[560] Zannis, VJ; Aliano, KM. The evolving practice pattern of the breast surgeon with disappearance of open biopsy for nonpalpable lesions. *Am J Surg,* 1998, Dec, 176(6), 525-528. PMID: 9926783.

[561] Bauer, RL; Sung, J; Eckhert Jr, KH; et al. Comparison of histologic diagnosis between stereotactic core needle biopsy and open surgical biopsy. *Ann Surg Oncol,* 1997 Jun;4(4), 316-320. PMID: 9181231.

[562] Britton, PD; Flower, CD; Freeman, AH; et al. Changing to core biopsy in an NHS breast screening unit. *Clin Radiol,* 1997, Oct;52(10), 764-767. PMID: 9366536.

[563] Helbich, TH; Mayr, W; Schick, S; et al. Coaxial technique: approach to breast core biopsies. *Radiology*, 1997, Jun, 203(3), 684- 690. PMID: 9169689.

[564] Khattar, SC; Torp-Pedersen, S; Horn, T; et al. Ultrasound-guided biopsy of palpable breast masses. *Eur J Ultrasound*, 1997, 6(1), 1-7.

[565] Liberman, L; Dershaw, DD; Glassman, JR; et al. Analysis of cancers not diagnosed at stereotactic core breast biopsy. *Radiology*, 1997, Apr, 203(1), 151-157. PMID: 9122384.

[566] Pitre, B; Baron, PL; Baron, LF; et al. Stereotactic core biopsy of the breast: Results of one-year follow-up of 101 patients. *Am Surg,* 1997, 63(12), 1 124-1127. PMID: 9393264.

[567] Stolier, AJ. Stereotactic breast biopsy: A surgical series. *J Am Coll Surg*, 1997, 185(3), 224-228. PMID: 9291397.

[568] Sutton, S; Dahlstrom, JE; Jain S. Stereotactic large-gauge core biopsy: its role in the diagnosis of non-palpable mammographic abnormalities presenting to a screening service. *Australas Radiol*, 1997, May;41(2), 103-108. PMID: 9153803.

[569] Walker, TM. Impalpable breast lesions: Stereotactic core biopsy with an 'add-on' unit. *Breast*, 1997, Jun;6(3), 126-131.

[570] Frazee, RC; Roberts, JW; Symmonds, RE; et al. Open versus stereotactic breast biopsy. *Am J Surg,* 1996, Nov, 172(5), 491-493, 494- 495. PMID: 8942551.

[571] Fuhrman, G; Cederbom, G; Champagne, J; et al. Stereotactic core needle breast biopsy is an accurate diagnostic technique to assess nonpalpable mammographic abnormalities. *J La State Med Soc*, 1996, Apr, 148(4), 167-170. PMID: 8935619.

[572] Head, JF; Haynes, AE; Elliott, MC; et al. Stereotaxic localization and core needle biopsy of nonpalpable breast lesions: two- year follow-up of a prospective study. *Am Surg,* 1996, Dec, 62(12), 101 8-1023. PMID: 8955240.

[573] Mainiero, MB; Philpotts, LE; Lee, CH; et al. Stereotaxic core needle biopsy of breast microcalcifications: correlation of target accuracy and diagnosis with lesion size. *Radiology*, 1996, Mar, 198(3), 665-669. PMID: 8628852.

[574] Meyer, JE; Christian, RL; Lester, SC; et al. Evaluation of nonpalpable solid breast masses with stereotaxic large- needle core biopsy using a dedicated unit. *AJR Am J Roentgenol,* 1996, 167(1), 179-1 82.

[575] Nguyen, M; McCombs, MM; Ghandehari, S; et al. An update on core needle biopsy for radiologically detected breast lesions. *Cancer*, 1996, Dec 1, 78(11), 2340-2345. PMID: 8941004.

[576] Pettine, S; Place, R; Babu, S; et al. Stereotactic breast biopsy is accurate; minimally invasive; and cost effective. *Am J Surg,* 1996 May; 171 (5), 474-476. PMID: 8651388.

[577] Rosenblatt, R; Fineberg, SA; Sparano, JA; et al. Stereotactic core needle biopsy of multiple sites in the breast: efficacy and effect on patient care. Radiology 1996 Oct;201(1), 67-70. PMID: 8816522.

[578] Scopa, CD; Koukouras, D; Spiliotis, J; et al. Comparison of fine needle aspiration and Tru-Cut biopsy of palpable mammary lesions. *Cancer Detect Prev*, 1996, 20(6), 620-624. PMID: 8939348.

[579] Cross, MJ; Evans, WP; Peters, GN; et al. Stereotactic breast biopsy as an alternative to open excisional biopsy. *Ann Surg Oncol,* 1995, May, 2(3), 195-200. PMID: 7641014.

[580] Doyle, AJ; Murray, KA; Nelson, EW; et al. Selective use of image-guided large-core needle biopsy of the breast: accuracy and cost-effectiveness. *AJR Am J Roentgenol,* 1995, Aug, 165(2), 281-284. PMID: 7618540.

[581] Hamed, H; De Freitas, Jr R; Rasbridge, S; et al. A prospective randomized study of two gauges of biopty-cut needle in diagnosis of early breast cancer. *Breast*, 1995, 4(2), 135-136.

[582] Burbank, F; Kaye, K; Belville, J; et al. Image- guided automated core biopsies of the breast; chest; abdomen; and pelvis. Radiology 1994 Apr;191(1), 165-171. PMID: 8134564.

[583] Gisvold, JJ; Goellner, JR; Grant, CS; et al. Breast biopsy: a comparative study of stereotaxically guided core and excisional techniques. *AJR Am J Roentgenol,* 1994 Apr; 1 62(4), 81 5-820. PMID: 8140997.

[584] Parker, SH; Burbank, F; Jackman, RJ; et al. Percutaneous large-core breast biopsy: a multi-institutional study. *Radiology*, 1994, Nov, 193(2), 359-364. PMID, 7972743.

[585] Smyth, AT; Cederbom, GJ. Core biopsy of breast lesions. *J La State Med Soc,* 1994, Nov, 146(1 1), 499-501. PMID: 7806950.

[586] Elvecrog, EL; Lechner, MC; Nelson, MT. Nonpalpable breast lesions: correlation of stereotaxic large-core needle biopsy and surgical biopsy results. *Radiology*, 1993, Aug, 188(2), 453-455. PMID: 8327696.

[587] Parker, SH; Jobe, WE; Dennis, MA; et al. US- guided automated large-core breast biopsy. *Radiology*, 1993, May, 187(2), 507-511, PMID: 8475299.

[588] McMahon, AJ; Lutfy, AM; Matthew, A; et al. Needle core biopsy of the breast with a spring-loaded device. *Br J Surg*, 1992, Oct, 79(10), 1042-1045. PMID: 1422715.

[589] Barreto, V; Hamed, H; Griffiths, AB; et al. Automatic needle biopsy in the diagnosis of early breast cancer. *Eur J Surg Oncol,* 1991, Jun, 17(3), 237-239. PMID, 2044776.

[590] Cusick, JD; Dotan, J; Jaecks, RD; et al. The role of Tru-Cut needle biopsy in the diagnosis of carcinoma of the breast. Surg Gynecol Obstet 1990 May;170(5), 407-410. PMID: 2183373.

[591] Parker, SH; Lovin, JD; Jobe, WE; et al. Stereotactic breast biopsy with a biopsy gun. *Radiology*, 1990, Sep; 176(3), 741-747. PMID: 2167501.

[592] Friese, CR; Neville, BA; Edge, SB; et al. Breast biopsy patterns and outcomes in Surveillance; Epidemiology, and End Results-Medicare data. *Cancer*, 2009, Feb 15, 115(4), 716-724. PMID: 19152430.

[593] Verkooijen, HM, Borel Rinkes, IH, Peeters, PH, et al. Impact of stereotactic large-core needle biopsy on diagnosis and surgical treatment of non-palpable breast cancer. *Eur J Surg Oncol,* 2001, 27(3), 244-249.

[594] Kettritz, U; Rotter, K; Schreer, I; et al. Stereotactic vacuum-assisted breast biopsy in 2874 patients: a multicenter study. *Cancer*, 2004, Jan, 15, 100(2), 245-251. PMID: 14716757.

[595] Whiting, P; Rutjes, AW; Reitsma, JB; et al. The development of QUADAS: a tool for the quality assessment of studies of diagnostic accuracy included in systematic reviews. BMC Med Res Methodol 2003, Nov 10;3(1), 25. PMID: 14606960 (Note: There is a separate set of references at the end of Appendix G whose reference numbers are different from those in the text of the report.).

Chapter Sources

Chapter 1 - This is an edited, reformatted and augmented version of a U.S. Department of Health and Human Services publication, Agency for Healthcare Research and Quality, 10-EHC007-EF, dated December, 2009.

Chapter 2 - This is an edited, reformatted and augmented version of a U.S. Department of Health and Human Services publication, Agency for Healthcare Research and Quality, 10-EHC007-EF, dated December, 2009.

Index

A

B

C

D

E

N

O

P

Q

R

S

T